Chemotherapy of Gynecologic Cancer

Chemotherapy of Gynecologic Cancer

Editor

Gunter Deppe
Department of Obstetrics and Gynecology
Wayne State University School of Medicine
Detroit, Michigan

Alan R. Liss, Inc., New York

Address all Inquiries to the Publisher
Alan R. Liss, Inc., 150 Fifth Avenue, New York, NY 10011

Printed in the United States of America.

Library of Congress Cataloging in Publication Data
Main entry under title:

Chemotherapy of gynecologic cancer.

Includes Index.
1. Generative organs, Female—Cancer—Chemotherapy.
2. Antineoplastic agents. I. Deppe, Gunter. [DNLM:
1. Genital neoplasms, Female—Drug therapy. WP 145 C517]
RC280.G5C44 1984 616.99'465061 83-26779
ISBN 0-8451-0232-X

This book is dedicated to Lori, Nina, Marc, Erik, and my parents with affection and appreciation for all their support and patience.

Contents

Contributors

David S. Alberts, Section of Hematology and Oncology, College of Medicine, University of Arizona, Tucson, AZ 85724 **[301]**

Jonathan S. Berek, Division of Gynecologic Oncology, UCLA School of Medicine, Jonsson Comprehensive Cancer Center, Los Angeles, CA 90024 **[363]**

John A. Blessing, Gynecologic Oncology Group Statistical Office, Roswell Park Memorial Institute, Buffalo, NY 14263 **[49]**

Philip D. Bonomi, Section of Medical Oncology, Department of Internal Medicine, Rush-Presbyterian-St. Luke's Medical Center, Chicago, IL 60612 **[85, 103]**

Howard W. Bruckner, Departments of Medicine and Neoplastic Diseases, Mount Sinai School of Medicine of the City University of New York, New York, NY 10029 **[151]**

Gunter Deppe, Division of Gynecologic Oncology, Department of Obstetrics and Gynecology, Wayne State University School of Medicine, Detroit, MI 48201 **[xiii, 139, 203, 341]**

Thomas E. Dolan, Division of Gynecologic Oncology, Department of Obstetrics and Gynecology, Lutheran General Hospital, Park Ridge, IL 60068 **[31]**

Robert M. Galbraith, Departments of Basic and Clinical Immunology and Microbiology, Medicine, and Biochemistry, Medical University of South Carolina, Charleston, SC 29425 **[331]**

S.B. Gusberg, Department of Obstetrics and Gynecology, Mount Sinai School of Medicine of the City University of New York, New York, NY 10029 **[xi]**

Neville F. Hacker, Division of Gynecologic Oncology, UCLA School of Medicine, Jonsson Comprehensive Cancer Center, Los Angeles, CA 90024 **[363]**

James F. Holland, Department of Neoplastic Diseases, Mount Sinai School of Medicine of the City University of New York, New York, NY 10029 **[257]**

Allan J. Jacobs, Department of Obstetrics and Gynecology, Washington University School of Medicine, St. Louis, MO 63110 **[351]**

John R. Lurain, Division of Gynecologic Oncology, Brewer Trophoplastic Disease Center, Northwestern University Medical School, Chicago, IL 60611 **[231]**

Vinay Malviya, Division of Gynecologic Oncology, Department of Obstetrics and Gynecology, Wayne State University School of Medicine, Detroit, MI 48201 **[341]**

Rodrigue Mortel, Department of Obstetrics and Gynecology, The Milton S. Hershey Medical Center, Pennsylvania State University, Hershey, PA 17033 **[125]**

Hyman B. Muss, Department of Medicine, Bowman Gray School of Medicine of Wake Forest University, Winston-Salem, NC 27103 **[1]**

George A. Omura, Department of Medicine, University of Alabama in Birmingham, Birmingham, AL 35294 **[213]**

Lawrence S. Perlow, Department of Neoplastic Diseases, Mount Sinai School of Medicine of the City University of New York, New York, NY 10029 **[257]**

Sydney E. Salmon, Cancer Center, College of Medicine, University of Arizona, Tucson, AZ 85724 **[301]**

P.G. Satyaswaroop, Department of Obstetrics and Gynecology, The Milton S. Hershey Medical Center, Pennsylvania State University, Hershey, PA 17033 **[125]**

Robert E. Slayton, Section of Medical Oncology, Department of Internal Medicine, Rush-Presbyterian-St. Luke's Medical Center, Chicago, IL 60612 **[195, 199]**

Earl A. Surwit, Division of Gynecologic Oncology, Department of Obstetrics and Gynecology, College of Medicine, University of Arizona, Tucson, AZ 85724 **[301]**

Leslie A. Walton, Division of Gynecologic Oncology, Department of Obstetrics and Gynecology, University of North Carolina School of Medicine, Chapel Hill, NC 27514 **[321]**

Gregory W. Warr, Departments of Basic and Clinical Immunology and Microbiology, Medicine, and Biochemistry, Medical University of South Carolina, Charleston, SC 29425 **[331]**

George D. Wilbanks, Section of Gynecologic Oncology, Rush-Presbyterian-St.-Luke's Medical Center, Chicago, IL 60612 **[85]**

Edgardo L. Yordan, Jr., Section of Gynecologic Oncology, Rush-Presbyterian-St. Luke's Medical Center, Chicago, IL 60612 **[85, 103]**

Richard J. Zaino, Department of Pathology, The Milton S. Hershey Medical Center, Pennsylvania State University, Hershey, PA 17033 **[125]**

Foreword

The disciplines that utilize cytotoxic agents in their antitumor therapy have come into a new era: We have now the possibility of cure as well as palliation. Indeed, the past history of life extension with chemotherapeutic agents frequently posed a moral problem for the therapist, that of administering a harsh treatment that had the possibility of extending life for a brief period, but this was commonly interspersed with debility and pain for the subject together with emotional and financial disability for her family.

Current evidence indicates increasing rates of cure with chemotherapeutic adjuvants for many tumors, as new strategies are devised almost weekly and new anticancer drugs are introduced. Combination therapy, with surgery of irradiation therapy preceded or followed by chemotherapy, has become increasingly successful in eradicating disease, for the surgery or its equivalent can reduce the tumor burden, while the cytotoxic agents "mop up" so to speak. This should not be surprising for we know now that surgery or irradiation, no matter how radical, are local treatments while cancer is frequently a general disease. Only chemicals programmed to seek out the cancer cell and destroy it can be effectual in such instances.

Gynecologic oncologists are no strangers to this form of treatment for one of the earliest and most successful chemotherapeutic regimens has been that for choriocarcinoma. Those old enough to remember the total mortality of young women afflicted with this disorder can appreciate the change to almost total cure now available by cytotoxic agents. This dramatic change, unfortunately, has not as yet been seen in other advanced cancers of the female reproductive tract, where the past thirty years have brought more improvement from screening and early diagnosis than by treatment. However, recent advances have been made in the medicinal treatment of gynecologic cancer and the era of formal training for gynecologic oncologists has accelerated its use and effectiveness.

Because new agents and new protocols of treatment are introduced continually, clinical trials have become the norm of advancing this form of therapy and gynecologic oncologists have frequently collaborated in this type of clinical investigation. The bewildering array of new agents and combinations has made it difficult for the generalist and even for the specialist to stay current. For this reason this volume, edited and authored by experts in special areas, will make an important contribution to the understanding and utilization of modern anticancer treatment. Gathering in this monograph the experience of many scholars and investigators is especially important for it presents the state of the art for gynecologic cancer treatment in the present, and a chemotherapeutic baseline for the future.

S.B. Gusberg, M.D., D.Sc., F.A.C.S., F.A.C.O.G., F.R.C.O.G.
Distinguished Service Professor and
Chairman of Obstetrics and Gynecology Emeritus
The Mount Sinai School of Medicine
New York, New York

Acknowledgments

The editor of this book would like to express his profound gratitude to all contributing authors who meticulously prepared their chapters and thereby made this book possible.

I also wish to thank my teachers, outstanding leaders in the field of gynecologic and medical oncology, Saul B. Gusberg, M.D., James F. Holland, M.D., Carmel J. Cohen, M.D., and Howard W. Bruckner, M.D., at the Mount Sinai School of Medicine, New York, New York, for the standards of excellence they taught me.

I am indebted to Paulette Cohen, Randi Laisi, and the staff at Alan R. Liss for their valuable assistance in the preparation of this book, as well as my secretary, Jane Wittersheim, for all her help, support, suggestions, and handling of the manuscripts from each author.

A final, special tribute is due to my wife, Lori, who has helped me in so many ways, not only with this project, but with many others over the years.

Principles of Cancer Chemotherapy

Hyman B. Muss

Department of Medicine, Bowman Gray School of Medicine, Wake Forest University, Winston-Salem, North Carolina 27103

The explosive growth of oncology as a medical discipline, coupled with a rapidly expanding knowledge and technology of tumor biology, frequently obscures the humble and very recent beginnings of cytotoxic anticancer chemotherapy. In 1942 Gilman and co-workers [Gilman and Philips, 1946] treated a patient with lymphoma with nitrogen mustard and noted objective tumor regression. This historic event demonstrated the potential for cytotoxic agents to treat malignancies and began the modern era of cancer chemotherapy. Soon after, Farber demonstrated antitumor activity of the antifolate compounds in children with leukemia [Farber et al., 1948]. This was followed by the synthesis of methotrexate in 1949 which proved to be the first drug capable of curing an advanced malignancy—gestational choriocarcinoma in women [Hertz et al., 1961]. This latter event demonstrated conclusively that chemotherapy had the potential for curing human malignancy. The 1950s and 1960s were an exciting period of drug development, and by 1970 there were more than 20 active compounds available for cancer chemotherapy, including numerous alkylating agents, antimetabolites, antitumor antibiotics, plant alkaloids, nitrosoureas, and hormones. Such developments preceded another major milestone—the demonstration by DeVita and colleagues [DeVita and Serpick, 1967] that a combination of drugs (nitrogen mustard, vincristine, procarbazine, and prednisone; MOPP) used concurrently was capable of curing a majority of patients with advanced Hodgkin's disease. The importance of this achievement was the demonstration that the combination chemotherapy program could result in cure in at least half of the patients, whereas the same drugs used individually, although capable of causing objective responses, rarely resulted in

Chemotherapy of Gynecologic Cancer, pages 1–30

cure. The success of the MOPP program stimulated interest in the development of combination chemotherapy trials for almost all types of human cancer and ultimately led to the development of curative programs in non-Hodgkin's lymphoma, childhood leukemia, Wilms tumor, and testicular cancer.

This chapter will introduce the reader to basic biologic and pharmacologic principles related to the use of cancer chemotherapy and summarize the mechanisms of action, metabolism, and toxicity of the most commonly used agents.

CELL AND TUMOR BIOLOGY

Cell Kinetics and the Cell Cycle

Although cancer cells differ from the normal human cells from which they are derived, there are no unique attributes of cancer cells that distinguish them from their normal counterparts. Cancer cells do not proliferate faster than some normal cells [Baserga, 1981], and both malignant and normal cells proceed through a specific series of steps or phases in the process of cell division. For broad purposes of classification, cytotoxic agents can be divided into two classes: 1) those that work exclusively or preferentially during a specific phase of the cell cycle (cell cycle, specific), and 2) those that are able to induce cell death during any portion of the cycle (cell cycle, nonspecific). The planning of single agent and combination regimens and the optimal scheduling and sequencing of drugs rest on the knowledge of such cellular reproductive biology and drug–cell cycle specificity.

The specific phases of the cell cycle are illustrated in Figure 1. The cell cycle is divided into four unequal phases. During G_1, the intermitotic phase, cell machinery is primed for DNA synthesis. This phase is generally the longest phase of the cell cycle in mammalian cells but is highly variable in duration. The initiation and completion of DNA synthesis takes place during the S-phase which generally lasts 10–20 h. During this phase, normal 2N (diploid) DNA is copied in preparation for cell division. Following the S-phase there is a short premitotic or G_2 phase lasting 2–10 h during which the machinery necessary for mitosis such as the spindle apparatus is synthesized. Finally mitosis occurs during the M-phase. During this very short phase, which generally lasts 30 min to 1 h, cells proceed through the four classic steps of mitosis: prophase, metaphase, anaphase, and telophase, resulting in cell division and the formation of two new daughter cells. New cells may then go back into cycle or become resting G_0 cells. While it is controversial whether there are any substantial differences between G_0 and

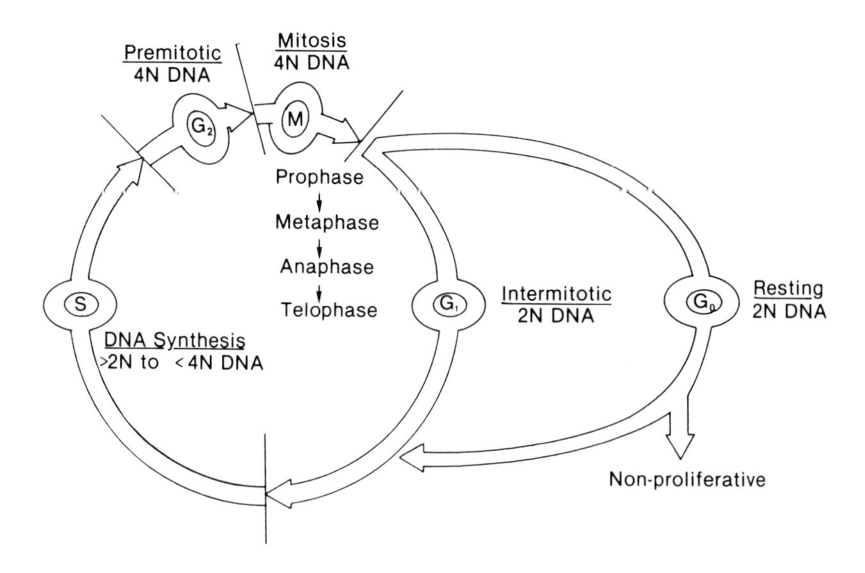

Fig. 1. The cell cycle. G_0, resting cells; G_1, intermitotic phase; S, DNA synthesis; G_2, postmitotic phase; M, mitosis; 2N, normal diploid number for DNA. Non-proliferative cells are not capable of reentering the cell cycle and will ultimately die.

G_1 cells, it is clear that in most clinically detectable human tumors most cells are not actively cycling. Some of these noncycling cells may be incapable of proliferating and eventually die, and others may go back into cycle after spending variable amounts of time in the resting state. In addition, cells that are in cycle may be in any phase of the cycle at any given time. Thus a cytotoxic agent that is specific for only one phase of the cycle might be expected at any given time to exert maximal effects only on a very small proportion of cells.

The growth of the tumor mass depends on the percentage of cells actively cycling (growth fraction), the cell doubling time (cycle time), and the rate of cell death. A tumor with a short cell doubling time, a large growth fraction, and a low rate of cell loss would be expected to increase rapidly in size, whereas one with a long cell doubling time, a small growth fraction, and a high rate of cell loss may change minimally over a long time interval. These factors are responsible for the great variability in clinical behavior that is frequently observed even in histologically similar tumors.

Most experiments in animal and human tumor systems have shown that tumor growth is critically related to the proportion of cells that are actively in cycle, and that the growth fraction is usually inversely related to the size of the tumor. Gompertz, a 19th century actuary, derived a mathematical formula for predicting age-related mortality that fits the observed growth rates for most animal and human tumors that have been studied (Fig. 2). An initial rapid growth phase (log phase) is followed by a slower phase (plateau). Experimental data from a variety of tumor systems reveal that the major factor responsible for these growth characteristics is the amount of cells proliferating in the tumor at a given time, and not a change in individual cell doubling time (cell cycle time). During the log phase of growth when the tumor is clinically undetectable, the proliferative index is high. About the time the tumor becomes clinically detectable (about 1 cm^3), tumor growth slows and enters the plateau phase.

In addition there is a growing number of investigations that indicate great heterogeneity of cancer cells within the same individual tumor [Tsuruo and Fidler, 1981]. Within a tumor exist subpopulations of cells with different growth characteristics, metastatic potential, and susceptibility to therapy. These observations have profound implications not only for drug trials but also for the investigation of neoplasia in general.

From these concepts the chemotherapist should recognize the following: 1) Since most chemotherapeutic agents are effective in destroying proliferating cells, the smaller the tumor the higher the probability for a larger growth fraction, and the better the chance for a good therapeutic result. 2) At the time of clinical detection (1 cm^3), a malignant tumor has already completed 75% of the doublings that it will need to destroy the host (33 of

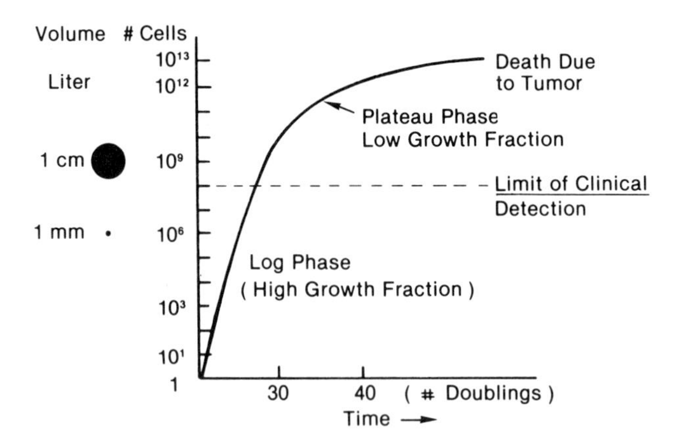

Fig. 2. Gompertzian curve. Size and number of cells in the tumor are plotted on the Y-axis, time and number of doublings on the X axis. A period of increased growth, the log phase, is followed by a slower or plateau phase.

approximately 40). 3) Substantially decreasing the tumor volume ("debulking"), whether by surgery, radiation therapy, chemotherapy or other treatment, may enable one to further improve therapeutic efficacy by bringing resting (G_0) cells into the cell cycle (recruitment). 4) Within a given tumor there is likely to be cellular heterogeneity, resulting in variable sensitivity of individual tumor cells to specific agents.

The doubling times of several human tumors are shown in Table I. The concepts above are supported by the observation that cytotoxic therapy has had its greatest success in tumors with rapid doubling times and hence high growth fractions.

FUNDAMENTAL CONCEPTS OF CANCER CHEMOTHERAPY

Cancer chemotherapy is based on the following fundamental concepts: 1) For a given malignancy the potential for cure is inversely related to the tumor burden—that is, the smaller the tumor the more likely the probability for response; 2) in general there is dose-response effect for most cancer chemotherapeutic agents; 3) the development of cancer cell resistance to chemotherapy is a frequent event, and increases directly with the number of cancer cells (size of the tumor) and the length of time it takes to complete treatment; and 4) chemotherapy kills a constant fraction (%) of cells after each given dose, and *not* a specific number of cells (the log-kill hypothesis).

The first principle derives directly from the observation that smaller tumors have higher growth fractions and are consequently more sensitive to cytotoxic agents.

TABLE I. Tumor Doubling Time, Response, and Potential Curability With Chemotherapy

Tumor type	Doubling time (days)	Percent CR to chemotherapy	Percent curable with chemotherapy
Gestational choriocarcinoma	1.5[a]	85–100	75–95
Acute lymphoblastic leukemia	4–6[b]	80–90	60
Testicular (excludes teratocarcinoma)	21[c]	75	60
Hodgkin's disease	38[c]	75	50–60
Squamous carcinoma	58[d]	30–40	Rare
Lung—small cell	67[e]	30–60	0–10
Adenocarcinomas	83[d]	20–40	Rare
Lung—adenocarcinomas	134[c]	20–40	Rare

From [a]Zubrod, 1972; [b]Henderson and Jones, 1982; [c]Shackney et al., 1978; [d]Tubiana and Malaise, 1977; [e]Charbit et al., 1972.

Although dose-response effects for chemotherapeutic agents vary, in most systems the larger the dose the greater the cell kill. The importance of the dose-response curve is illustrated in Figure 3. With a steep dose-response curve as noted in A, a small change in dose may have major therapeutic effects. With B, the response could be intermediate, and with C tremendous increases in dosage would be required to achieve even modest gains in therapeutic results. These data have broad implications concerning the potential toxicity of the drug or drugs being used. For single-agent therapy, early attainment of the maximally tolerated dose is of main importance since if response is not observed, it is assured that further alterations in dose will not be beneficial. For combination chemotherapy, the assumptions become more complex. In general, except for nonmyelosuppressive agents, maximally tolerated doses of drugs cannot be given in combination without risking major toxicity and a decrease in the therapeutic index. Thus for combination regimens the potential benefit of each drug included must be carefully weighed since toxicity from relatively inactive drugs may necessitate suboptimal doses of active drugs.

Dramatic responses to chemotherapy are frequently followed by relapse. Numerous mechanisms of drug resistance have been defined including

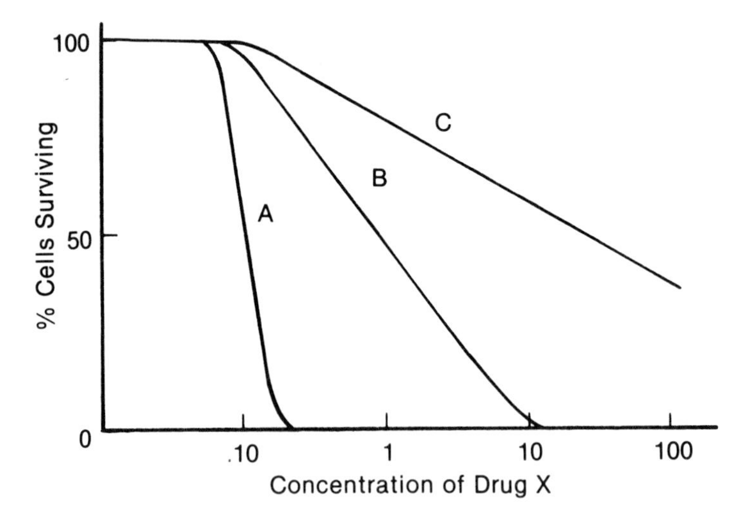

Fig. 3. Dose-response curve. The percent cell survival is plotted against the concentration of a drug, X. A) A steep dose-response curve indicates marked enhancement of cytotoxicity with a small change in drug concentration. B) A substantial change in drug concentration is needed to enhance cytotoxicity. C) Even extremely great changes in concentration extending over several orders of magnitude are unlikely to obtain maximum cytotoxicity.

alterations in the cell membrane and induction of new enzymes resulting in salvage pathways which bypass key cytotoxic effects. The work of Goldie has suggested strategies for overcoming potential resistance to chemotheraphy [Goldie et al., 1982]. In this hypothesis resistant cells are considered to arise from spontaneous mutations in the cancer cell population, and these mutations occur with a measurable frequency. Fundamental to this hypothesis is the premise that the probability for cure is related to the product of the mutation rate as well as the tumor size.

There are at least two main means to attack the problem of cell resistance. First, one can use several drugs with different mechanisms of action concurrently, in an effort to destroy the maximum number of tumor cells in the shortest period of time. Resistance would be less likely with several agents than with a single agent. Second, one can treat the tumor at the earliest possible time, since the smaller the tumor the smaller the number of potentially resistant cells. This hypothesis is an important correlate to the principles above and supports the concepts that the most beneficial therapeutic results are obtained when tumor volumes are small, that for almost all curable human tumors maximal responses to chemotherapy are seen early in the course of treatment, and that failure to see a complete response is synonymous with treatment failure. It also questions the value of "maintenance chemotherapy," which has not proved to be necessary in most curable malignancies. Therapy if directed at cure should therefore be maximal at the time of initial tumor presentation. Another important hypothesis relevant to the design of treatment programs is that put forth by Norton and Simon [1977]. This hypothesis questions several commonly held concepts and considers the possibility that as tumors respond to effective therapy, the growth fraction may actually decrease. Small microscopic tumors will then be less sensitive and not more sensitive to chemotherapy. This hypothesis, like Goldie's, questions the value of continuous low-dose "maintenance" therapy and suggests that large doses of treatment be given even after maximal response (complete remission) is obtained, so-called "late intensification." Both these hypotheses are currently being tested in clinical trials.

The last observation describes the kinetics of cell kill for anticancer agents and has been elegantly described by Skipper and colleagues [Skipper et al., 1964]. These data indicate that when a dose of an effective agent is given, a constant fraction (percent) of cells are destroyed and not a specific number of cells. This concept, termed the "log-kill hypothesis," is illustrated in Figure 4 and leads to the following conclusions: 1) After only several courses of chemotherapy a tumor may become undetectable, yet therapy will have

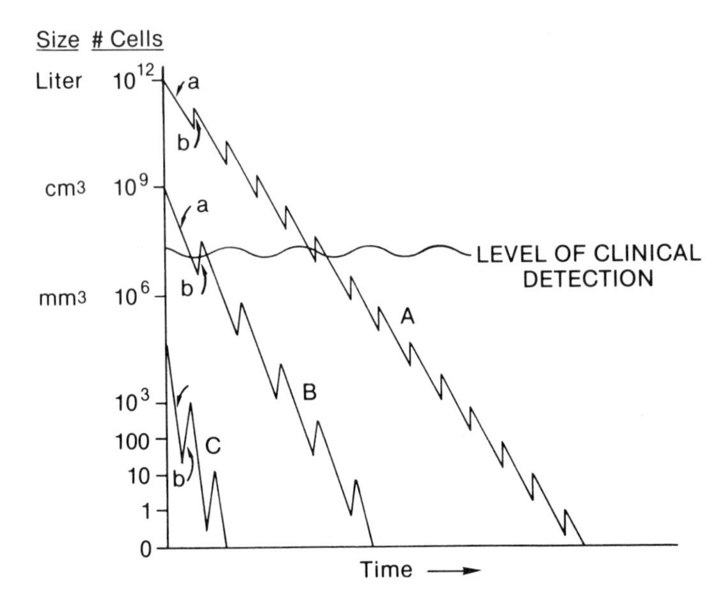

Fig. 4. Log-kill hypothesis. The number of cells and tumor size are plotted versus time. In curve A only a small fraction of cells are destroyed with each dose of drug administration. Line *a* indicates the extent of the log kill each time the specific drug is given. Line *b* indicates the regrowth of the tumor prior to the next course. Tumor resistance and subsequent regrowth are most probable in this situation. Curve B pertains to a smaller malignancy where a dosage of drug results in a larger cell kill each time it is administered. The percent of cells destroyed each time the drug is administered (line *a*) is larger, and because the tumor is smaller there is a higher probability of tumor eradication. Curve C pertains to therapy of a small, clinically occult malignancy that is assumed to be rapidly growing. A large percentage of cells is destroyed each time the drug is given, and because the tumor is smaller a short course of treatment is likely to result in cure.

to be continued to obtain total tumor eradication; 2) a tumor has the ability to regrow and ultimately destroy the host as long as there is even one viable cell, only total eradication of the tumor can lead to cure; 3) by increasing the percentage of cell kill for each dose, or by starting treatment with the tumor at a smaller volume, one is more likely to achieve total tumor eradication.

The concepts above are fundamental to the understanding of tumor biology and the effects of cytotoxic agents on both malignant and normal tissue. Having precise details such as the growth characteristics of an individual tumor as well as information suggesting which cytotoxic agents are most likely to be beneficial, the oncologist is best able to design promising therapeutic trials.

CLINICAL PHARMACOLOGY

Response to chemotherapy is dependent on numerous factors all related to the final step of drug administration—the reaction of the drug or its active metabolite with the appropriate target. Before this is achieved, the agent(s) must be administered to the patient by one of several routes, must equilibrate with plasma or other tissue fluids, may require activation in a normal host tissue, must be transported to the tumor site, must permeate the tumor bed and be transported across the tumor cell membrane, and must react with the target site before being metabolized. The numerous steps involved in this process underlie its complexity.

At the cellular level, membrane transport remains a crucial factor and both active (carrier-mediated) and passive transport processes may be involved. These processes are influenced by the molecular size and configuration of the drug, its concentration, lipid solubility, the pH of the milieu, temperature, and other factors. In addition, other agents may enhance or compete with the chemotherapeutic agent at the membrane level. Recently, attempts at modifying the cell membrane to facilitate drug delivery have been made. Agents such as amphotericin may alter cell membranes and allow enhanced transport of active drugs [Presant et al., 1980]. The use of liposomes to facilitate drug delivery to individual cells has also been shown to be a potentially feasible method of drug delivery [Weinstein et al., 1979].

In addition, preliminary data suggests that tumor oxygenation may play a major role in drug sensitivity. In a system utilizing mouse mammary tumor cells in culture, bleomycin, streptonigrin, procarbazine, dactinomycin, and vincristine were preferentially cytotoxic to cells under oxygenated conditions whereas mitomycin and doxorubicin had greater effects on hypoxic cells. The nitrosoureas, cisplatin, methotrexate, and fluorouracil displayed no preferential cytotoxity either under hypoxic or oxygenated conditions [Teicher et al., 1981]. Hypoxic cells can also be modified by electron-affinic agents such as misonidazole to make them more sensitive to chemotherapeutic agents, most notably melphalan, cyclophosphamide, fluorouracil, and cisplatin [Adams, 1981]. Such cell "sensitizers" are currently being studied in conjunction with irradiation therapy and, more recently, chemotherapy. Early trials are also in progress studying compounds capable of protecting normal host tissues from the potential toxic effects of chemotherapeutic agents, thus allowing higher dosage.

Other methods are also being investigated which may enhance the therapeutic index. Hyperthermia, ultrasound, and other physical methods may change tumor characteristics and enhance drug uptake. These approaches, which attempt to modify the normal or malignant tissue of the host, hold great promise and are likely to be the focus of many new clinical trials.

The route of drug delivery is another crucial variable. When feasible, oral administration is preferred by most patients, but is associated with the major drawback of variable absorption. The intravenous route is usually preferred since drug delivery is more predictable and factors such as patient compliance are minimized. More recently there has been renewed interest in regional and organ infusions. An example is hepatic artery infusion with fluorodeoxyuridine (FUdR), which has been shown to be associated with high response rates in patients with isolated hepatic metastasis from colon cancer. Such systems of drug delivery frequently allow one to increase the therapeutic index of the drug used. In addition, new methods for infusing drugs such as totally implantable pumps (Infusaid™) have made such techniques more acceptable to patients [Ensminger et al., 1981]. Intraperitoneal, intrapleural, and intrathecal administration of agents may also enhance the therapeutic index by leading to increased local concentrations of drugs that would not be achieved with systemic treatment without the risk of increased toxicity. Recently, intraperitoneal treatment for ovarian cancer has attracted considerable interest. Doxorubicin, cisplatin, fluorouracil, and methotrexate have been given to selected patients using an intraperitoneal or "belly bath" technique with encouraging preliminary results [as discussed by Walton in this volume].

Regardless of the method of administration, the goal is to achieve an effective drug level of the agent(s) selected for the longest period of time, with the least toxicity. Determining the therapeutic level of an agent by following its concentration over a period of time ($C \times t$) enables one to compare different dosages and schedules. In order to apply such information for drug selection, three major factors must be considered: 1) the lowest concentration of drug needed to achieve cytotoxicity; 2) the peak concentration of drug expected according to the route, schedule, and dose selected; and 3) the pharmacokinetic properties of the drug including rate of excretion and metabolism.

Effective concentrations of drugs needed for cytotoxicity can be approximated from pharmacologic data in vivo, as well as from in vitro cytotoxic studies using such methods as the human tumor stem cell (clonigenic) assay. Information related to pharmacologic principles relies on carefully done studies in human and animal tumor systems.

Crucial data obtained from pharmacologic evaluation relate to drug distribution, rate of elimination, and mode of excretion. The distribution measurements define the dispersion of the drug into body tissues. The rate of elimination is best defined by the half-life of the drug ($T_{1/2}$). Most cytotoxic drugs are eliminated by having a specific fraction (or %) of the drug metabolized or excreted per unit time, a first order kinetic process. Detailed analysis of urine, biliary, and fecal contents as well as other body fluids will clarify routes of drug excretion; such data are necessary so as to minimize toxicity which might result from giving standard doses of drugs to patients who have damage to an organ system that is the dominant site of drug excretion or metabolism (e.g., doxorubicin in patients with hepatic disease).

Lastly, host factors that influence response to treatment must be considered in program planning. The performance status, a semiquantitative means of describing patient function, has been related to response in most studies. In general, the sicker the patient the less likely the response to treatment. Age, number of metastatic sites, and other patient variables may also be of prime importance depending on the type of malignancy being treated.

CHEMOTHERAPEUTIC AGENTS

Continued development of cancer chemotherapeutic agents has resulted in a large list of active agents comprising several drug classes. In Table II, the most commonly used agents are listed according to generic name, common name, registered trademark, and effectiveness in gynecologic and breast cancer. The sections below describe specific classes of drugs with agents active in the treatment of gynecologic malignancy discussed in more detail. Pharmacologic data, unless otherwise specified, have been compiled from reviews and texts by Carter et al. [1982], Chabner and Myers [1982], Chabner [1982], Dorr and Fritz [1980], Holland and Frei [1982], and Pratt and Ruddon [1979]. These sources all provide excellent, in-depth reviews of the anticancer agents.

Alkylating Agents

The alkylating agents consist of six major classes of drugs: 1) nitrogen mustards—mechlorethamine, cyclophosphamide, ifosfamide,* melphalan, chlorambucil, and uracil mustard; 2) nitrosoureas—carmustine (BCNU), lomustine (CCNU), semustine,* streptozotocin, chlorozotocin;* 3) ethyleneimines—triethylene thiophosphoramide (thiotepa); 4) methane sulfonic acid esters—busulfan; 5) triazines—dacarbazine; and 6) miscellaneous—cisplatin, galactitol,* dibromodulcitol.*

*Investigational use only.

TABLE II. Commonly Used Chemotherapeutic Agents: Efficacy in Breast and Gynecologic Malignancy

Generic	Common name	Trademark	Therapeutic efficacy[c]					
			Breast	Cervix	Endometrium	Ovary	Sarcoma	Germ cell
Alkylating agents								
Mechlorethamine	Nitrogen mustard, HN_2	Mustargen	++[f]			++		
Chlorambucil		Leukeran	++	+/++	–[d]	++	++	+/++
Melphalan	Phenylalanine mustard, L-PAM	Alkeran	++	+/++		++	+[e]	
Cyclophosphamide		Cytoxan	++	+/++		++	++	+
Carmustine	BCNU	BicNU	+					
Lomustine	CCNU	CeeNU	–/+					
Semustine	Methyl-CCNU	I[b]	–/+					
Chlorozotocin	DCNU	I						
Streptozotocin	STZ	Zanosar						
Busulfan		Myleran						
Dacarbazine	DTIC, DIC	DTIC-DOME	–/+				+/++	
Triethylene thiophosphoramide	Thiotepa	Thiotepa	++			++		
Cisplatin	Platinum, CPDD, CDDP	Platinol	+	++	+	++	+/++	++
Antimetabolites								
Fluorouracil	5-Fluorouracil, 5-FU	Fluorouracil, Adrucil	++	+	+/++	++		
Methotrexate	Amethopterin, MTX	Methotrexate, Mexate	++	+/++		++		+/++
Citrovorum factor[a]	Folinic acid, 5-formyl-FH_4	Leucovorin Calcium						
Mercaptopurine	6-Mercaptopurine, 6-MP	Purinethol	+					
Thioguanine	6-Thioguanine, 6-TG	Thioguanine	–/+					
Cytarabine	Cytosine arabinoside, ara-C	Cytosar	+					

Antibiotics								
Dactinomycin	Actinomycin D	Cosmegen	+				+	+/++
Daunorubicin	Daunomycin, rubidomycin	Cerubidine						
Doxorubicin		Adriamycin	++		++	++	++	
Bleomycin		Blenoxane		+				++
Mithramycin		Mithracin	−/+					+/++
Mitomycin	Mitomycin C	Mutamycin	++					
Plant alkaloids								
Vincristine		Oncovin	++	−/+			+/++	+/++
Vinblastine		Velban	++			+		
Etoposide	VP-16	VePesid	−/+	−	+	+	−	++
Miscellaneous								
Hydroxyurea		Hydrea	−/+	−				
Procarbazine		Matulane	−					
Hexamethylmelamine		I	+/++	+		++		
L-asparaginase		Elspar						

[a]Used as rescue for high-dose MTX.
[b]I = investigational use only.
[c]Blank = none or not enough data.
[d]Inactive.
[e]+ = 10–20% response.
[f]++ = >20% response.
Data concerning response is approximation only; compiled from Livingston and Carter, 1970, and major text references cited.

Alkylating agents possess one to several reactive alkyl groups capable of forming an ionized, highly reactive, positively charged intermediate that binds covalently to a negatively charged nucleophilic group such as the amino or carboxyl group on a protein or nucleic acid. Those agents with more than one reactive group may, after forming a covalent bond with one molecule, form a covalent bond with the same molecule or another molecule resulting in cross-linking of protein or nucleic acid strands. The alkylating agents are not phase-specific; however, most exert their maximal cytotoxicity on cells that are actively in cycle and synthesizing DNA.

The most commonly used alkylating agents used in gynecologic malignancy include chlorambucil, cyclophosphamide, melphalan, and most recently cisplatin. Nitrosoureas, although displaying modest activity in some gynecologic tumors, have not added to current treatment programs. Thiotepa may be used in place of mustardlike agents but is not commonly prescribed. Dacarbazine is used in sarcoma therapy but its activity appears modest at best. Several of the investigational drugs such as galactitol have activity, but their role in improving current treatment modalities is yet to be determined.

Cyclophosphamide. Cyclophosphamide is unique among the alkylating agents since it requires activation by the hepatic microsomal mixed-function oxidase system to its active metabolite phosphoramide mustard. Although the drug can be given orally or intravenously, it has variable oral absorption. Its metabolism can be affected by other compounds, especially those that may stimulate the liver microsome system, but there is no convincing evidence that this alters therapeutic efficacy or toxicity. In addition, although renal elimination remains a major route of drug excretion, especially for the more polar and ionized metabolites, there is no evidence that severe renal impairment increases hematologic toxicity. In patients with markedly diminished hepatic function, cyclophosphamide can still be converted to its active metabolite, phosphoramide mustard. The plasma $T_{1/2}$ of 3–12 h is somewhat longer than most other mustards.

Short-term toxicity includes myelosuppression, nausea and vomiting, and drug-induced hemorrhagic cystitis. Myelosuppression primarily consists of leukopenia, and marked thrombocytopenia is uncommon. The nadir is usually seen between days 8 and 14 with recovery within 2–3 weeks. Gastrointestinal toxicity consisting of nausea and vomiting can be substantial with large intravenous doses but is also common, although milder, with the smaller oral doses frequently used in breast and ovarian cancer. It may be ameliorated by changes in time of administration and antiemetics. Drug-induced hemorrhagic cystitis is an infrequent but major complication. Patients may complain of frequency or urgency hours to weeks after administration, and urine analysis reveals microscopic hematuria with negative bacterial cultures; definitive diagnosis requires cystoscopy and biopsy. Continued utilization in patients with cystitis may result in cumulative bladder damage and the development of a small fibrotic bladder. Recent evidence has suggested that the cellular dysplasia that is commonly found can lead to bladder carcinoma. A high oral fluid intake may minimize cystitis. Patients who have recurrent cystitis should not be given further cyclophosphamide; another alkylating agent such as chlorambucil, thiotepa, or melphalan should be substituted. On rare occasions, and after large dosages, patients have been reported to have inappropriate antidiuretic hormone secretion. Pulmonary or cardiac toxicity is rare. Alopecia is usually minimal at lower doses, but may be moderate at higher dosage.

Chlorambucil. Chlorambucil, another member of the mustard class of alkylating agents, is available for use by the oral route. Unlike cyclophosphamide and melphalan, however, the drug is well absorbed orally with a $T_{1/2}$ of approximately 1.5 h. Except for myelosuppression with a nadir of 2–4 weeks, chlorambucil is relatively devoid of toxicity. Pulmonary fibrosis is rare, and nausea and vomiting are uncommon.

Melphalan. Melphalan, another mustard compound, is generally given by oral administration, although intravenous forms are available for investigational use. The drug has variable oral absorption and unless myelosuppression is noted it is not clinically possible to determine if adequate drug has been given. The mean $T_{1/2}$ is approximately 2 h and in man, fecal excretion appears to be the main method of elimination of the drug.

Like chlorambucil, melphalan is relatively devoid of substantial toxicity except for myelosuppression. Nadir counts are usually seen 2–3 weeks after oral administration with recovery taking 1 to several weeks. Continued administration may lead to cumulative bone marrow toxicity and longer times to recovery. Nausea and vomiting are uncommon. Pulmonary fibrosis has been reported but is extremely rare.

Cisplatin. Cisplatin, considered an alkylating agent, exerts its principal action by embedding itself between DNA base pairs (intercalation) with subsequent cross-linking of DNA nucleic acid strands. The drug is given intravenously and has a short initial $T_{1/2}$ of 30–60 min followed by a long secondary $T_{1/2}$ of 2–3 days. The drug is excreted mainly in the urine.

Cisplatin, although effective in many solid tumors, must be used cautiously because of its potential toxicity. Moderate to severe nausea and vomiting are seen in almost all patients although newer antiemetics such as metoclopramide will alleviate these symptoms in more than half the patients. Nephrotoxicity due to proximal tubular damage, previously dose-limiting, has generally been eliminated by vigorous hydration. Hypocalcemia, hypokalemia, and hypomagnesemia occur frequently and produce arrhythmias or tetany in a small percentage of patients. Myelosuppression is usually mild to moderate, and usually occurs only after large cumulative doses or in combined drug regimens. Peripheral neuropathy and CNS symptoms are occasionally seen after large doses and may be severe, including profound loss of motor function, seizures, and visual disturbances. Ototoxicity has been noted, and while clinical hearing loss is unusual, patients receiving a large cumulative dose should be questioned concerning hearing loss, and an audiogram should be performed if such toxicity is suspected. Uncommonly allergic reactions including anaphylaxis have been noted. Low doses of cisplatin up to 50 mg/m^2 can generally be given in the outpatient setting after adequate hydration is ensured. Larger doses generally require hospital admission and close monitoring.

Dacarbazine. Dacarbazine, although a structural analogue of a precursor for purine bases, exerts its main activity as an alkylating agent. The drug is only available for intravenous use and has an average plasma $T_{1/2}$ of 5 h. Most of the drug is metabolized by the liver although urinary excretion can account for 30–45% of the administered dose.

Toxicity includes severe nausea and vomiting in most patients, and may be difficult to control with antiemetics. In addition, a flu-like syndrome characterized by low-grade fever, myalgia, and malaise is occasionally noted, especially with large doses. These symptoms may last several weeks and usually occur several days after completion of the treatment program. Myelosuppression is generally moderate, occurs 3–4 weeks after administration, and usually is not dose-limiting in commonly used schedules.

Antimetabolites

The antimetabolites are structural analogues of nucleic acid bases, whose major action is competition with normal metabolic substrates for key enzymes involved in DNA and RNA synthesis. Antimetabolites can be divided into three major groups: 1) folate antagonists—methotrexate, triazinate,* dichloromethotrexate*; 2) pyrimidine antagonists—fluorouracil, fluorodeoxyuridine, cytarabine, ftorafur,* 5-azacytidine*; and 3) purine antagonists—azathioprine, mercaptopurine, thioguanine.

Antifols. The folate antagonist methotrexate represents the prototype for this group although other folate antagonists such as triazinate (Baker's antifol) and dichloromethotrexate are available for investigational use. Methotrexate inhibits the key enzyme, dihydrofolate reductase, which catalyzes the conversion of folic acid to its active tetrahydrofolate metabolites. Enzyme blockage leads to inhibition of transfer of one-carbon moieties which are needed to synthesize thymidylic acid and purine rings, with subsequent arrest of DNA, RNA, and protein synthesis. The antifols are cell cycle–specific and have their greatest activity in cells in S-phase. Triazinate has been studied in human tumors and seems to offer no advantages when compared with methotrexate. Dichloromethotrexate, unlike methotrexate, is excreted in the bile and may prove to be of value in combination chemotherapy programs using potentially nephrotoxic agents.

Methotrexate. Methotrexate may be administered by oral, intramuscular, or intravenous routes and can also be used for intrathecal therapy. Oral doses less than 30 mg/m^2 are well absorbed. The average initial plasma $T_{1/2}$ of methotrexate is 2 h followed by a secondary $T_{1/2}$ of 10 h. Methotrexate is excreted unchanged in the urine. Since it is a weak acid in its plasma form, its urinary excretion can be diminished by salicylates, probenecid, and other drugs that diminish the renal excretion of weak acids. Salicylates, sulfonamides, phenytoin (Dilantin), and other compounds displace methotrexate from its protein-binding sites, resulting in increased serum levels, and may enhance toxicity.

Methotrexate can also be given in very high intravenous doses followed by the administration of calcium leucovorin (citrovorum factor)—"high-dose methotrexate with rescue." Citrovorum factor, a tetrahydrofolate, bypasses the enzymatic block produced by methotrexate, resulting in salvage of the affected metabolic pathways. Protocols utilizing high doses of methotrexate with rescue may use doses of several hundred milligrams to 15–25 g. The therapeutic advantage of high-dose therapy rests on the assumption that malignant cells have different membrane characteristics or inadequate salvage pathways rendering them less susceptible to rescue. Convincing evidence that high-dose methotrexate with rescue is therapeutically superior to conventional dosage is lacking, and several trials comparing conventional and high-dose therapies have not shown significantly different results. High-dose therapy does yield cytotoxic CSF levels which may be efficacious in malignancies such as leukemia and lymphoma, where tumor meningitis is a common event. Patients receiving high-dose programs must be adequately hydrated, their urine alkalinized, and closely monitored. Although uncommon, nephrotoxicity can be a major complication of high-dose treatment, and pooling of methotrexate in effusions may lead to markedly elevated serum levels for prolonged periods, increasing the likelihood of toxicity. At present, high cost and potential toxicity preclude the routine use of high-dose therapy; it is still considered investigational.

Myelosuppression is frequent but with standard clinical doses is generally mild to moderate. The time to the nadir is slightly shorter than with alkylating agents and averages 1–2 weeks followed by rapid recovery. Nausea and vomiting are usually absent or mild, but mucositis can be disabling, involve the entire oral and gastrointestinal mucosa, and poses the risk for secondary superinfection and, rarely, perforation. Diarrhea is also occasionally seen. Patients may infrequently have transient elevation of liver function tests, but hepatic damage is uncommon except in patients receiving long-term, low, oral dosage where fibrosis and cirrhosis have been reported. Pulmonary complications, allergic reactions, and significant alopecia are uncommon.

Pyrimidine antagonists. Pyrimidine antagonists include fluorouracil, fluorodeoxyuridine (FUdR), cytarabine, and investigational agents such as 5-azacytidine, cyclocytidine, and ftorafur. It is unlikely that these newer compounds will prove to be of major value in the therapy of gynecologic malignancy.

Fluorouracil. Fluorouracil, by acting as a "false" pyrimidine base, competes with uracil deoxyribotide for the active site on thymidylate synthetase, the enzyme essential for the conversion of uridylic to thymidylic acid. Fluorouracil exerts its maximal cytotoxic effect in S-phase and impedes DNA synthesis; it can, however, inhibit RNA synthesis and other metabolic events within the cell. The drug is generally given by IV bolus, although recently the use of continuous infusions have aroused interest and have been used in several single-agent and combination chemotherapy protocols. To date, however, there is no role for continuous intravenous infusion except for investigational use. Fluorouracil is mainly metabolized intracellularly and in the liver with a small percentage excreted unchanged in the urine. Its $T_{1/2}$ in the plasma is short, lasting 10–15 min.

Major toxicity relates to the gastrointestinal tract and bone marrow. Nausea and vomiting are generally not severe; however, large doses can result in severe stomatitis and diarrhea. These latter toxicities if prolonged can become life-threatening. Leukopenia and thrombocytopenia are generally mild, usually seen within 1–2 weeks, and recovery is usually rapid. Significant alopecia is rare. The drug is occasionally associated with hyperpigmentation of the nailbeds and superficial veins. An unusual but significant complication of fluorouracil seen after very large doses or infusions is cerebellar ataxia, which usually spontaneously subsides after discontinuation of therapy.

Fluorouracil has been given orally although its variable gastrointestinal absorption precludes recommending this route for routine use. Solutions and creams containing fluorouracil are also available and have been used for patients with premalignant keratoses and malignant lesions of the skin. In addition, fluorouracil and its closely related analogue fluorodeoxyuridine (FUdR) have been used for intra-arterial therapy, most notably in patients with hepatic metastasis from colorectal carcinoma. Intraperitoneal administration of fluorouracil to patients with ovarian cancer may be beneficial, and the drug can be used as an intracavitary agent in the treatment of effusions. Such therapy will be discussed in subsequent chapters.

Purine antagonists. The purine antagonists, although highly active in several human malignancies, have no firmly established role in the treatment of gynecologic or breast cancer. By today's standards, however, most of these compounds have not had adequate clinical trials in untreated or minimally treated patients with metastatic disease. Further investigation is needed to define conclusively the role of these agents in patients with gynecologic malignancy.

Antitumor Antibiotics

This group consists of agents obtained from microbial fermentation processes that have a wide variety of effects and activity in human tumors. They tend to have long plasma half-lives and many behave like alkylating agents, cross-linking DNA and RNA strands. The antibiotics that have established roles in gynecologic cancer are discussed below. Many new agents are currently undergoing investigation.

Bleomycin. Bleomycin consists of a mixture of several different peptide subtypes, is cell cycle–specific, and exhibits major activity in the G_2 and M-phases. The drug can be given only by intravenous or intramuscular administration although it is occasionally used as an intracavitary agent in patients with malignant effusions.

Bleomycin is rapidly metabolized in all tissues except for the skin and lung, the two organs most likely to be involved in toxic reactions. Of importance is the fact that up to 20–40% of the drug is excreted in the urine over a 24-h period and dose modifications are recommended in patients with severe compromise of renal function. The drug has a short initial $T_{1/2}$ of 10–20 min followed by a terminal $T_{1/2}$ of about 2–3 h.

Toxicity includes febrile reactions which are commonly seen and usually occur several hours after drug administration. Concurrent use of corticosteroids may prevent this toxicity. Anaphylactic reactions have been reported but seem rare. Nevertheless, appropriate precautions should be taken in patients receiving bleomycin; epinephrine, hydrocortisone, and diphenhydramine (Benedryl) should be available at the bedside. Skin reactions are common and occasionally account for dose-limiting toxicity. Erythema and inflammation are frequently seen in the hands and over pressure points such as the elbows. Hyperpigmentation is also common although this rarely results in protocol modification. Severe stomatitis may occur. The most serious complication is pulmonary toxicity, which is most common in patients over age 70, those with prior chest or mediastinal irradiation, or those who have received more than 500 mg of drug; however, a small percentage of patients may develop lethal damage even after very small doses. Early detection rests on the clinical finding of fine basilar rales on chest auscultation which frequently precede chest x-ray evidence of disease. Pulmonary function tests commonly show a decreased vital capacity, with the diffusion capacity being the first and most sensitive indicator of alveolar damage. Patients requiring surgery who have had prior bleomycin must have the inspired oxygen content closely monitored as high pO_2 levels may enhance subclinical pulmonary damage, increasing the probability of serious or fatal pulmonary toxicity.

Dactinomycin. Dactinomycin, a cell cycle–specific agent with optimum activity in the G_1 and S-phases, interferes with DNA as well as RNA synthesis. The drug is given intravenously and after equilibrating in body tissue is slowly cleared from the plasma and excreted in the bile and urine. Dose modifications should be considered for patients with severe hepatic or renal disease. The drug has a long serum half-life of 36 h and whereas previously, small daily doses were given, many protocols now incorporate single large doses with similar antitumor activity.

The major toxicity is myelosuppression which is generally seen 1–2 weeks after treatment with the nadir occurring at 3 weeks. Thrombocytopenia may be profound and precede leukopenia. The drug must be given with caution since skin infiltration causes severe necrosis. Nausea and vomiting are moderate to severe. Large doses may result in substantial mucositis involving the entire alimentary tract. Skin changes are frequent with acne-like rashes most commonly observed. An unusual property of dactinomycin is its ability to cause erythema and occasional skin ulceration in skin sites that have received prior radiation therapy ("radiation recall reaction"). This may occur as long as several months after treatment. Alopecia is moderate.

Doxorubicin. Doxorubicin (adriamycin) exerts its effect by intercalating between DNA base pairs, resulting in inhibition of DNA and RNA synthesis. It is cell cycle–nonspecific, but its maximum effects are seen during the S-phase. The drug must be administered intravenously and is metabolized predominantly by the liver. Dose modifications are required for patients with hepatic dysfunction. The initial plasma $T_{1/2}$ is short at 30 min to 4 h, with a long terminal $T_{1/2}$ of 24 h.

The major toxicity of doxorubicin is myelosuppression, with granulocytes being much more severely affected than platelets. The nadir count usually occurs 1–2 weeks after the drug has been administered, and there is usually rapid return to normal pretreatment levels. Total alopecia is almost always observed. The use of scalp hypothermia may diminish this complication. The most serious potential complication of doxorubicin is a cardiomyopathy, which is rarely seen in patients who have received less than 450 mg/m^2 of drug, and clinically presents as congestive heart failure that is generally refractory to standard medical management. Older patients, those who have received mediastinal irradiation, or those who have a preexisting history of heart disease are at highest risk. Techniques that measure left ventricular function such as echocardiography and radionuclide scanning (MUGA scanning) may be used to monitor cardiac function, although their role in predicting and preventing toxicity is not precisely defined. Endomyocardial biopsy techniques have also been developed and may be helpful in selecting patients at high risk for toxicity [Bristow et al., 1978]. Keeping the total dosage below 450 mg/m^2 should prevent this complication in most patients. Nausea, vomiting, and stomatitis are usually moderate. The drug must be administered with great caution since leakage into the tissue can cause severe necrosis which on occasion has led to limb loss. In a small percentage of patients a reddish hue and "flare" may be noted in the vein used for drug administration, a rapidly resolving side effect that is not indicative of a drug leakage. Hyperpigmentation has also been noted. An insignificant but frequently alarming side effect is the passage of red urine due to renal excretion of the parent drug. This usually occurs within hours of drug administration and is not of clinical consequence. Radiation recall reactions similar to dactinomycin are occasionally seen.

Mitomycin. Mitomycin probably functions as an alkylating agent resulting in cross linking of DNA strands. It is cell cycle–nonspecific but appears most active in the G_1 and S-phases. It must be given intravenously and is mainly metabolized in the liver although a small percent is excreted in the urine. In spite of its very short $T_{1/2}$, probably 30–40 min, large boluses appear as clinically effective as small daily doses [Carter and Crooke, 1979].

The major toxicity is myelosuppression, which is cumulative. Nadirs are generally seen at 3–4 weeks and once toxicity is observed, recovery may be very slow, possibly as long as 4–6 weeks. Nausea, vomiting, and stomatitis are generally not a major problem. As with doxorubicin and dactinomycin, severe skin damage may result from drug leakage and meticulous administration is necessary. On rare occasions patients may develop severe alopecia, liver function abnormalities, or pulmonary toxicities. Nephrotoxicity is uncommon but has been reported. The current use of mitomycin in several adjuvant programs, mainly for gastrointestinal carcinoma, has been associated with reports of an adult "hemolytic-uremic" syndrome, consisting of microangiopathic hemolytic anemia and progressive glomerular damage [Kressel et al., 1981]. This syndrome, although uncommon, has usually been progressive and has resulted in death in most patients reported. Caution must be recommended for the use of mitomycin in patients with a favorable long-term prognosis until the pathophysiology of this unusual but frequently reported syndrome is defined.

Plant Alkaloids

The plant alkaloids include vincristine and vinblastine, naturally occurring substances derived from the periwinkle plant (*Vinca rosea*); semisynthetic compounds such as etoposide (VP-16), Tenoposide (VM-26), and vindesine; and maytansine derived from the mandrake plant. Although some of these compounds are structurally related, they vary substantially in their spectrum of antitumor activity and toxicity.

The most commonly used agents are vincristine and vinblastine, discussed in detail below. Etoposide shows great promise in the treatment of a variety of malignancies including germ cell tumors. Tenoposide is similar in activity to etoposide and, like vindesine and maytansine, is currently being investigated.

Vinblastine. Vinblastine, cell cycle–specific for the M-phase, must be administered by intravenous injection and has a short initial $T_{1/2}$ of 30–60 min and long terminal $T_{1/2}$ of 19 h. The drug is metabolized and excreted primarily via the liver.

The major toxicity of vinblastine is myelosuppression, with white cells being more profoundly affected than platelets. The nadir usually occurs 7–14 days after treatment, with rapid recovery. Nausea and vomiting are usually mild as is neurotoxicity, the latter much less common than noted with vincristine. Large doses of vinblastine, as used in germ cell tumors, can result in severe constipation, myalgia, jaw pain, and peripheral neuropathy.

Vinblastine must be administered with great care as extravasation may lead to severe skin necrosis. Alopecia is generally mild.

Vincristine. Vincristine, although differing only slightly in structure from vinblastine, has a different spectrum of antitumor activity and toxicity. The drug must be given intravenously and has a short initial $T_{1/2}$ of 1–10 min followed by a long terminal $T_{1/2}$ of 2–3 h. Like vinblastine, most of drug is excreted via the liver into the bile.

The major toxicity associated with vincristine administration is peripheral neuropathy which can progress to severe motor loss. Paresthesias and loss of deep tendon reflexes are usually the first manifestations of neurotoxicity, and occur in almost all patients treated with more than several full courses of drug. Fortunately, cranial nerve and CNS abnormalities are extremely uncommon. Ileus and constipation are occasionally seen but are rarely severe. Nausea and vomiting are mild to absent and myelosuppression is extremely rare. Inappropriate secretion of antidiuretic hormone (ADH) is a rare complication. Alopecia is mild to moderate. As with vinblastine, extravasation may cause severe skin damage.

Miscellaneous Agents

The miscellaneous agents include compounds that do not fit the standard classes defined above. Drugs in this category include hydroxyurea (Hydrea), an oral S-phase–specific agent which has no defined role in gynecologic malignancy except possibly as a radiation potentiator [Hreshchyshyn et al., 1979]; procarbazine (Matulane), an active agent in lymphoma whose mechanism of action is unclear; L-asparaginase (Elspar), an enzyme that depletes asparagine, an amino acid usually essential to tumor but not normal cells in patients with acute lymphoblastic leukemia; and hexamethylmelamine (described below), an investigational agent with activity in gynecologic malignancy.

Hexamethylmelamine. Hexamethylmelamine, initially thought to be an alkylating agent, probably exerts its activity as an antimetabolite by inhibiting the incorporation of nucleotides into DNA and RNA. It probably is cell cycle–specific with its maximum activity noted during the S-phase. Hexamethylmelamine is administered orally and rapidly metabolized in the liver, with the bulk of metabolites being excreted in the patient's urine. Its initial $T_{1/2}$ is approximately 13 h with a prolonged terminal half-life.

The major toxicity of hexamethylmelamine is nausea and vomiting, which occur in almost all patients when the drug is given in high doses. Some patients develop tolerance to the drug after continued usage although nausea remains a major problem for most patients. Dividing the daily dosage, utilizing antiemetics, and taking the drug after meals may help alleviate these symptoms. Myelosuppression is usually mild to moderate, with nadirs usually occurring 3–4 weeks after a 2- to 3-week course of drug. A potentially severe but uncommon side effect is peripheral neuropathy which may be prevented by the utilization of pyridoxine. On rare occasions central nervous system toxicity may be noted. Alopecia, skin rash, and other toxicity is rare.

HORMONAL THERAPY

Hormonal agents, although only of modest importance in the treatment of most gynecologic malignancy, play a major role in the therapy of advanced breast cancer. Hormonal manipulation, whether achieved by using pharmacologic doses of agents, removing endocrine tissue responsible for the secretion of hormones, or utilizing antihormones, is based on the principle that the malignancy to be treated contains cells whose normal growth is dependent upon endogenous hormones. Recently, refinements in these concepts have led to the discovery of hormone receptors which act as the target site for hormone-cell interactions [O'Malley and Schrader, 1976]. Such receptors may be on the cell surface as is the case with polypeptide hormones, or in the cytoplasm for steroid hormones. The utilization of hormones in the treatment of breast cancer is a complex subject that will be dealt with later in this text. In gynecologic malignancy, endometrial carcinoma and less commonly ovarian carcinoma may respond to hormonal manipulation. A complete discussion of polypeptide and steroid hormones is beyond the scope of this discussion, which will confine itself to progestins and antiestrogens.

For most hormone-responsive malignancies there is a direct correlation of response and steroid receptor activity, with estrogen and progesterone receptor being the most common receptor proteins analyzed [Friedman et al., 1978]. However, techniques are available for the measurement of androgen and corticosteroid receptors. In general, patients whose tumors display no receptor activity rarely respond to hormonal manipulation, observations which pertain to both breast and endometrial carcinoma. Patients whose tumors contain both estrogen and progesterone receptors are most likely to respond to hormonal therapy, although the relationship of response rate to receptor activity is still not precisely defined for endometrial carcinoma. In patients with breast cancer, those whose tumors contain both estrogen and progesterone receptors are more likely to respond than those whose tumors contain estrogen receptors alone, as are patients with high levels when compared to patients with low levels. Measurement of estrogen and progesterone receptors should be done in all patients with breast and endometrial carcinoma and possibly in patients with ovarian malignancy.

Only progestins and the antiestrogen tamoxifen will be described here. Progestins comprise the most commonly used agents in the treatment of endometrial carcinoma. Tamoxifen shows promise in the treatment of gynecologic malignancy, and is probably the most widely used form of hormonal manipulation currently used for breast cancers. Estrogens, androgens, corticosteroids, and aromatase inhibitors such as aminoglutethimide also play a role in the treatment of breast cancer.

Progestins

Progestins are synthetic compounds structurally related to the naturally occurring human steroid progesterone. Commonly used progestin derivatives are noted below:

Generic:	Trademark:
Medroxyprogesterone acetate	Provera (oral), Depo Provera (IM)
Megestrol acetate	Megace
Hydroxyprogesterone caproate	Delalutin

Progestins can be given by both the oral and intramuscular route, are rapidly metabolized by the liver, but may display prolonged biologic activity. The longest activity is seen after administration of intramuscular hydroxyprogesterone acetate and may last 4–6 weeks; megestrol acetate appears to have the shortest duration, 1–3 days.

Progestins are virtually devoid of serious side effects. Patients may report a gain in body weight, fluid retention, and increased appetite. On occasion progestins cause impaired hepatic function with enzyme changes characteristic of cholestasis. Upon withdrawal, all the agents may cause vaginal bleeding and they should be used with caution in patients with previous phlebitis. Uncommonly, patients with breast cancer and bone metastases may develop hypercalcemia after progestin administration.

Tamoxifen

Tamoxifen (Nolvadex™), an antiestrogen whose mechanism of action has still not been precisely defined, is capable of blocking cytoplasmic receptors for estrogen but also has other actions related to cytotoxicity. The drug is given orally and is excreted mainly via the liver. It has an initial $T_{1/2}$ of 7–14 h followed by a long secondary $T_{1/2}$ which lasts days to weeks. Low levels of tamoxifen may be detectable for long periods of time, and receptor measurements done in patients taking this drug may be difficult to interpret unless several months have elapsed since discontinuation.

Unlike the estrogens and androgens which may result in substantial toxicity, tamoxifen is generally well tolerated and associated with only minimal side effects. A small percentage of patients have gastrointestinal disturbances but this rarely leads to discontinuation. Some patients, especially those who are premenopausal, experience hot flushes, which usually resolve even when the drug is continued. Breast cancer patients may experience a "flare" reaction consisting of an increase in bone pain, inflammation of locally recurrent lesions, and occasional hypercalcemia. These flare reactions usually occur soon after treatment has started and tend to subside in 1–2 weeks. Patients who have flare reactions frequently respond excellently to treatment. It may be difficult to separate tumor progression from the flare reaction, and careful observation is mandatory to prevent discontinuation of a potentially beneficial treatment modality.

NEW DRUG DEVELOPMENT

Continued success in the treatment of malignant tumors rests on the development of new and more effective agents as well as the continued exploration of innovative approaches using established drugs. The National Cancer Institute (NCI), the pharmaceutical industry, and other sources are continually developing and screening new drugs for anticancer activity. Each year the NCI evaluates approximately 15,000 new compounds, screening them for antitumor activity in the P388 mouse leukemia as well as other biologic and biochemical systems. After screening, the most promising compounds are studied in panels of mouse tumors, human tumor xenografts, and most recently with the human tumor stem cell assay. After toxicity testing in larger animals the most promising are released for clinical trials.

USES OF CANCER CHEMOTHERAPY

Combination Chemotherapy

With the exception of gestational choriocarcinoma, single-agent therapy rarely results in cure and most successful programs utilize combinations of active agents. The use of combination regimens is supported by the concepts discussed above and by recent discoveries concerning tumor heterogeneity.

Using several drugs concurrently, especially if members of different drug classes, allows the oncologist to attack the malignant cell via several mechanisms making response more likely. For many agents, synergistic as opposed to additive effects are noted which even further enhance therapeutic results. In human tumors, the utilization of drugs in combination has led to curative programs in acute lymphoblastic leukemia, Hodgkin's and non-Hodgkin's lymphoma, and germ cell tumors of the testes. In addition, small numbers of patients with ovarian and small cell lung carcinoma appear curable.

Combination regimens must be carefully planned. Concurrent use of agents frequently requires downward dose modification and the oncologist must concern himself that decreased dosage of potentially useful agents will not lead to decreased response. He must also observe the patient carefully for unanticipated toxicity secondary to drug interactions.

Adjuvant Chemotherapy

The basic principles of cancer chemotherapy discussed above indicate that ideally the physician should treat a patient with malignant disease at the earliest possible time. Unfortunately, many patients are seen with advanced metastatic disease and in most instances cure is unlikely. Careful study of the natural history of cancer has allowed us to determine precisely the risk of recurrence for most patients and has led to the concept of preventive or "adjuvant" chemotherapy. Since it is impossible to accurately predict recurrence in an individual patient, specific high-risk groups have been selected to receive adjuvant programs.

The use of adjuvant therapy assumes that if metastases do exist they are very small and likely to have a higher growth fraction. In this setting drugs that cannot cure patients with advanced disease might cure those with microscopic metastases. This appears true in breast cancer, where preliminary data indicate that several adjuvant programs are capable of significantly enhancing disease-free survival and curability. Successful adjuvant therapy is likely only in diseases where curative or substantially beneficial programs exist for patients with overt metastatic diseases. For those malignancies where chemotherapy has only been marginally effective, adjuvant trials have almost always been negative [Weiss and DeVita, 1979].

Recently there has been interest in the utilization of chemotherapeutic agents prior to surgery or radiation therapy in patients with advanced but locally confined malignancy such as carcinoma of the head and neck, breast, or bone (osteogenic sarcoma). Chemotherapy given prior to radiation or surgery has several advantages. First, the tumor vasculature has not been disturbed by surgery, radiation therapy, or other local procedures. Second, the patient generally has maximum performance status and is not recovering from the side effects of other treatment. Lastly, the physician may assess in vivo, using the patient's primary tumor as a measurable indicator, the results of treatment. In osteosarcoma such an approach has generated impressive preliminary results and has demonstrated prolonged survival in patients who have little or no evidence of malignancy after histological examination of their resected primary lesion [Rosen et al., 1979]. The impact of such therapy has yet to be determined, but conceptually such "neoadjuvant" therapy has great promise.

Finally, the physician must consider the immunologic impact of cytotoxic agents as well as their direct effect on tumor tissues. Previously, the immunosuppressive activity associated with the use of most if not all antineoplastic agents was considered detrimental. Recent data, however, suggest otherwise, and in fact chemotherapeutic agents may alter the host's immune system in a beneficial manner [Berd et al., 1982]. Technologic advances have enabled us to precisely measure subtle alterations in lymphocyte subpopulations and immune function, and it is possible that some of the effects attributed to the cytotoxic properties of chemotherapeutic agents may actually be due to changes in immunologic function which enable the host to destroy or suppress the tumor.

CONCLUSIONS

The impressive gains in the treatment of malignancy and the potential for curing advanced malignant tumors utilizing chemotherapeutic agents have had a major impact on modern medicine. In spite of these achievements only a small portion of human tumors are curable, and the major malignancies affecting man such as colon, breast, lung, and gastrointestinal malignancy remain incurable. Even for patients with potentially curable tumors, relapse is frequent and many eventually succumb to their cancer. Those treatment regimens capable of curing substantial percentages of patients should not be considered "fixed," and the physician should always be flexible, open-minded, and willing to participate in clinical trials designed to improve patient treatment. Future gains in cytotoxic cancer chemotherapy must rest on strong collaborative efforts between scientists involved in basic and clinical research and the practicing physician. Only through such efforts can we maintain continued development of new and potentially effective agents, design and complete clinical trials for those regimens most promising, and finally realize these gains in the communities where most of our patients receive their care.

REFERENCES

Adams GE (1981): Hypoxia-mediated drugs for radiation and chemotherapy. Cancer 48:696–707.

Baserga R (1981): The cell cycle. N Engl J Med 304:453–459.

Berd D, Mastrangelo MJ, Engstrom PF, Paul A, Maguire H (1982): Augmentation of the human immune response by cyclophosphamide. Cancer Res 42:4862–4866.

Bristow MR, Mason JW, Billingham ME, Daniels JR (1978): Doxorubicin cardiomyopathy: Evaluation by phonocardiography, endomyocardial biopsy, and cardiac catheterization. Ann Intern Med 88:168–175.

Carter SK, Crooke ST (1979): "Mitomycin C: Current Status and Developments." New York: Academic Press.

Carter SK, Glatstein E, Livingston RB (1982): "Principles of Cancer Treatment." New York: McGraw-Hill.

Chabner B (1982): "Pharmacologic Principles of Cancer Treatment." Philadelphia: WB Saunders.

Charbit A, Malaise EP, Tubiana M (1971): Relation between the pathological nature and the growth rate of human tumors. Eur J Cancer 7:307–315.

DeVita VT Jr, Serpick A (1967): Combination chemotherapy in the treatment of Hodgkin's disease. Proc Am Assoc Cancer Res 8:13.

DeVita VT Jr, Hellman S, Rosenberg SA (1982): "Cancer Principles and Practice of Oncology." Philadelphia: JB Lippincott.

Dorr RT, Fritz WL (1980): "Cancer Chemotherapy Handbook." New York: Elsevier.

Ensminger W, Niederhuber J, Dakhil S, Thrall J, Wheeler R (1981): Totally inplanted drug delivery system for hepatic arterial chemotherapy. Cancer Treat Rep 65:393–400.

Farber S, Diamond LK, Mercer RD, Sylvester RF, Wolff JA (1948): Temporary remissions in acute leukemia in children produced by folic acid antagonist, 4-aminopteroyl-glutamic acid (Aminopterin). N Engl J Med 238:787–793.

Friedman MA, Hoffman PG, Jones HW (1978): The clinical value of hormone receptor assays in malignant disease. Cancer Treat Rev 5:185–194.

Gilman A, Philips FS (1946): The biological actions and therapeutic applications of the B-chloroethyl amines and sulfides. Science 103:409–436.

Goldie JH, Coldman AJ, Gudausakas GA (1982): Rationale for the use of alternating non-cross-resistant chemotherapy. Cancer Treat Rep 66:439–449.

Henderson ES, Jones B (1982): Acute lymphoblastic leukemia. In Holland JF, Frei ET III (eds): "Cancer Medicine." Philadelphia: Lea and Febiger, pp 1379–1406.

Hertz R, Lewis J Jr, Lipsett MB (1961): Five years' experience with the chemotherapy of metastatic choriocarcinoma and related trophoblastic tumors in women. Am J Obstet Gynecol 82:631–640.

Holland JF, Frei ET III (1982): "Cancer Medicine." Philadelphia: Lea and Febiger.

Hreshchyshyn MM, Aron BS, Boronow RC, Franklin EW III, Shingleton HM, Blessing JM (1979): Hydroxyurea or placebo combined with radiation to treat stages IIIB and IV cervical cancer confined to the pelvis. Int J Radiat Oncol Biol Phys 5:317–322.

Kressel BR, Ryan KP, Duong AT, Berenberg J, Schein PS (1981): Microangiopathic hemolytic anemia, thrombocytopenia, and renal failure in patients treated for adenocarcinoma. Cancer 48:1738–1745.

Livingston RB, Carter SK (1970): "Single Agents in Cancer Chemotherapy." New York: IFI/Plenum.

Norton L, Simon R (1977): Tumor size, sensitivity to therapy, and design of treatment schedules. Cancer Treat Rep 61: 1307–1317.

O'Malley BW, Schrader WT (1976): The receptors of steroid hormones. Sci Am 234:32–43.

Pratt WB, Ruddon RW (1979): "The Anticancer Drugs." New York: Oxford University Press.

Presant CA, Hillinger S, Klahr C (1980): Phase II study of 1,3 bis (2-chloroethyl)-1-nitrosourea (BCNU, NSC# 409962) with amphotericin B in bronchogenic carcinoma. Cancer 45:6–10.

Rosen G, Marcove RC, Caparros B, Nirenberg A, Kosloff C, Huvos AG (1979): Primary osteogenic sarcoma: The rationale for preoperative chemotherapy and delayed surgery. Cancer 43:2163–2177.

Shackney SE, McCormack GW, Cuchural GJ Jr (1978): Growth rate patterns of solid tumors and their relation to responsiveness to therapy. Ann Intern Med 89:107–121.

Skipper HE, Schabel FM Jr, Wilcox WS (1964): Experimental evaluation of potential anticancer agents. XII. On the criteria and kinetics associated with "curability" of experimental tumors. Cancer Chemother Rep 35:1–111.

Teicher BA, Lazo JS, Sartorelli AC (1981): Classification of antineoplastic agents by their selective toxicities toward oxygenated and hypoxic tumor cells. Cancer Res 41:73–81.

Tsuruo T, Fidler IJ (1981): Differences in drug sensitivity among tumor cells from parental tumors, selected variants, and spontaneous metastases. Cancer Res 41:3058–3064.

Weinstein JN, Magin RL, Yatvin MB, Zaharko DS (1979): Liposomes and local hyperthermia: Selective delivery of methotrexate to heated tumors. Science 204:188–191.

Weiss RB, DeVita VT Jr (1979): Multimodal primary cancer treatment (adjuvant therapy): Current results and future prospects. Ann Intern Med 91:251–260.

Zubrod CG (1972): Chemical control of cancer. Proc Natl Acad Sci USA 69:1042–1047.

Management of Toxicities and Complications of Gynecologic Cancer Chemotherapy

Thomas E. Dolan

Division of Gynecologic Oncology, Department of Obstetrics and Gynecology, Lutheran General Hospital, Park Ridge, Illinois 60068

In order to understand the management of toxicities and complications of gynecologic cancer chemotherapy, a full understanding of the specific natural history of the disease entity as well as the disease response to chemotherapy is imperative.

There must always be a balance between the therapeutic benefit goal and the complications or toxicity risks which must be taken to reach that goal. Ultimately, the goal is to eradicate the disease completely but the reality is that this is rarely completely achieved. This fact must be kept in mind when treating with a specific drug in any given disease entity. More commonly, the disease either is put into a complete or partial remission, remains static or progresses. Patients who do get a partial or complete remission may do so for a period of time and then relapse, but sometimes the remission will be sustained for a considerable period of time. Hence, the balance between therapeutic benefit and risk is so important to bear in mind when treating the individual patient. At all times, the goal should be to maintain a quality of life that is understandable and acceptable to the patient.

Predominantly, the chemotherapy used in clinical practice consists of phase IV and phase III drugs in which the toxicities are readily understood. However, patients who have failed treatment are often treated with phase II or phase I drugs in which the possibility of toxicity is less well understood for the particular treatment and, hence, the chance of toxicity is greater.

Many regimens utilize combination drug treatments to obtain a synergistic or additive therapeutic goal. Unfortunately, increased toxicity may well

Chemotherapy of Gynecologic Cancer, pages 31-47

ensue requiring a decreased dosage and hence an actual decrease in the therapeutic benefit. It is therefore imperative that the therapist understand the side effects of any and all drugs used as some of the side effects are minor and some are major. Doses for a given tumor are not always understood, and even though there is usually a standard dose in a given situation that dose may need to be exceeded in some patients and decreased in others to maximize the therapeutic gain and minimize the toxic losses.

As was pointed out in the chapter "Principles of Cancer Chemotherapy" by Muss, one must understand the cell cycle and kinetics to appreciate the therapeutic goals—likewise, the toxic side effects are related in a similar manner. Certainly if the tumor has a marked growth fraction that is responsive to a lower dose of drug, there will be fewer side effects. Likewise, it must be appreciated that as the tumor cell's doubling increases, threatening the body's vital systems, any increased toxicity may do likewise to the body's vital systems. If tumor volume can be reduced either by surgical or radiotherapeutic means, then a lower dose of drug and lesser toxicity can be achieved. Just as tumors are heterogeneous with sensitive cells and nonsensitive cells, the remainder of the body's systems are heterogenetically sensitive or nonsensitive to the drug's toxicities.

The fundamental principles of chemotherapy are that 1) cure is inversely proportional to tumor burden; 2) there is a drug-dose-related responsiveness; 3) cancer cell resistance is proportional to the size of the tumor; and 4) chemotherapy drugs that will kill a constant fraction percentage (log kill hypothesis) will also proportionally affect the overall toxicity of normal sensitive body cells in a similar fashion.

The one danger of combination chemotherapy is the loss of potential benefit by the potentially best drug using a lowered dose to decrease overall combined toxicity. This becomes ever more detrimental when a relatively suboptimal dose of the most active drug has to be given because of a combination with a relatively inactive drug.

Very often a dramatic response is followed by a relapse and this is attributed to tumor cell resistance. Despite the tumor's ability to undergo cell mutations and develop resistance, the body's other sensitive cells are not necessarily so fortunate and continue to become toxic. This is the major reason that maintenance chemotherapy has a limited value. Despite the toxicity, treatment should be maximal initially to get the best response.

The log kill hypothesis for tumor cell kill should be understood to appreciate the problems of toxicity. Just as it will take 2–3 courses of chemotherapy to detect tumor kill response, it will often take 2–3 courses to appreciate maximum toxicity. Despite this fact, because a single tumor cell can allow the entire tumor to regrow, one must accept the potential toxicity to get maximum tumor response from therapy.

The complexity of toxicity has to also be understood in relationship to the particular route of a given drug or drugs, its ability to equilibrate with plasma, activators in host tissue (i.e., exposure to UV light, hyperthermia, cell sensitizers, Flagyl), transportation to site, permeation of normal cells as well as the tumor bed and across cell membranes, and finally, specific reactions. Toxicity is related to any and all steps along the way.

In an attempt to minimize toxicity at all times, one must understand: 1) the lowest concentration of drug to obtain a therapeutic goal with the least cytotoxicity; 2) peak concentrations relative to route, schedule, and dose; and 3) the pharmacokinetic properties—i.e., rate and location—of excretion and metabolism. This may require analysis of urine, bile, feces, plasma, spinal fluid, sputum, etc.

SPECIFIC SYSTEM TOXICITIES AND COMPLICATIONS

Having discussed the development of drug toxicities in general, the remainder of this chapter will be devoted to management of specific system toxicities and complications.

Three symposia in the fall of 1982 were held to discuss cancer chemotherapy and controlling the side effects. They listed the complications of therapy of neoplastic disease using cytotoxic chemotherapy as usual and unusual (see Fig. 1).

Previously, the Gynecologic Oncology Group in December 1980 developed a grading system of adverse effects criteria (see pp. 68–72). This outline specifically grades the toxicities from 0 to 4 (none to life-threatening or most severe) in an objective way to evaluate and quantitate toxicity and facilitate corrective measures. The management will be taken system by system with specific reference to the causative drugs and corrective measures to be taken. The table consists of the following criteria: No criteria (0) represents the lower limits of normal where a chemotherapy should be initiated. Mild (1) represents a minimal toxic effect for which one can appreciate an effect of the therapy, but no interruption of treatment and only minimal countermeasures need be taken. Moderate (2) or severe (3) will most often require corrective measures including prolongation and/or reduction of the treatment cycle. The most severe or life-threatening adverse effects will require cessation or marked reduction of therapy and extensive corrective and supportive measures. Ideally, therapy will be directed to achieve only grade 1 or 2 toxicity at the nadir period with return to complete normalcy by the time of the next therapy cycle.

Fig. 1. Complications of therapy of neoplastic disease using cytotoxic chemotherapy.

Usual
- Nausea, vomiting
- Alopecia
- (Pan)cytopenia—transfusion requirement
- Hemorrhage, sepsis
- Cellulitis (if extravasation occurs)
- Stomatitis
- Hyperpigmentation, generalized
- Thrombophlebitis at intravenous site

Unusual
- Peripheral neuropathy (vincristine)
- Cystitis (cyclophosphamide)
- Obstipation (vinblastine)
- Cardiomyopathy (doxorubicin, daunomycin)
- Vein pain (carmustine, dacarbazine)
- Renal failure (cisplatin, methotrexate, mitomycin, nitrosoureas [?])
- Pulmonary fibrosis (bleomycin, carmustine, cyclophosphamide, busulfan)
- Yellow nails (bleomycin)
- Meningoencephalitis (methotrexate)
- Anaphylaxis (bleomycin, L-asparaginase)
- Ototoxicity (cisplatin)
- Hypocalcemia (mithramycin)
- Sterility, male and female (alkylating agents)
- Premature ovarian failure (alkylating agents)
- Abortion (all agents, especially methotrexate)
- Fetal malformations (any agent in first trimester)

Hematologic

Bone marrow suppression and fatal complications from neutropenia and thrombocytopenia from chemotherapy have been decreased but not eradicated. Virtually all the chemotherapeutic alkylating agents, antibiotics, less so with the plant alkaloids, antimetabolites cause myelosuppression. Maximum myelosuppression usually occurs 10–14 days after therapy has been initiated. Combinations such as hexamethylmelamine, cyclophosphamide, 5-fluorouracil, and doxorubicin, CHAP, HAD, CMF, CAP CHAD, MECY, FUCY, PAC-1, PAC-5, and CHEX VP produce severe marrow suppression 10–28% of the time. Initial measures to decrease the adverse effects require modification of subsequent treatment cycles as outlined in Table I.

If after the first cycle there has been grade 3 WBC or platelet toxicity, at the nadir count, but recovery occurs by the time of the second cycle, the

TABLE I. Toxicity Grade-Dose Adjustment

Lowest WBC (grade)	Lowest platelet count (grade)				
	0	1	2	3	4
0	No change	No change	No change	Dec 1 level	Dec 2 level
1	No change	No change	No change	Dec 1 level	Dec 2 level
2	No change	No change	No change	Dec 1 level	Dec 2 level
3	Dec 1 level	Dec 1 level	Dec 1 level	Dec 1 level	Dec 2 level
4	Dec 2 level	Dec 2 level	Dec 2 level	Dec 2 level	Dec 2 level

drug should be reduced by one level or 25%. Usually, cis-platinum can be maintained at the same level.

If after the first cycle there has been grade 4 WBC or platelet toxicity, but recovery by the time of the second cycle, alkylating agents and antibiotics need to be reduced by two levels or 50% and cis-platinum should be reduced one level or 25%. If dosage of chemotherapy has been diminished because of nadir count in the first cycle and no further myelosuppression has been noted, then subsequent drug doses should be escalated by one level or 25% with each subsequent course until the maximum dose is reached. While this adjustment is being carried out, weekly WBC and platelet counts should be obtained and observed for a nadir value. If, at any time, CBC or platelet counts drawn show grade 3 or 4 toxicity, dose modifications should be made.

No subsequent treatment course is to begin until the WBC exceeds 3,000/cc and the platelet count 100,000/cc. The next course should be delayed week by week until these levels are exceeded. If at the end of 6 weeks these levels have not been reached, the following dose modification will be used: If the platelet count is at least 75,000/cc and WBC at least 2500/cc, drug doses should be reduced by two levels. If the platelet or WBC count is lower than these values, patients should not receive further chemotherapy until the counts recover.

The effective use of transfusion techniques including erythrocytes, platelet replacement therapy, and granulocytes in conjunction with antibiotics has reduced the threat of myelosuppression with fatal complications. The following transfusion guidelines are useful for commonly encountered hematologic problems.

Chronic anemia. 1) No significant cardiopulmonary compromise; stable patient. No absolute indication for transfusion when hemoglobin is above 6–7 g/100 ml. Consider transfusion in the presence of otherwise unexplained lassitude, malaise, tachycardia, dyspnea, in association with hemoglobin less than 9–10 g/100 ml.

2) Cardiopulmonary disease; fever; surgery; radiation therapy. Maintain hemoglobin level at 10 g/100 ml.

3) If management protracted (years), transfusion reactions with WNBC antibodies are frequent and require the use of washed RBC. Secondary hemochromatosis should be monitored for. Anemia is most commonly seen with prorated cisplatin therapy—more so than with other agents.

Thrombocytopenia due to failure of platelet production. 1) Platelet count greater than 20,000/cc; stable patient without retinal hemorrhages. Platelet transfusion probably not necessary.

2) Platelet count less than 20,000/cc; patient not bleeding. Provide prophylactic platelet transfusion once daily.

3) Platelet count less than 50,000/cc; patient clinically bleeding or surgery anticipated. Use local measures to control bleeding; look for defects in coagulation pathways; maintain platelet counts at 50,000/cc or above with transfusion every 12–24 h.

4) Platelet count less than 20,000/cc; patient refractory to random platelet transfusion. Consider transfusion for evidence of bleeding, when retinal hemorrhages are noted or when platelet count is less than 10,000/cc; consider use of leukocyte-poor or HLA-matched platelets.

Platelet transfusions differ from red cell transfusions in several important aspects under normal circumstances; red cells have a mean survival time of 120 days whereas platelets survive only 9–10 days.

Granulocytopenia. Patient candidate for aggressive supportive care.

1) Granulocytes less than 1,000/cc; afebrile, stable patient; no established indication for granulocyte transfusion.

2) Granulocytes less than 1,000/cc; patient febrile, but cultures negative and no clinical evidence of infected area or tissue. No established indication for transfusion, but may want to initiate prophylactic IV antibiotics and reverse isolation.

3) Gram-negative sepsis, fever, and granulocytes less than 500/cc. Granulocytes indicated as well as IV antibiotics and reverse isolation.

4) Local infection, thought to be due to gram-negative organisms, not responsive to appropriate antibiotic therapy occuring in a patient with a granulocyte count below 500/cc. Granulocytes probably indicated along with antibiotic and isolation measures.

Gastrointestinal Toxicities

Gastrointestinal toxicities include nausea and vomiting, anorexia, cachexia, mucositis, diarrhea, constipation, mechanical bowel problems, stomatitis, esophagitis, and abnormalities in liver function as manifested by blood chemistries, bleeding, GI infection, perforation, stricture (see Fig. 2).

The most common and troublesome toxicity encountered is nausea and vomiting. This appears to be a direct result from stimulation of a distinct medullary center in the fourth ventricle of brain called the chemoreceptor trigger zone (CTZ) (see Fig. 3).

Stimulation of this center apparently can occur directly or via afferent input from several sources.

When vomiting can be anticipated, prophylactic therapy is much more effective than after vomiting ensues. Table II shows the emetogenic potential of chemotherapeutic agents commonly used in gyn cancers.

Patients most commonly suffer from nausea and vomiting as a direct result of therapy, but other causes should also be assessed and treated. These include GI inflammation or obstruction, infection, heart failure, metabolic problems, and psychological status of the patient. Consequences of nausea and vomiting may lead to poor compliance which will interfere with the possibility of care or optimal therapy. Complications of emesis such as dehydration and hypokalemia, malnutrition, violent wretching, and depression must also be dealt with. Some patients suffer from conditioned response, such as vomiting upon arrival at the setting (either outpatient department or hospital) or the disastrous effect of another patient vomiting in the same area. These problems are difficult to control, but if the patient

Fig. 2. Gastrointestinal toxicity of chemotherapy.

Nausea	Constipation
Vomiting	Hepatotoxicity
Anorexia	Bleeding
Cachexia	GI infection
Mucositis	Perforation
Malabsorption	Stricture
Diarrhea	

Fig. 3. Emetic trigger mechanisms.

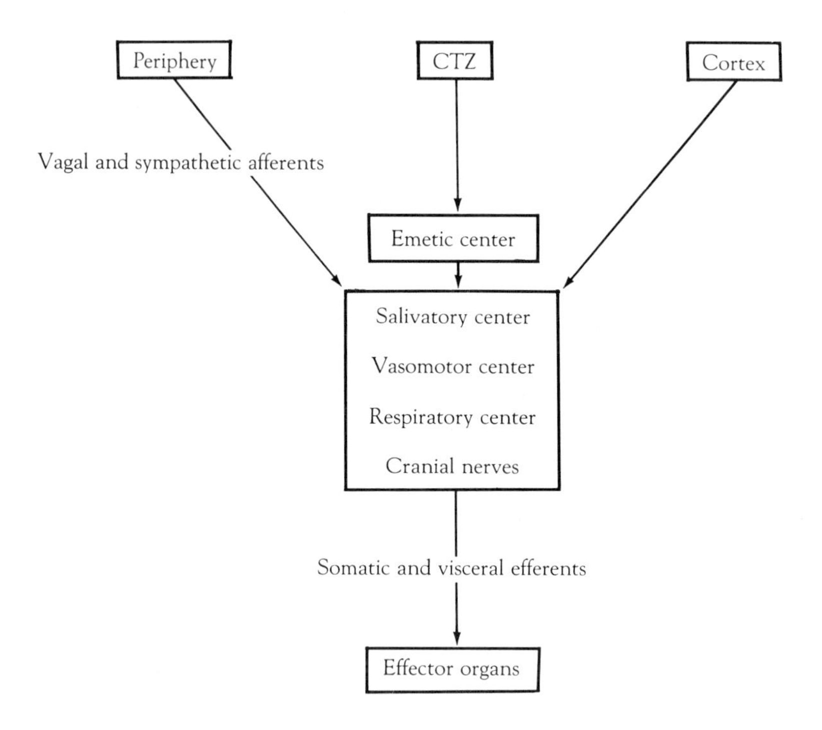

TABLE II. Classification of Chemotherapeutic Agents According to Emetic Potential

Class I: Greatest emetic potential
Combinations of agents including nitrogen mustard, cyclophosphamide (>1,300 mg/m^2), dactinomycin, dacarbazine (300 mg/m^2), carmustine 300 mg/m^2, lomustine (>60 mg/m^2), cisplatin in doses >60 mg/m^2
Class II: Moderate emetic potential
Combinations of agents including cyclophosphamide (500–900 mg/m^2), doxorubicin (>50 mg/m^2), carmustine (100–200 mg/m^2), or lomustine (<60 mg/m^2), cisplatin in doses <60 mg/m^2
Class III: Least emetic potential
Combinations including methotrexate, 5-fluorouracil, vinblastine, cyclophosphamide (<500 mg/m^2), or doxorubicin (<40 mg/m^2)

is kept free of noxious sites or smells in a quiet and private setting, this will at least decrease the anxiety that stimulates nausea. Antiemetic drugs fall into several categories. At the recent symposium in the fall of 1982, they were classified pharmacologically as well as by their proposed site of action (Figs. 4, 5).

The most commonly used drugs are the phenothiazines (Thorazine), chlorpromazine from the aliphatic class (Compazine), prochlorperazine (Torecan), thiethylperazine, or Trilafon perphenazine from the piperazine class. Although the piperazine class has the more pronounced antiemetic activity, it is often associated with an increased problem with extrapyramidal side effects. Many antihistamines have antiemetic properties. Among the most common used are dimenhydrinate (Dramamine), tumethobenzamide (Tigan), and diphenhydramine (Benadryl); the last is used in combination with other antiemetics for best results. The active ingredients of marijuana, the cannabinoids, delta-9-tetra-hydrocannabinol (THC) has been shown to have active antiemetic properties. THC is distributed for use as an antiemetic by the National Cancer Institute, but thus far has not been shown to be as good as other, more common antiemetics in use. Another class of antiemetics include haloperidol (Haldol), benzquinamide (Emete-con), sropolamine, and metoclopramide (Reglan). Sedation from antiemetics should be understood, and patients should be cautioned regarding the dangers of driving an automobile.

Selection of an antiemetic has to be individualized depending on the specific chemotherapy—drugs, dose, and medical setting (inpatient or outpatient).

Fig. 4. Pharmacologic classification of antiemetics.

Dopamine antagonists
- Metoclopramide
- Domperidone
- Phenothiazines
- Butyrophenones
- Antihistamines
- Anticholinergics
- Cannabinoids

Miscellaneous agents
- Corticosteroids
- Trimethobenzamide
- Diazepam
- Nortriptyline

Fig. 5. Classification of antiemetics by their proposed sites of action.

Emetic center
- Antihistamines*
- Anticholinergics*

Chemoreceptor trigger zone
- Phenothiazines
- Butyrophenones
- Trimethobenzamide
- Metoclopramide**

Cerebral cortex
- Cannabinoids
- Diazepam
- Antihistamines*

Periphery
- Domperidone
- Metoclopramide**

Unknown
- Corticosteroids

*Proposed but unsubstantiated.
**Dual sites of action.

Perhaps the most difficult chemotherapeutic drug that universally causes nausea and vomiting in use today is cis-platinol, which is commonly used for gyn malignancies. At the UCLA symposium, Dr. Strum pointed out the antiemetic efficacy of metoclopramide. Recently a combination of metoclopramide (Reglan), diphenhydramine (Benadryl), and cortisone has been the most effective in reducing or eliminating emesis in these group chemotherapy patients (see Table III). Sedation with lorazepam (Ativan) 2 mg IV along with metoclopramide 2 mg/kg IV, diphenhydramine 25-50 mg IV, and cortisone 20 mg IV, one half hour prior to chemotherapy and continued with metoclopramide injections every 2 h for five doses after chemotherapy has been very effective. Table IV lists the common antiemetic drugs by trade and generic names as well as the recommended adult doses, regimens, and routes.

Drug dose reduction or temporary discontinuance of one level should be initiated for severe or life-threatening emesis.

Diarrhea is a less common side effect and can be most often controlled by Lomotil or Motrin tablets. Adriamycin, actinomycin D, methotrexate, and

TABLE III. Prior Chemotherapy Exposure (with or without prior nausea and/or emesis) Versus Incidence of Total Antiemetic Protection with Intravenous Metoclopramide: Current Study

	Prior treatment				No prior			
	Emesis		No emesis		treatment		Total	
Protection	No.	(%)	No.	(%)	No.	(%)	No.	(%)
Yes	3	(50)	10	(91)	26	(80)	39	(78)
No	3	(50)	1	(9)	7	(20)	11	(22)
Total	6	(100)	11	(100)	33	(100)	50	(100)
Emesis score	1.67		0.18		0.33		0.46	
P value	<0.001		<0.10		>0.10			

TABLE IV. Antiemetic Drugs in Common Use

Trade	Generic	Routes	Doses	Regimen
Reglan	Metoclopramide	IV, PO	1–2 mg/kg	½ h pre then every 2 h × 6
Benadryl	Diphenhydramine	IV, IM, or PO	10–50 mg	q.i.d.
Ativan	Lorazepam	IV, IM, or PO	IV 2–4 mg 0.02 mg/lb	given 1 or 2 times
Cortisone[a]				
Compazine	Prochlorperazone	IV, IM, or PO	10 mg	q 6 h
Torecan	Thiethylperazine	IV, IM	10 mg	q 6 h
Trifalon	Perphenazine	IV, IM, or PO	5 mg IV or IM; 4 mg PO	q 4–6 h
THC[a]	Delta-9-tetra-hydro cannabinol			
Dramamine	Dimenhydrinate	IV, IM, or PO	50–100 mg	q 4 h IV given over 15 min
Haldol	Haloperidol	IM or PO	0.5–0.1 mg	q 8 h
Emete-con	Benzaquinamide	IV, IM	25 mg IV	3–4 h 50 mg IM

[a]Usually used as a combination.

5FU are drugs that can cause diarrhea. Occasionally, diarrhea with methotrexate or 5FU will limit the dose. Mechanical problems such as constipation or an ileus is less often seen, but is most common with the plant alkaloids. Cathartics are usually corrective. Electrolyte imbalance, especially hyponatremia or hypokalemia, is usually due to incomplete replacement of fluids lost because of diarrhea or vomiting, which can be corrected by adequate replacement.

Stomatitis or mucositis is seen with adriamycin, bleomycin, actinomycin D, methotrexate, 5FU, and less so with Velban, vincristine, and cytoxan. Toxicities with the former drugs may require dose limitation, whereas with later drugs this is usually less severe. Ulceration of oral, vaginal, or vulvar mucosa may occur. Repeated chemotherapy drug treatments should not be resumed until mucositis has resolved. The dose should be reduced by 50% for grade 3 mucositis. It should be remembered that mucositis may be a mirror image of ulcers along the entire GI tract.

Esophagitis will sometimes accompany problems with nausea, vomiting, or mucositis. These patients will often benefit by the temporary use of Cimetidine (Tagamet) 300 mg by mouth or IV every 6 h.

Hepatic toxicity is seen with methotrexate, adriamycin, Cytoxan, and mithramycin and less so with other drugs used in gyn/oncology. Serum bilirubin, SGOT, SGPT, and alkaline phosphatase should be followed for evaluation of hepatotoxicity. If the total bilirubin level, SGOT/SGPT, or alkaline phosphatase exceeds 2.5 times normal, then future doses should be decreased by 50%; if the levels exceed 5 times normal, then treatment should be discontinued with the causative drug or drugs.

Genitourinary

Genitourinary complications include renal toxicity as measured by serum BUN, creatinine, creatinine clearance, proteinuria, or hematuria. Bladder toxicity problems appear less frequently, but may be both acute and chronic.

Cis-platinum is a unique drug in that it is the only heavy metal compound in use as a cancer chemotherapeutic agent. It is also one of the most active compounds in use for ovarian cancer in particular and in gyn cancers in general. It is also one of the most toxic to GI and GU systems. Twenty to seventy-five percent of the drug is excreted in the urine within 24 h after administration. It is excreted in the urine as the result of glomerular filtration of unbound platinum. Because of its primary renal toxicity and excretion, attempts to reduce the renal toxicity have been made by hydration. Usually, patients are hydrated 4–6 h prior with 1 liter of fluid either by mouth or IV. Often 25–50 mg of Mannitol or 40 mg of Lasix is used and hydration is continued after the drug is given for 12–24 h with 1–2 liters. In the absence of hydration, the incidence of nephrotoxicity has been reported to be as high as 30% when doses of Platinol 50–75 mg/m^2 are given. Hypocalcemia, hypokalemia, and hypomagnesemia are also reported, but are rare and need to be corrected. These can be severe, but replacement therapy is usually effective. Severe renal tubular defects, although rare, may require chronic replacement therapy and discontinuance of therapy. If the

BUN exceeds 30 or creatinine 2.0 mg%, the drug must be withheld and restarted only when the parameters return to these levels or normal. If delay of therapy is more than 6 weeks from the start of previous treatment because of renal insufficiency, the drug may have to be discontinued.

Cystitis as measured by dysuria, frequency, hematuria, and pyuria can be seen commonly. Cytoxan (cyclophosphamide) has a tendency to concentrate in the bladder after administration and is the leading agent for causing bladder toxicity. It must be kept in mind that patients who have previously been irradiated may compound this problem. This is especially true with recall phenomena that is seen with the use of adriamycin and Cytoxan. Cytoxan-related moderate to severe cystitis is an indication to stop the drug until the cystitis has cleared. After the cystitis has cleared, the drug should be restarted at half dose. Increased fluid intake prior to administering cyclophosphamide may aid in preventing cystitis. Hemorrhagic cystitis that requires blood transfusion or intravesical instillation of 1/4% formalin solution may require discontinuance of therapy.

Infection and Fever

Infection problems usually occur at the time of the drug nadir. Mild infections such as nonbacteremic UTI, bronchitis, cellulitis, URI are often able to be treated with oral antibiotics. Fever is a common occurrence in cancer patients and may be a result of tumor, necrosis, inflammation, transfusions, and drugs (both chemotherapeutic and antimicrobial). A presumed infection with fever as the only sign despite negative blood culture should be treated with antibiotics, especially in the granulocytopenic patient. The morbidity and mortality of infection are reduced from 50% to less than 20% when empiric broad sprectrum antibiotic therapy is initiated immediately after fever evaluation is performed. An empiric antibiotic regimen should "cover" major pathogens isolated at the particular institution, be synergistic, bactericidal, and should have the least possible organ toxicity. Serum levels of the antibiotic should be monitored closely to regulate the dosage and control potential side effects. Most common usage today is a two- or three-drug combination that includes cephalosporins or a semisynthetic penicillin and an aminoglycoside. It must be remembered that the antibiotic side effects such as nephron and ototoxicity can compound the side effects of the chemotherapeutic drugs and, therefore, must be used cautiously.

Fever itself should be treated with antipyretics and cooling measures when temperature exceeds 40°C that lasts for more than 24 h. Fevers of 39°C or greater should have workups that include blood and urine cultures.

Cultures of wounds, oral, or anal orifices should also be considered as well as chest x-rays where indicated to accurately determine the cause of fever. The granulocytopenic patient is especially at risk as was outlined above under Hematologic Toxicities.

Allergic and Cutaneous

True allergic reactions from chemotherapeutic drugs to the point of anaphylaxis are rare. Bleomycin has been reported to cause anaphylaxis, and is therefore recommended to be skin tested 1–2 units prior to initial use. Anaphylactic reactions with cis-platinol presenting symptoms of tachycardia, hypotension, erythema, facial edema, and wheezing have been reported. Treatment may well require antihistamines, Solu-Cortef, epinephrine, and intubation.

Skin reactions include erythema, pigmentation, dry desquamation, vesiculation, pruritis, phlebitis, and/or induration at injection site. Extravasation of an agent especially adriamycin or actinomycin D can cause severe tissue reaction. Measure to decrease toxicity include: 1) immediate termination of an infusion and removal of the needle; 2) ice pack to induce local vasoconstriction and continue for 24 h; 3) ethyl chloride to anesthetize the skin; 4) 50–100 mg hydrocortisone sodium succinate directly into the infiltrated area using a 25-gauge straight needle with multiple injections into the affected site; 5) covering the area with 1% hydrocortisone cream; 6) applying cortisone b.i.d. until the erythema has subsided; and 7) continuing exercise with the affected extremity.

Probably the most distressing side effect after nausea and vomiting is alopecia. It is seen with adriamycin, actinomycin-D, Velban, vincristine, 5FU, methotrexate, and Cytoxan. The use of a scalp tourniquet was first proposed for patients using vincristine since the plant alkaloids are rapidly cleared from the bloodstream. It was felt that if the superficial veins were occluded temporarily during administration of the drug, then the drug would not have direct contact with hair follicles. The pneumatic tourniquet technique was used on patients using Cytoxan, 5FU, and methotrexate and was reported to have prevented alopecia in 20 patients, but studies have not been able to produce comparable results. The use of the scalp tourniquet is limited to drugs that are able to achieve plasma concentration below epilation levels but within the maximum tolerance time of a tourniquet, approximately 20 min.

Scalp hypothermia can also achieve vasoconstriction. Ice turbans can reduce the scalp temperatures to 23–24°C. It is placed on the head 10 min prior to therapy and left in place for 30 min. Excellent results have been reported with adriamycin at doses under 50 mg/m^2/treatment. This was apparently able to be maintained for a 6- to 8-month cycle. Scalp hypothermia is less effective with doses greater than 60 mg.

Wound problems with chemotherapy tend to be infrequent and are usually self-corrective. Occasionally, patients will develop herpes Zoster or fungal infections. Fungal infections can be treated by imidazole derivatives such as miconazole and clotrimazole for mucocutaneous candidiasis. For more serious fungal infections, 5-fluorocytosine (5FC) or Amphotericin B is helpful. As for herpes Zoster, local skin care is important and observation for secondary infections has to be observed. Ara-A (Vidarabine), 10 mg/kg for 12 h/day for 5 days has been associated with accelerated skin healing. Interferon has recently been reported to help these patients also.

Neurotoxicity

Neurotoxicity can be divided into peripheral and central. CNS toxicity includes ototoxicity which is most significant with cis-platinol therapy. In patients with history of prior hearing loss, pretreatment audiometry is indicated. Patients who develop significant hearing loss or tinnitus may dictate interruption of cis-platinum therapy. Peripheral and central nervous toxicity such as weakness, paresthesia, change of mental status, mood, ideation, memory, consciousness, motor paresis, extrapyramidal symptoms, or seizures can occur with Velban, vincristine, methotrexate, Cytoxan, hexamethylmelamine, or cis-platinol. Most neurotoxicities are transient and reversible once the drug is discontinued. Unfortunately, interruption of therapy is often followed by progressive disease; hence one sometimes has to choose between continued and worsening toxicity versus progressive disease with discontinuance of the drug.

Pulmonary

Pulmonary toxicity by and large is a major problem with bleomycin and less so a problem with methotrexate. Pulmonary fibrosis can occur with bleomycin. Therefore, pulmonary function studies need to be monitored during treatment. The drug should be discontinued immediately if there is evidence of lung function impairment or x-ray changes. Methotrexate pneumonitis is uncommon but requires a change of medication.

Cardiovascular

Cardiotoxicity appears to be a unique problem of the anthracycline antibiotics—in particular, adriamycin—for gyn tumors. The biochemical effect is a complex interaction with sodium and potassium ATPase, direct membrane binding, generation of semiquinone radical, superoxide, hydrogen peroxide with peroxidation of membrane liquid, DNA intercalation, and alterations in myocardial calcium metabolism. The problem of assessment for cardiac damage has been done by two different paths. Billingham and co-workers depend on pathologic grading of cardiac tissue by endocardial needle biopsy. Most other workers have used various techniques from EKG to radionuclide cineangiography. Risk factors include mediastinal radiation therapy, uncontrolled hypertension, adriamycin doses greater than 450 mg/m^2, and coadministration with either Cytoxan or mitomycin C.

Adriamycin toxicity appears to be dose-related. While there is considerable difference in the rate at which the damage occurs, most patients will have moderate to severe pathologic damage and up to 50% will exhibit clear-cut functional impairment by the time they have received a total dose of 500 mg/m^2. Most gyn protocols therefore limit the dose to 400–450 mg/m^2 as a total dose. If congestive heart failure or any other life-threatening cardiac problem results, adriamycin should be discontinued.

Gonadal Dysfunction

Chemotherapeutic effect on ovarian function has been hampered by relative inaccessability of the ovary to biopsy and the inability to evaluate the germ cell population reliably. Most patients receiving chemotherapy either are in the postmenopausal age group or have had surgical removal or radiotherapy. A small number of patients are in the menstrual age group where fertility is still a question and a problem.

Overall, at least 50% of women treated with single alkylating agents develop permanent ovarian failure and amenorrhea. Recently, reports of young girls treated with combined therapy (vincristine, adriamycin, Cytoxan) have been able to become pregnant and deliver normal children.

CONCLUSIONS

The foregoing chapter has outlined the specific system toxicities and complications in a systematic way as outlined by the Gynecologic Oncology Group.

In general, when patients develop mild to moderate toxicity, grade 1 to 2 dosages should be reduced by 25–50%. Treatment should be discontinued for life-threatening or most severe grade 4 toxicities.

If dosage of chemotherapy has been diminished owing to toxicity and if no toxicity develops at the lower dose, then the dose can be increased one level or 25% with subsequent doses.

Physician judgment remains an important ingredient in cancer chemotherapy. Two or more unsuccessful treatment courses with several drugs are evidence that the tumor is refractory to the agents. Doubling a dose or adding one or two more agents often does not help. Therefore, a balance must be achieved between the cancer chemotherapy toxicity and what quality of life remains for the patient. Reason must prevail.

REFERENCES

Abrams RA, Deisseroth A (1982): The use of blood and blood products. In DeVita VT Jr, Hellman S, Rosenberg SA (eds): "Cancer Principles and Practice of Oncology," Ch 43, Sec 2. New York: Lippincott, pp 1640–1657.

Chary KK, Hisby DJ, Henderson ES, et al (1977): Phase I study of high dose cisplatinol with forced diuresis. Cancer Treat Rep 61:367–370.

Dean JC, Salmon SE, Griffith KJ (1979): Prevention of adriamycin hair loss with scalp hypothermia. New Engl J Med 301:1427–1429.

Gynecologic Oncology Group Gyn Management Committee (1980): Protocol Adverse Effects Criteria.

Herte JP (1982): Management of complications in gynecologic oncology. In "Chemotherapy Complications," Ch 12. New York: John Wiley & Sons.

Lyons A (1979): Better prevention of hair loss by headband during cytologic therapy. Lancet 1:354.

Madias NE, Harrington, JT (1978): Platinum nephrotoxicity. Am J Med 65:307–314.

Newberger PE, Sallarn SE (1979): Pain and vomiting. In "Care of Child With Cancer." New York: American Cancer Society.

O'Brien R et al (1970): Scalp tourniquet for lesser alopecia after vincristine. N Engl J Med 283:1409.

Sihimpf SC, Aisner J (1978): Empiric antibiotic therapy. Cancer Treat Rep 62:673–680.

Swartz AJ (1979): Chemotherapy extravasation. Cancer Nursing J 2:405–408.

Zweis J, Kaskow B (1978): An apparently effective countermeasure for adriamycin extravasation. JAMA 239:2116–2117.

Design, Analysis, and Interpretation of Chemotherapy Trials in Gynecologic Cancer

John A. Blessing

Gynecologic Oncology Group Statistical Office, Roswell Park Memorial Institute, Buffalo, NY 14263

A comprehensive presentation of the topics to be addressed in this chapter, would, of necessity, be a book in itself. Consequently, I will attempt to summarize concisely the key ingredients required to ensure statistically valid clinical trials and ensuing results.

Before embarking on a study of the marriage of statistics and medical research known as biostatistics, it would be productive to concentrate on the concept of statistics itself. Currently, views of this subject cover a broad spectrum—from witchcraft to a science. The word "statistics" is currently applied freely to any collection of numbers. How often we are subjected to "half-time statistics" in broadcasts of football games, "vital statistics" in beauty pageants, or "quarterly statistics" in business reports! As summary figures, each of the aforementioned statistics may be of interest, for they do indeed attempt to represent some past phenomena in a concise fashion. However, the science of statistics is concerned with more than the mere recapitulation of prior experience; of paramount importance is the statistical inference that can be drawn from such experience in an effort to project future experience under similar circumstances.

It would be of considerable benefit to both statistician and clinician to impart an appreciation of the complexity of statistical science to the clinician. A complete understanding of this subject matter is not necessary and in all likelihood impractical. Owing to the sophisticated mathematical background required prior to acquiring a statistical background, only the most rudimentary of statistics courses can be taken as an undergraduate in the

Chemotherapy of Gynecologic Cancer, pages 49-83

university. The trained statistician effectively begins his training in graduate school. On the other hand nonmathematicians, and in this context particularly clinicians, have quite often been exposed to service-type courses in statistics during their university education. These courses may do more harm than good. While they may give some intuitive feel for statistics, their oversimplification is noteworthy. Such courses give the erroneous impression that anyone with good "mathematical sense" can perform statistical analyses. Generally, these are one-semester courses and approximately two-thirds of this time must be spent attempting to develop a background in elementary probability theory before topics in "statistics" can even be broached. Unfortunately, individuals who successfully complete these elementary courses become well versed in such "vogue" phrases as "P value," "chi-square," and "t-test"; they may subsequently attempt to employ them, whether it is appropriate to do so or not. The relationship between this type of course and statistical science as applied to clinical research is roughly akin to that between high school biology and third-year medical school. A trained biostatistician, in addition to the basic graduate-level courses in probability theory and statistical inference, must at a minimum have studied such topics as design of experiments, testing of hypotheses, estimation theory, sampling theory, multivariate analysis, regression analysis, and biometry; each of these represents one or two semester graduate-level courses. Ideally, courses in nonparametric statistics, stochastic processes, and computer science would also be included. Beyond such study comes the practical experience to bridge the chasm between theory and appropriate application.

It may seem that I have strayed from the original topic. I think not. If an appreciation for the role of the statistician as a scientific collaborator is absent, the remainder of this chapter is of little value.This point is dramatically underscored in a provocative article by Bross [1974] entitled "The Role of the Statistician: Scientist or Shoe Clerk." In some instances investigators seek statistical consultation merely to give a seal of approval to their results and conversely minimize the importance of statistics if it fails to confirm what they are already certain is true. However, a substantial improvement in this situation has been noted in recent years. Hammond [1980] states:

> The role of the biostatistician in clinical investigation has evolved significantly. There has been an increasing recognition not only for the need for biostatistical expertise in helping to fathom the meaning of data at the end of a study, but also of an increasing dependence upon biostatistical methods for every step of clinical investigation, from clinical study design and feasibility testing to data analysis and reporting.

In national collaborative groups the interaction between statistical and clinical research is generally excellent. One such group, the Gynecologic Oncology Group (GOG), is devoted solely to the investigation of gynecologic malignancies. At the institutional level the degree and quality of collaboration varies with both the institution and the statistician.

Therefore, in the interest of good science as well as successful studies, statistical input should be sought before, during, and at the conclusion of clinical investigation.

DESIGN

Definition of a Clinical Trial

The clinical trial has been aptly defined by Zelen [1983] as "a scientific experiment to generate clinical data for the purpose of evaluating one or more therapies on a population." He further provides a clear distinction between the clinical trial and an observational study, noting that the former is characterized by a definite study design, describing both the patient population and the fashion in which treatments are allocated; the latter merely notes some phenomena. Clinical trials are the classical method for carrying out clinical investigations. But how does one learn to plan or design such a study? In 1978 Gordon wrote: "Unfortunately there is no standard textbook on clinical-trial methodology, and no courses on the subject are offered in schools of medicine or public health." Nonetheless, a method of procedure may be outlined. Initially the concept of the proposed study should be discussed with a competent biostatistician. Two key questions which should be addressed are: Is the study worth doing? Can the study be done? There is often a delicate balance between the two. However, it is better that the study die in the concept phase than be initiated with no chance of realizing its goals. The literature is replete with anecdotal articles that provide no valuable information regarding future patients from the same population.

Moreover, the casual reader of such an article may become convinced of the merit of a treatment method, when, in reality, the anecdotes are of no predictive value. In the next sections, factors to be considered by the statistician and clinical investigator in designing a clinical trial are outlined.

Types of Clinical Trials

There are various types of clinical trials for examining the efficacy of new chemotherapeutic agents. Following indication of possible therapeutic effects arising from animal studies, trials in man are desirable. The earliest study, called a phase I trial, is concerned with determining a tolerable dose and schedule which can be further examined in later trials.

Upon the determination of an appropriate promising regimen in a phase I study, a phase II study may be initiated to examine whether such a treatment plan is sufficiently active to warrant further study. Such a decision will be primarily based upon objective tumor response and observed adverse effects. Further study will generally be indicated if the rate of observed tumor response in the phase II study appears potentially higher than that of the current standard therapy. In some instances additional study could be indicated if the observed response rate was similar to that of the standard, but the agent in question demonstrated less toxicity. Agents satisfying neither of the above criteria, but demonstrating limited activity, might still be considered as a component of combination chemotherapy of a "salvage" regimen following treatment failure on the standard. It must be emphasized that the phase II study is not a comparative clinical trial, but rather the mechanism for identifying candidates for the comparative study.

Once a potentially efficacious regimen is identified, a controlled clinical trial comparing this regimen or regimens with the standard therapy is undertaken. It is this phase III study which must be judiciously planned and conducted with precision as the results may define a new standard or eliminate a mode of therapy from any further investigational use.

Other types of studies are sometimes conceived, but they nonetheless generally fall into the broad classification of phase I, II, or III studies. For example, follow-up studies are occasionally done on promising phase II trials. However, these are merely extensions of the phase II plan employed to enable more precise estimation of the true response rate by enrolling more patients. Also, confirmatory studies are less frequently developed in an attempt to independently reproduce or confirm results previously obtained by other investigators. It should be mentioned that confirmatory studies are not often popular and occasionally difficult to publish. However, as Zelen [1983] points out: "In nearly all scientific endeavors, a new experimental finding is regarded as tentative until it can be confirmed independently by other investigators." He further states that confirmation "should be done for clinical findings having major therapeutic impact." While this may not prove practical in many instances, it merits consideration whenever the results of an initial study are controversial or not readily accepted.

A detailed discussion of phase I, II, and III trials is found in Gehan and Schneiderman [1981]. The evolution of a new standard regimen is outlined in Figure 1.

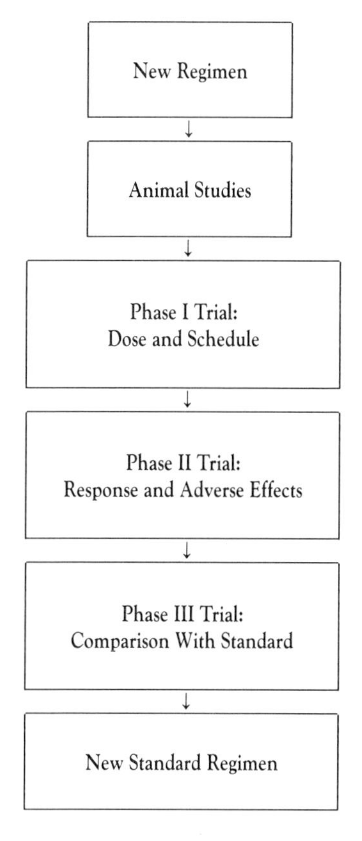

Fig. 1. The evolution of a new standard regimen.

Test of Hypothesis

A clinical trial can be viewed as a test of a particular hypothesis, called the null hypothesis, versus a particular alternative hypothesis. The ultimate decision resulting from the study will be to either reject or accept the null hypothesis. Table I shows that there are two types of error that might occur.

If the data from the clinical trial leads to a rejection of the null hypothesis, but in reality the null hypothesis is true, the resulting error is known as a type I error. Conversely, if the decision is to accept the null hypothesis, and in reality the alternative is true, the resulting error is known as a type II error.

In phase II trials the null hypothesis might be that the response rate to a particular chemotherapeutic agent is less than or equal to 20%; the alterna-

TABLE I. Possible Outcomes in a Test of Hypothesis

	Decision	
Reality	Accept null	Reject null
Null true	Correct decision	Type I error (false-positive)
Null false	Type II error (false-negative)	Correct decision

tive hypothesis would be that the response rate was greater than 20%. In a phase III study a possible null hypothesis is that the response rate of regimen A does not differ from that of regimen B, while one alternative hypothesis is that the response rate of A is greater than that of B. Note that for both the phase II and phase III trials, the alternative hypothesis is what would be considered a positive result. Therefore, the *erroneous* rejection of the null hypothesis (with its implied acceptance of the alternative hypothesis) constitutes a false endorsement of a positive conjecture. For this reason the type I error is often referred to as a "false-positive" error. Similarly, the type II error, accepting the negative null hypothesis when it is in fact false, is referred to as a "false-negative" error.

One of the primary goals of the statistician in designing the clinical trial is to minimize the probability of committing either error. Unfortunately, for a fixed number of patients it is mathematically impossible to minimize both types of errors simultaneously. When tests of hypothesis are designed the probability of a type I error is fixed at some level (called the level of significance) and denoted by α; it is customary to chose $\alpha = 0.05$ (5 chances in 100). The chance of committing a type II false-negative error is denoted by β. Although some trials are conducted with $\beta = 0.10$, a more customary choice is $\beta = 0.20$. A phrase often heard, but not always understood, is "the power of the test." This refers to the probability that a declared positive finding is in reality true. Reflecting upon Table I, we see that this probability is equal to $1-\beta$.

When designing a clinical trial the clinician and statistician should pay special attention to the level of significance and power of the test. As mentioned $\alpha = 0.05$ and $\beta = 0.20$ are common choices. However, the impact of such choices are not always appreciated. A false-positive probability of only 0.05 may be quite acceptable as the chance of erroneously declaring a significant treatment difference in a phase III study is quite small. However, one might ask: Need we be so stringent, as a false-positive result would certainly be discovered in later trials? Conversely, having a false-negative rate of 0.20 might be too lax in certain circumstances. If no significant treatment difference was found in a phase III study, there would be a one-in-five chance that this conclusion was wrong. Moreover, since the results would be considered negative, it would be unlikely that the study would ever be repeated; thus, this error would be more likely to go undetected than a false-positive error. The purpose of this presentation is not to suggest that the use of $\alpha = 0.05$ and $\beta = 0.20$ are inappropriate; on the contrary, most of the Gynecologic Oncology Group studies feature such choices. However, the principals involved in study design must be aware of the possible consequences of various choices of α and β and discuss this aspect in light of ethical considerations, available patients for study, and the background and current status of the disease entity to be studied.

Determination of appropriate level of significance and power *prior to onset* of the study is but one important aspect which underscores the need for medical and biostatistical interaction during all phases of study design. Many clinicians have a vague notion regarding the notion of level of significance since, in some ways, it seems similar to the "P value." (Having been trained to "worship at the altar of 0.05," they know that a P value of less than 0.05 is indicative of positive results.) However, the concept of "power" is even less understood; if it is ever seen at all, it is in the "statistical considerations" section of the written protocol. Here it is generally regarded as some statistical jargon required by the National Cancer Institute to activate the study. A clear understanding of the false-negative and false-positive errors is an important factor in sound design.

The Phase I Study

Little can be said about the appropriate design of a phase I study. As no prior human experimentation has been performed, there is scant information about the agent to draw upon. Patient safety must be a prime consideration. The knowledge and experience of an expert medical oncologist is therefore a key ingredient. Such a study should be conducted under a constant environment; a single investigator at a single institution is the ideal setting. Moreover, the selection of patients should be monitored closely. There is sometimes a tendency to reserve such "experimental" treatment for terminal cases, thereby introducing considerable bias. In general, only a small number of cases will be required in this phase of study.

Phase II Studies

As mentioned earlier, in the phase II study, the therapeutic effect of a regimen will be examined employing response and toxicity as primary parameters. In gynecologic cancer, separate trials must be conducted for distinct disease categories. For a particular disease entity, the clinician can determine what level of activity would constitute a significant finding. For example, suppose a phase II study investigating a new drug was to be designed for epithelial tumors of the ovary and an objective complete response rate of 20% was felt meaningful. A test of hypothesis could be envisioned. The null hypothesis would be that the response rate is $\leqslant$ 20%. The alternative hypothesis would obviously be that the response rate is $>$ 20%. A statistical test of the hypothesis with specification for α and β could certainly be carried out. However, the current trend is not to conduct such a test of hypothesis which concludes that the true response rate lies about or below a particular point, but rather to estimate the true response rate with some predetermined degree of precision. The key question of the clinician is "How many patients will be required?"

If it is desired to estimate the true response rate and be 90% certain that this estimate is within $\pm$ 15% of the true population rate, a sample size of 30 patients will suffice. To increase the confidence level to 95% or to tighten the 15% restraint to 10% would increase the sample size to 68 or 43 patients, respectively.

In designing a phase II trial a quandary is faced. Requiring too much precision can deplete the available patient population and consequently limit the number of agents that can be tested. Conversely, relaxing the restraints on a trial greatly increases the chance of passing minimally effective agents on to further study. In general practice, phase II trials requiring 30 patients as outlined above are considered feasible and scientifically valid. However, sound judgment must be employed in interpreting the results. Tannock and Murphy [1983] caution that there is a need "to set a higher threshold of effectiveness for a drug deemed worthy of further testing and for earlier decisions to abandon minimally effective agents." In this regard stopping rules are often employed to terminate investigations of inactive agents early. One popular stopping rule introduced by Gehan [1961] has been frequently misinterpreted. Gehan essentially sought to test the null and alternative hypothesis defined at the beginning of this section inherently involving a 20% response rate. He noted that if a drug "were 20% effective or more, there would be more than a 95% chance that one or more successes would be obtained in 14 consecutive cases." Thus, if 14 consecutive nonresponses were observed at the outset, one would conclude that the agent was unlikely to produce response in 20% of the patients or more, and be correct in this action more than 95% of the time. This example was used to substantiate one entry into a table in the paper.

Unfortunately, many oncologists missed the point of the example and erroneously believed that consecutive failures among the first 14 cases is always an indication to terminate the study. This is true only if the initial hypotheses to be tested were that the response rate was $\leqslant 20\%$ versus that the response rate was $>20\%$. His paper also shows, for example, that, if the hypotheses centered around a true response rate of 5%, 59 initial failures, not 14, would be required. Similarly, if the hypotheses centered around 50%, only five consecutive initial failures would be required. Thus, the so-called "rule of 14" pertains *only* to the hypothesis introduced earlier. This is by no means suggesting that stopping rules should not be employed; rather, inappropriate use of stopping rules must be avoided. Correctly used, a stopping rule enables more efficient allotment of patients when inactive agents are studied; incorrectly used, they can negate the value of a study.

One final word about Gehan's stopping rule: It is designed to "reject ineffective agents quickly." The number of consecutive initial failures required to terminate represents the minimal number of patients that will be entered. As such, it may prevent excessive testing of an ineffective agent. However, it is not always a safeguard against further testing of an ineffective agent. There is always a certain nonnegligible chance that an agent of low-order effectiveness will produce at least one response. Stopping rules may be employed to terminate early if warranted by the initial results. Once the results indicate that early termination is not warranted, the clinical trial should proceed to its originally determined end point.

Phase III Studies

The key factor in designing a phase III trial is generally considered to be feasibility; if the study is not practical, other considerations are of little importance. However, feasibility can be envisioned as having two components—statistical and medical. As will be discussed later, there can be a delicate balance between the two.

In order to discuss the number of patients necessary to conduct a clinical phase III trial, it is necessary to examine the types of parameters upon which sample size determination is based. In gynecologic cancer one of the most frequently employed parameters is objective tumor response for patients with measurable disease. Four categories are generally employed: complete response, partial response, stable disease, and increasing disease. Results of major chemotherapeutic phase III studies in gynecologic malignancies by Omura et al. [1983], Cohen et al. [1983], and Bonomi et al. [1982] have demonstrated that patients who achieve a complete response have significantly longer survival than all other patients and also that there is essentially no difference between the survival of patients achieving partial response and those with stable disease. This background indicates that for purposes of determining sample sizes, one should focus on the objective complete response rate rather than combined complete and partial response rate. Thus, in this context, response essentially may be considered to be a binary variable—one with only two possible outcomes. This is in marked contrast to two other oft-employed variables—survival and disease-free survival (often called progression-free interval). Both of these are continuous variables measured in time, thus conceptually having an infinite number of possible outcomes. Also, at any particular time, the outcome for some patients on study will be censored by time (i.e. some patients still alive or disease-free). Suffice it to say that response as a parameter differs dramatically from the time variables. Consequently, sample size determination methodology differs according to the primary parameter employed.

If objective complete tumor response is the primary parameter of interest, there are essentially four factors to be taken into account. Often an investigator will inquire how many patients will be required to demonstrate a 15% difference between two regimens. While this sounds like a reasonable inquiry, it addresses only one factor—magnitude of the difference.

While it is not readily apparent, demonstration of a difference of 15% will require different numbers of patients depending on the baseline or starting point of the standard treatment. That is, to demonstrate a 15% improvement from 5% to 20% will require a different number of patients than to demonstrate a 15% difference from 35% to 50%.

The third factor has already been discussed in some detail—specification of α and β, the probability of committing a type I or type II error, respectively. The more these are to be reduced the more patients required. The fourth factor will now be developed.

In discussing tests of hypotheses an example was given testing the null hypothesis that the response rate of regimen A does not differ from regimen B against *one* alternative that the response rate of A is greater than that of B. Note that neither hypothesis included the contingency that the response rate for B could be greater than that for A. This is called a "one-sided alternative" and is used in circumstances where the logistics of the study, the composition of the regimens, and prior experience essentially rule out the notion that the response rate for B could be superior to that for A.

As an example, consider Figure 2, which depicts the schema of GOG protocol 47. The two regimens differ by the presence of cis-platinum in one regimen. Previous experience in phase II studies had documented the activity of cis-platinum in advanced ovarian cancer [Thigpen et al., 1979], while

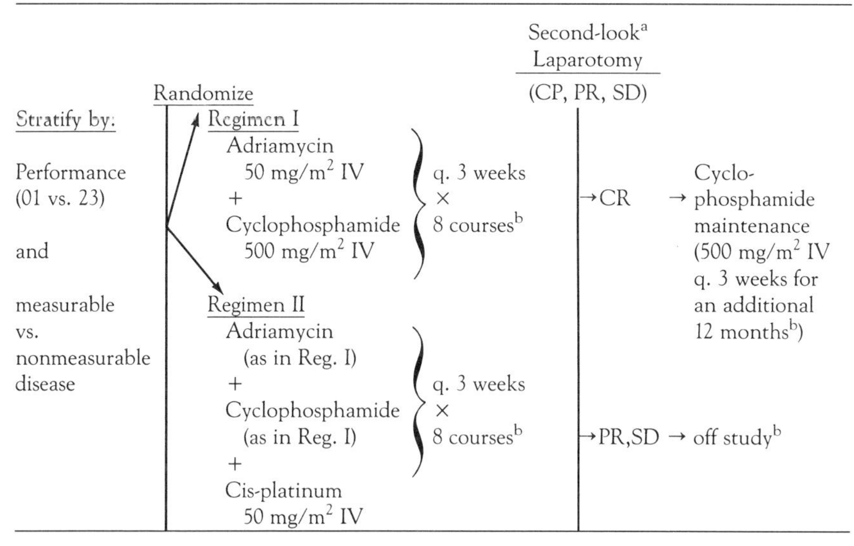

[a]PR or SD to have second look only in selected cases.
[b]Patients with progressive disease at any time will be removed from further chemotherapy on this study and will continue to be followed.

Fig. 2. Schema of GOG protocol 47.

a previous phase III study had documented the activity of the adriamycin-cytoxan regimen [Omura et al., 1983]. Thus, there was absolutely no reason to incorporate into the design the possibility of the two-drug regimen proving more active than the three-drug regimen. Thus, a "one-sided" test was called for.

On the other hand, if the composition of treatment regimens indicate that either might prove superior, then a "two-sided alternative" is warranted. In terms of the initial example in this section it would be stated: The response rate for regimen A is greater than that for regimen B or the response rate for regimen B is greater than that for regimen A. Figure 3 depicts the schema for GOG protocol 28, "A randomized comparison of melphalan, 5FU, and megace versus adriamycin, cytoxan, 5FU, and megace in the treatment of patients with primary stage III, primary stage IV, recurrent or residual endometrial carcinoma (phase III)," which is an example of a study requiring a two-sided alternative. It should be intuitively clear that the number of patients required for a two-sided test is greater than that for a similar study featuring a one-sided test.

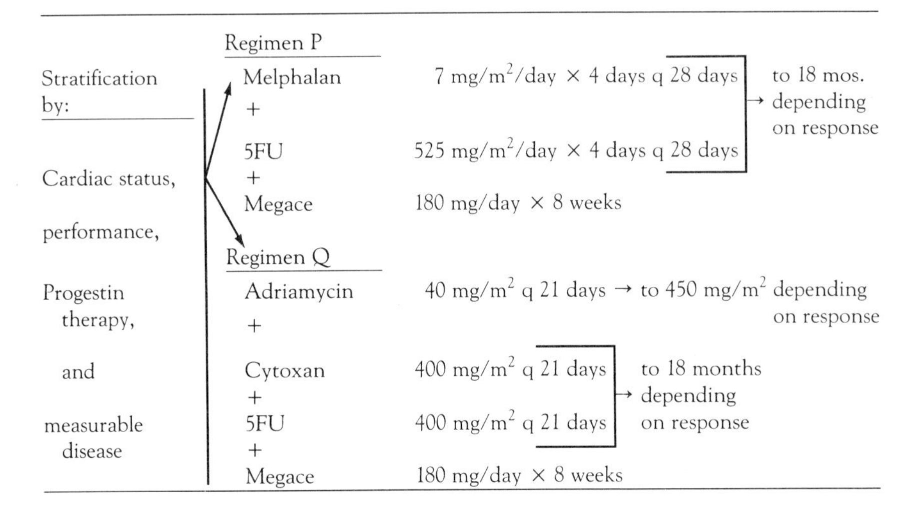

Fig. 3. Schema for GOG protocol 28.

TABLE II. Number of Patients Required in Each Regimen to Detect a 15% Treatment Difference (α = 0.05)

		No. patients	
Difference	β	One-sided	Two-sided
5–20%	0.2	55	69
	0.1	76	93
20–35%	0.2	110	135
	0.1	150	185
35–50%	0.2	135	175
	0.1	185	230

To recap, the factors needed for sample size determination are the magnitude of the treatment difference, baseline response rate, the specification of α and β, and the type of test required.

Table II shows the number of patients required *in each regimen* to demonstrate a 15% treatment difference for various combinations of starting point α and β, and type of test based on the methodology of Cochran and Cox [1957]. Revisions in these figures for the one-sided test have been developed by Casagrande et al. [1978], resulting in slight increases in patient requirements. However, to facilitate comparison of one-sided and two-sided tests the figures of Cochran and Cox are employed. Clearly the question as initially posed was insufficient to enable accurate sample size determination; without further specifications the required number of patients to carry out such a study was between 110 and 460.

One other aspect requires mention—the size of the difference. It is a mathematical reality that if all other factors are held constant, recognition of larger differences requires fewer patients than recognition of small differences. In this context we must now consider medical feasibility. Suppose we wish to design a study in which the current standard therapy has a known response rate of 25%, the nature of the new regimen is such that a "one-sided test" is warranted and we choose $\alpha = 0.05$ and $\beta = 0.20$. Table III gives the number of patients required according to Casagrande et al. [1978] for different magnitudes of difference to be sought.

Clearly the number of patients necessitated varies dramatically with the magnitude of the difference sought. Mathematical practicality (available patients) must not dictate to medical feasibility. While in this example seeking an improvement of 40% might be quite easy to perform, if there is no medical reason to imagine such a large difference might exist, such a study would be a waste of time. In addition to having sufficient patients to do the study, there must be sufficient reason to do it. Allowing potential accrual of patients to determine the medical aspects of a study is a classic example of letting the tail wag the dog. The risk of sacrificing biological

TABLE III. Number of Patients per Regimen Required to Detect an Increase in Response Rate of Various Magnitudes (one-sided test, $\alpha = 0.05$, $\beta = 0.20$, and response rate of standard therapy fixed at 25%)

Magnitude of difference in response rates (%)	No. patients per regimen
5	1,026
10	277
15	132
20	78
25	54
30	37
35	30
40	23
45	18
50	15
55	12
60	10
65	9
70	8

significance for mathematical practicality must also be minimal. Again we return to a recurrent theme—there is much to be gained through early collaboration of clinical investigator and biostatistician.

In all deliberations sample size projections should be considered merely as guidelines to study feasibility. The previous discussion emphasizes the triviality of published studies featuring multiple regimens of 25 patients. Unfortunately such poorly designed studies represent an enormous waste of resources and available patients.

For trials in which survival or progression-free interval (PFI) is the primary parameter upon which statistical considerations will be based, the size of the difference between regimens in median survival or PFI must be specified. Again, particular attention must be paid to the choice of α and β. Statistical methodology for clinical trials involving time variables is sophisticated and not particularly intuitive to those not trained in this area. Research into sample size determination has been carried out by George and Desu [1974], who have formulated the number of *failure* observations (not patient entries) required in each regimen to observe a significant difference in two survival distributions. In the context of their paper, "survival time" may also be viewed as "progression-free interval" or "remission duration." Table IV presents the required number of failures per regimen.

It is difficult for a nonstatistician to use Table IV properly and he would be ill advised to do so. It is presented here to illustrate the large number of failures (and larger number of entries) required to conduct most phase III time-variable studies. Those studies which mathematically require few pa-

TABLE IV. Number of Patients (d) Required to Detect a Significant Difference in Two Survival Distributions

	Δ													
$1-\beta$	1.1	1.2	1.3	1.4	1.5	1.6	1.7	1.8	1.9	2.0	2.5	3.0	3.5	4.0
0.95	3,479	951	460	280	193	144	113	92	77	66	38	27	21	17
	2,384	652	315	192	132	98	77	63	53	46	26	18	14	12
0.90	2,870	785	379	231	159	118	93	76	64	55	32	22	17	14
	1,884	515	249	152	105	78	61	50	42	36	21	15	11	9
0.80	2,213	605	292	178	123	91	72	59	49	42	24	17	13	11
	1,360	372	180	110	76	56	44	36	30	26	15	11	8	7

Abbreviations: Δ–the ratio of the median survival for the experimental treatment group to the median survival for the control treatment group (the ratio of means could be substituted for the ratio of medians); $1-\beta$–the probability of detecting a significant difference at the 0.01 level (upper figure) or the 0.05 level (lower figure) when the true ratio is Δ; d–the number of patients required for each treatment group, all followed until failure.

tients are seeking differences so large that they are apt to be of minimal medical interest.

As an example, suppose the median survival for patients having advanced squamous cell carcinoma of the cervix treated with cis-platinum is 7.0 months and we wanted to test this standard against a regimen consisting of cis-platinum plus some other new drug. If we accept as reasonable $\alpha = 0.05$ and $\beta = 0.20$ and find it medically plausible to seek an improvement in median survival to 10.5 months, then we would require 76 failures per regimen.

Recently, Schoenfeld and Richter [1982] have introduced a nomogram method for calculating the number of patients needed for a clinical trial featuring survival. This methodology considers the duration of the accrual period as well as the duration of the follow-up period in determining the sample size. If in the previous example we desire to accrue patients for 2 years and have 1 additional year of follow-up, then approximately 97 entries per treatment arm are required.

These examples illustrate that, as was the case for studies based on comparison of the response rates, published trials featuring comparison of time variables based on small numbers of patients should be read skeptically.

Randomization

Randomization assignment of patients to treatment regimens is occasionally employed in phase II studies. If two phase II trials are being conducted simultaneously, randomization may be an effective means of reducing investigator bias, and consequently the method for selection of patient might be improved. This process is quite simple and has no implications beyond patient entry as treatment comparisons are not the focus of phase II studies.

As previously mentioned, the primary purpose of the phase III clinical trial is a comparison of treatment efficacy. If the results of such a trial indicate that one treatment regimen did better than the others, there are two possible scenarios: Either one regimen is more efficacious, or the one regimen had more "good prognosis" patients who probably would have done just as well if treated on the other regimen. The aim of prospective randomization is to minimize the possibility of the latter contingency. It is essential that the study be designed such that the only plausible rationale for an observed difference in efficacy between regimens is the therapy itself. To ensure this each regimen must consist of comparable patients. Any selection bias, whether intentional or unintentional, will cause the final results to be tainted and suspect. Randomization will not guarantee complete patient comparability, but it will improve the likelihood of its occurring, while eliminating bias. Moreover, following randomization, adjustment for differences in patient characteristics among regimens can be performed in the analysis.

Design of the randomization scheme varies with the nature of the study. The usual concept features equal allocation of patients to all treatment regimens. Often stratification is incorporated into this basic scheme. Mutually exclusive subsets of patients are defined by various prognostic factors taken at different "levels." A separate randomization is then prepared for each stratum. For example, if a randomization were to be designed stratifying by prognostic factors prior chemotherapy (yes vs. no) and tumor size ($\leqslant$ 2 cm vs. $>$ 2 cm), four distinct strata would result: 1) no prior chemotherapy, $\leqslant$ 2 cm; 2) no prior chemotherapy, $>$ 2 cm; 3) prior chemotherapy $\leqslant$ 2 cm; and 4) prior chemotherapy $>$ 2 cm.

Such a randomization attempts to allocate patients evenly to the regimens within each strata, thereby improving patient comparability. There are two schools of thought regarding stratification. Peto et al. [1976] consider stratification unnecessary as sophisticated statistical methodology exists allowing adjustment for any imbalanced distribution of prognostic factors in regimens. While this view is quite acceptable from a purely statistical point of view, it has little intuitive appeal to the medical audience who must digest the published reports. Consequently, an appropriately analyzed study may not be readily publishable, let alone widely accepted.

> The use of prospective stratification also tends to avoid situations in which conclusions of a study are not convincing to the medical community because of suspicion of an analysis used to adjust for a lack of comparability. This is a very real concern, for the term "adjustment" itself often elicits skepticism. [Simon 1979]

This opinion was substantiated in one Gynecologic Oncology Group publication. Omura et al. [1983] published a paper on chemotherapy of ovarian cancer featuring such statistical analysis only after a detailed explanation was provided to the reviewers, who did not understand the methodology employed.

It should be noted that overstratification can easily produce undesired effects. As stratification variables at various levels are incorporated into the design, the number of individual strata and associated randomization schemes increases. This increases the likelihood that many strata will have few patients entered, leading to possible imbalance within the strata. Consequently, there is a small, but definite, chance that overall treatment arm imbalance will result. In order to avoid the situation a method of adaptive stratification has been developed for use when there are several prognostic factors [cf. Simon, 1979]. Hannigan and Brown [1982] have refined randomization techniques using a biased-coin design, which simultaneously examines all stratification variables and then determines the regimen to which a patient should be assigned to improve patient balance.

If the response is quantified in some subjective fashion, it might be wise to consider a double-blind study in which both the patient and the investigator are unaware of the regimen to which the patient is randomized. Obviously, this type of study cannot be done if surgery or radiotherapy is involved or if the study features a "no-treatment" arm. However, for certain types of chemotherapeutic studies it is occasionally possible.

In large-scale multi-institutional collaborative studies the need for double-blind studies may be obviated by a system of independent study chairman review which can be quite effective in eliminating subjectivity.

The last type of design to be introduced is the crossover. Brown [1980] described this design which uses "each patient as his own control by trying both drugs on each patient at different times and comparing the results, patient by patient." There are certain potential drawbacks to this type of trial and they are quite possible in gynecologic trials. Among those cited by Gehan and Schneiderman [1982] are the following: 1) Patients may not survive long enough to receive the second treatment; 2) second sequence delayed by a sustained response to first therapy; 3) markedly different responses on each sequence invalidating any comparison of response duration; and 4) interaction of effect of first response with the response to the second treatment, such that the two are not independent. In summary, one should be aware of the existence of the crossover design; but, as was the case with double-blind studies, the opportunity to employ this design appropriately will not often arise.

Alternatives to randomized clinical trials have been considered and are endorsed by some statisticians. Generally the pitfalls outweigh the gains. The first of these alternatives is the use of historical controls. Gehan and Freireich [1974] advocate the use of nonrandomized controls "when the primary purpose of the study is to estimate effectiveness of treatment; when large differences in response rate are expected on the basis of preliminary studies." In phase III trials involving gynecologic malignancies, neither of these contingencies can be expected to occur very often. In contrasting use of randomization in clinical trials with nonrandomized controls, Green [1982] stated: "With randomization, bias (whether conscious or unconscious) is avoided, prognostic factors (both known and unknown) tend to be balanced across treatment groups, the validity of statistical tests of significance is guaranteed, and problems with time trends are avoided.

Similarly Byar [1980] argues against the use of data bases to replace randomized phase III studies: "A review of the methodological problems likely to arise in analyzing such data for the purpose of comparing treatments suggests that sound inferences would not generally be possible because of difficulties with bias in treatment assignment, non-standard definitions, definitions changing in time, specification of groups to be compared, missing data, and multiple comparisons."

These are compelling arguments favoring randomized comparisons in gynecologic studies.

Patient Data and Data Collection Forms

It is not always readily apparent to investigators that considerations of patient data and appropriate data collection forms are pertinent to the design phase of clinical trials. Nonetheless, decisions must be made prior to the initiation of the study which can have a substantial effect on realization of study objectives. As mentioned previously, the nature of the primary parameters is necessary to determine the feasibility of the trial. However, more precise specifications must be developed to guarantee unambiguous data and objective interpretations.

As an example, we focus on tumor response. First, it is necessary to specify how response will be gauged. If the patient population consists of only patients with measurable disease, it is possible to quantify response objectively. Determination of response categories and their definitions is essential prior to patient accrual to enhance objectivity. This is not always a trivial matter: More than one mass may be involved; a minimal period of time to sustain the response must be defined; the method of tumor measurement must be provided. If the population contains patients with nonmeasurable tumors, a subjective interpretation of response may be possible. Is so, this must be clearly defined. In a similar fashion, definitions of recurrence or progression of disease must be presented as response duration will also be of interest.

Although this example has focused on response, similar considerations must take place for adverse effects, laboratory tests, pathology, patient history data, follow-up data, etc. Tables V and VI give examples of possible response and adverse-effects definitions, respectively.

In addition to determination and definition of parameters of interest, it is necessary to design appropriate data collection forms. Retrospective collection of data should be avoided. It is not only difficult and time-consuming

TABLE V. GOG Response Criteria

Complete response is a disappearance of all gross evidence of disease for at least 1 month.
Partial response is a 50% or greater reduction in the product obtained from measurement of each lesion for at least 1 month.
Increasing disease is a 50% or greater increase in the product from any lesion documented in two separate examinations at least 2 weeks apart or the appearance of any new lesion within 3 months of entry into study.
Stable disease is defined as disease not meeting any of the above three criteria.

to attempt to retrieve data, it is less accurate and less objective to do so. Data integrity is appreciably enhanced by the completion of well-designed data forms at the time the patient is seen.

The Written Document

It is imperative that a well-written document, called a protocol, detailing the plan of investigation, be prepared. All collaborative groups and cancer centers have a general format to their particular protocols. Table VII displays the elements of all protocols prepared by the Gynecologic Oncology Group.

Objectives of the study should be succinctly and unambiguously stated. The background and rationale behind these objectives must be provided. Patient population must be accurately defined so that those sampled are in fact representative of the true population. Method of patient entry must be described. If it is a randomized study, will stratification be involved and how will randomization by accomplished? Study agents must be described fully. For chemotherapeutic agents exact dosage and schedule should be clearly stated as well as provisions for treatment modification following adverse effects. Required observations such as tumor measurements, blood work, laboratory tests, etc. should be noted regarding both frequency and reporting. Methodology and a timetable for reporting of data must be included. Lastly, a statistical documentation of the feasibility and duration of the study is mandatory.

Following final preparation of the written protocol and its subsequent review and approval, patient entry and data acquisition may proceed.

ANALYSIS

Statistical analysis of clinical trials is a complex issue. The purpose of this section is not to teach statistical methodology, but rather to discuss several very important concepts and their relationship to a successful, meaningful presentation of a study.

TABLE VI. Gynecologic Oncology Group Adverse Effects Criteria (December 1980)

System	0	1 = Mild	2 = Moderate	3 = Severe	4 = Life-threatening/ most severe
Hematologic	≥11.0	9.5–10.9	8.0–9.4	6.5–7.9	<6.5
HGB (/mcl)	≥4,000	3,000–3,999	2,000–2,999	1,000–1,999	<1,000
WCB (/mcl)	≥1,999	1,500–1,999	1,000–1,499	500–999	<500
Granulocytes (/mcl)	≥150,000	100,000–149,999	50,000–99,999	25,000–49,999	<25,000
Platelets (/mcl)	No transfusion	Drop in HGB of <2 g	Transfusion 1 or 2 units	Transfusion 3 or 4 units	Reexploration to control bleeding, transfusion 5 units or hypovolemic shock
Anemia/blood loss (cumulative)		Not requiring transfusion			
Gastrointestinal					
Nausea and vomiting	None	Nausea only	Vomiting controlled by antiemetics	Vomiting 6×/day in spite of antiemetics requiring hospitalization	Life-threatening dehydration and/or bleeding
Diarrhea	None	Watery, semisolid; no therapy needed	Watery; responds to therapy	Watery, ≥5/day; unresponsive to therapy	Hemorrhagic, severe dehydration/electrolyte loss
Mechanical problems	None	Temporary ileus of 3 days or less duration	Ileus requiring tube decompression; narrowing of intestinal segment on x-ray, or moderate mucosal edema on procto exam	Surgically correctable defect—no stoma	Fistula, perforation, chronic bleeding requiring diversion
Stomatitis	None	Erythema and/or enanthema	Ulcers, unable to eat	Ulcers, unable to eat	Life-threatening dehydration; hemorrhage, ulceration sepsis, aspiration

Esophagus	None	Transient—no therapy required	Odynophagia, dysphagia, antacids or viscous xylocaine needed	Odynophagia, dysphagia, lasting longer than 14 days in spite of symptomatic treatment < 10% body weight loss, unable to eat solids	Odynophagia, dysphagia, > 10% loss of body weight, dehydration, hospitalization required
SGOT/SGPT	N (SGOT only)	Up to 2.5 N	2.6—5.0 N	5.1—10 N	> 10 N
Bilirubin	None	Up to 2.5 N	2.6—5.0 N	5.1—10 N	> 10 N
Alkaline phosphatase	None	Up to 2.5 N	2.6—5.0 N	5.1—10 N	> 10 N
				Precoma	Hepatic coma
Genitourinary					
Renal					
BUN	None	> N–40 mg%	41–60 mg%	> 60 mg%, reversible without dialysis	Irreversible without dialysis, life-threatening renal failure
Creatinine	None	> N–2.5N	2.6–5.0 N	5.1–10 N	> 10 N
Creatinine clearance	None	N–50%↓	50%↓–80%↓	80%↓–90%↓	> 90%↓
Proteinuria	None	1 + < 300 mg%	2–3 + 300–1,000 mg%	4 + > 1,000 mg%	Renal failure, Nephrotic syndrome
Hematuria	None	Microscopic	Gross	Gross and clots requiring transfusion	Obstructive uropathology
Bladder and ureter					
Acute	No problems	Dysuria, frequency and/or microscopic hematuria; injury of bladder with primary repair	Bacterial infection; gross hematuria not requiring transfusion (less than 2 g% decrease in HGB); injury requiring reanastomosis or reimplantation	Gross hematuria requiring transfusion (greater than 2 g% decrease in HGB); sepsis, obstruction or fistula requiring secondary operation; loss of one kidney	Life-threatening hematuria or septic shock; obstruction of both kidneys or vesicovaginal fistula requiring diversion

(continued)

TABLE VI. Gynecologic Oncology Group Adverse Effects Criteria (December 1980) *(Continued)*

System	0	1 = Mild	2 = Moderate	3 = Severe	4 = Life-threatening/ most severe
Bladder and ureter					
Chronic	None	Dysuria; frequency; minimal telangiectasia with edema on cystoscopy	Superficial ulceration; moderate telangiectasia; gross hematuria (less than 2 g% decrease in HGB); bladder volume less than 150 cc	Deep ulceration; severe pain; gross hematuria requiring transfusion (greater than 2 g% decrease in HGB); permanent unilateral loss of function of kidney	Decreased bladder volume requiring diversion or catheter drainage; fistula; necrosis, permanent bilateral obstruction or loss of renal function requiring dialysis
Infection	None	Minor infection (nonbacteremia UTI, bronchitis, cellulitis, URI) treated responding to oral antibiotics	Presumed infection with fever as only sign; blood cultures negative; parenteral therapy antibiotics	Infection with chills and/or fever of grade 3; blood cultures positive	Fulminant; local or visceral infection with sepsis, shock, or other system failure
Fever (note: if drug induced)	<38°C	38–40°C less than 24 h duration	38–40°C greater than 24 h duration	>40.1°C	Fever with hypotension
Allergic	None	Dermatitis or urticaria	Bronchospasm, oral therapy required	Bronchospasm, parenteral therapy required; serum sickness	Anaphylaxis
Cutaneous					
Skin	None	Erythema, pigmentation	Dry desquamation; vesiculation; pruritus; phlebitis and/or induration at injection site	Moist desquamation; ulceration	Exfoliative dermatitis, necrosis; requiring grafting

Hair	None	Minimal hair loss	Moderate patchy loss	Total reversible	Total nonreversible
Wound	None	Wound seroma; cuff hematoma	Abscess or superficial separation	Fascial disruption with evisceration	Necrotizing fasciitis
Peripheral neurologic					
Reflex	Normal	Decreased DTRs	Absent DTRs		
Strength	Normal	Mild weakness	Moderate weakness	Severe weakness, paresis; cannot squat or sit up in bed unassisted	Paralysis; transverse myelitis
Sensory	Normal	Mild pain; mild paresthesia	Moderate pain; moderate paresthesia	Severe pain; severe paresthesia, trophic ulcers	
GI mobility (constipation)	None	Mild constipation requiring laxatives	Moderate constipation	Obstipation, requiring enemas, manageable without surgery	Obstipation requiring surgery, perforation
Central neurologic					
Mental status; mood, ideation, memory, consciousness	Normal	Transient alteration and/or minimal lethargy	Alteration substantially affecting function <50% of time or of function	Alteration substantially affecting function >50% of time or of function	Comatose, acute toxic psychosis, suicide attempt
Motor paresis	None	Mild or transient	Substantially affects function, <50% decrement in baseline capabilities	Substantially affects function, >50% decrement in baseline capabilities	Paralysis
Cerebellar	Normal	Mild or transient alteration	Substantially affects function, <50% decrement in baseline capabilities	Substantially affects function, >50% decrement in baseline capabilities	Confined to bed
Seizure disorder	Normal	None	Transient or satisfactorily controlled medical therapy	Seizure disorder not controlled by medical therapy	Status epilepticus

(continued)

TABLE VI. Gynecologic Oncology Group Adverse Effects Criteria (December 1980) *(Continued)*

System	0	1 = Mild	2 = Moderate	3 = Severe	4 = Life-threatening/ most severe
Pulmonary					
Cough/dyspnea/fever	None	Minimal or transient symptoms	Moderate symptoms; no specific treatment required	Severe symptoms, responsive to treatment (oxygen, steroids)	Irreversible; severe disability
X-ray changes	None	Early or localized findings	Mild bilateral infiltration	Moderate bilateral infiltration	Complete bilateral infiltration; opacification
Functional problems (PF tests)	None	Pulmonary functions impaired but patient asymptomatic and/or 25–50% decrement in D_{co} or VC	Pulmonary symptoms requiring therapy but not assisted ventilation and/or >50% decrement in D_{co} or VC	Assisted ventilation needed	Shock lung
Cardiovascular					
Dyspnea/fluid accumulation/energy/pain	Normal	Asymptomatic	Transient symptomatic dysfunction requiring no therapy	Symptomatic dysfunction responsive to therapy	Dysfunction not responsive to therapy
Cardiac rhythm, inflammation or performance (cardiac output or pressures) or peripheral resistance	Normal	Abnormal sign or test	Transient symptomatic dysfunction requiring no therapy	Symptomatic dysfunction responsive to therapy	Dysfunction not responsive to therapy; cardiac arrest
Venous problems	None	Superficial phlebitis	Pelvic or deep vein thrombophlebitis	Pulmonary embolus	Pulmonary embolus requiring embolectomy or caval ligation
Arterial problems	None	Spasm	Ischemia not requiring surgical treatment	Vascular thrombosis requiring resection with anastomosis	Myocardial infarction; resection of organ (bowel, limb, etc)
Lymphatics	None	Mild lymphedema	Moderate lymphedema requiring compression	Severe lymphedema limiting function	Severe edema limiting function with ulceration

TABLE VII. Protocol Elements

1. Objectives
2. Background and rationale
3. Patient eligibility
4. Study modalities
5. Treatment plan and randomization procedure
6. Treatment modifications
7. Study parameters and serial observations
8. Evaluation criteria
9. Duration of study
10. Study monitoring and reporting procedures
11. Statistical considerations
12. Bibliography

Eligibility and Evaluability

It would seem self-evident that to conduct an appropriate analysis of a clinical trial it is necessary to be able to evaluate patients. The definition of an evaluable patient can substantially alter the results. Unfortunately, no unequivocal definitions regarding "eligibility" and "evaluability" have been provided (indeed the two are often used interchangeably). By "eligible" patients, I am referring to those patients who are in the target population for the study as outlined in the written protocol. Possible reasons for ineligibility include wrong stage of disease, wrong histologic type, prior chemotherapy or prior radiotherapy (if so specified in the study), elevated blood counts *prior* to entry, no measurable tumor, etc. By "evaluability," I am referring to the value of the patient data in answering the questions posed in the study. Once a patient has been deemed "eligible" for the study a determination regarding evaluability can then be made. Ideally, no exclusions should occur in a clinical trial. In practice, however, they will arise.

Of the two types of exclusions, it would seem that ineligible patients are of somewhat less concern, as such patients are not part of the intended population. On the other hand, inevaluable patients are eligible, but not evaluable; consequently, in a certain sense they represent lost or missing data. Reasons for inevaluability must be clearly defined before a study begins. Very few patients should be deemed inevaluable. Variation from chemotherapy dosage or timing is not a sufficient reason to declare a patient inevaluable, nor is an early death if any therapy has been administered. Protocol violations may be noted and considered in the analysis, but to eliminate these cases induces definite bias.

Phase II Studies

Phase II studies requiring a minimal number of courses for a patient to be considered evaluable will quite likely produce inflated response rates. As an example, consider the hypothetical tabulation in Table VIII of tumor response (as defined in Table V) by number of courses administered. If all patients who received therapy are considered evaluable, the observed complete response rate is 16.7%; if administration of two courses of therapy are required for evaluability, the observed complete response rate jumps to 21.7%. If one were so restrictive regarding evaluability as to require three courses of therapy, the observed "response rate" would become 31.3%.

Although treatment comparisons are not involved in phase II studies, a decision regarding further study will be based upon the results. Therefore, some standard criteria are required. It is recommended that in phase II studies anyone receiving at least one course of therapy be considered evaluable.

If a substantial number of protocol violations exist, this can be noted in the analysis. Moreover, these cases should be compared with the remaining cases with respect to prognostic factors to determine if any selection bias has occurred. If the removal of major violations alters the study appreciably, the results of the analysis would apply only to that portion of the redefined population, rather than to the original target population.

Phase III Studies

As has been stressed earlier, the phase III comparative trial seeks differences in treatment efficacy. The usual parameters primarily involved are objective tumor response, progression-free interval, and survival. Ultimately, a conclusion regarding the existence of a "significant difference" in treatment effect is made based upon the "P value." Clinical investigators tend to "worship at the altar of 0.05." That is, if the mysterious, all-important P value is less than 0.05, a "statistically significant treatment difference" is pronounced. Just what does the P value represent? Suppose regimen A is being compared to regimen B and the results indicate that regimen A has a higher response rate than regimen B with $P < 0.05$. This

TABLE VIII. Hypothetical Tabulation of Observed Tumor Response by Number of Courses Administered in a Phase II Study

	Number of courses administered					
Response category	1	2	3	4	≥5	Total
Complete response	0	0	2	1	2	5
Partial response	0	1	0	1	0	2
Stable disease	1	3	5	3	2	14
Increasing disease	6	3	0	0	0	9
Total	7	7	7	5	4	30

does not mean that the probability that the two regimens are equivalent is 0.05. Rather it means that *if* the two regimens are equivalent, then the probability of getting a difference in response rate at least of this magnitude is less than 0.5. It should be stressed that, although P values are commonly employed to earmark such treatment differences, the technique employed varies substantially.

In examining response rates and other similarly categorized variables, data are often presented in the format of contingency tables. Statistical methodology for analyzing contingency tables has been developed by Pearson [1900], Yates [1934], and Fisher [1935]. Such analyses are often inappropriately applied by those unfamiliar with this area. Cox [1970] cautions that the "most frequent inadequacy of an analysis by a single 2 × 2 contingency table is the presence of further factors influencing the response; . . . To ignore such further factors can be very misleading." Efron [1978] presented a method of multiple logistic regression to enable prognostic factors such as prior therapy, performance status, stage of disease, histology, etc. to be incorporated into the analysis. These techniques have become possible owing to the development of high-speed computers.

As described in the introduction, time variables are very different from binary variables; consequently, the method of analysis is entirely different. Actuarial life-table analysis is employed to compare the regimens for treatment differences. A life table is a graph or table used to provide an estimate of the proportion of a group of patients living (or disease-free or progression-free) at any point in time after entry on a study. This technique takes into account not only how many have died (or recurred or progressed), but also how long after entry they did so. Moreover, information relating to censored observations (those patients who have not failed prior to the times of analysis) can be incorporated into the analysis.

Various investigators have developed life-table methodology. Kruskal and Wallis [1952] and Cutler and Ederer [1958] have been instrumental in research involving the construction and presentation of the life table itself, and Kaplan and Meier [1958], Gehan [1965], and Breslow [1970] have developed test statistics used in the actual comparisons of treatment regimens. A mere comparison of survival (or response duration or progression-free interval) by treatment often constitutes an oversimplified analysis. As was the case with response, the influence of prognostic factors must be considered in analysis of time variables. Cox [1972] presented techniques combining regression models with life-table analysis, thereby providing methodology for the examination of the effects of prognostic factors on possible treatment differences. This methodology was alluded to in an earlier discussion regarding stratification. A very readable presentation on life-table analysis may be found in Peto et al. [1977].

One final note on life-table analysis is prudent. It is not too difficult to understand the construction of a life table and to find a computer package featuring one or more of the above tests. It is far more complicated to comprehend the statistical assumptions involved in selecting the appropriate technique to apply.

Timing of Analyses

It may be surprising, but when and how often to analyze the data is just as important as the choice of methodology. Early analysis of a clinical trial can provide very misleading results. It has been shown previously that a substantial number of patients is required to conduct most phase III trials. Clearly then, small differences seen early in a study cannot be very compelling evidence that a true difference exists. Indeed subsequent data could easily negate such a difference or enhance it.

The cases evaluable in the early portion of a trial are often by nature not typical of the entire population. For example, final results are apt to be available on treatment failures while responders are likely to still be on study. Thus, response may be underestimated. Similarly, survival curves will be based primarily on early deaths until a reasonable period of time has passed. The nature of chemotherapeutic agents employed will govern the type of adverse effects expected and their ability to be accurately reported in the early phases of study. A number of early failures could easily underreport toxicity if the patients received minimal therapy. Conversely, if a number of patients were removed from study owing to drug-related toxicity, while the remainder were still on study, the problem could be overemphasized. Patient safety must be a prime concern, so adverse effects must be monitored. However, this can be accomplished independent of data analysis.

In addition to possibly producing misleading results, early analysis can have other deleterious effects. Small differences, though not significant, can produce a bias toward or against particular regimens by clinical investigators. Such a prejudgment can lead to improper randomization of cases with subsequent withdrawal of patients or a lack of enthusiasm for the study, jeopardizing its chance of fulfilling its objective. An early analysis can also lead to a desire to terminate the study prematurely. Consequences of such an action may be severe. An actual therapeutic difference may go unproved because of accrual of an insufficient number of cases. Worse yet, unproven differences may be publicized.

Ideally the data should not be analyzed until all data are collected. In practice this is virtually impossible. Ethical considerations require that the data be examined periodically; individual investigators will obviously know the results of their therapy, and cooperative groups will desire interim analyses to design replacement studies. Early analyses, if necessary, must be clearly labeled as such, and conclusions should not be drawn on the basis of these analyses. One might wonder what harm is done by repeated interim analyses. Most investigators believe a treatment difference is significant if $P \leqslant 0.05$. If one repeatedly analyzes a trial for treatment differences and in reality the treatments do not differ, the chance that *on any one* of these analyses the results will be significant is 0.05. However, the chance that significance will be obtained on *at least one* of these analyses is greater than 0.05. Peto et al. [1976] mention that if such a comparison were conducted on five occasions, "the chance that you will publish a 'significant ($P < .05$) difference' in a trial comparing two treatments which are, in fact, identical is probably more like 15% than the 5% which was claimed." It would therefore seem reasonable to limit the frequency of interim analysis and to require a lower P value before proclaiming statistical significance. Requiring a P value of < 0.01 particularly to justify early termination of a study would be an effective safe.

Prior to final analysis, the data themselves should be examined. All reviews such as pathology and chemotherapy quality control should be completed and a final determination made regarding each patient's evaluability. The investigator and statistician should meet, review the predetermined objective of the study, and discuss the analysis necessary to address these objectives. Upon completion of the final analysis an interpretation of the results is undertaken.

INTERPRETATION OF RESULTS

How does one interpret the results of a clinical trial? How should other studies summarized in journals be interpreted? Hopefully some light will be shed on both questions in the following sections.

Phase II Studies

It has been repeatedly mentioned in earlier sections that phase II trials are not comparative in nature and offer no definitive answers other than the estimates of treatment efficacy they provide. Nowhere is this more important to recall than in interpreting the results. Phase II trials designed as described earlier in this chapter can provide reliable estimates of true efficacy. While subconscious comparisons with other agents are inevitable, they are also inconclusive. In both presenting results and interpreting journal publications, the clinician is well advised to remember the limitations of the scope of this type of study.

Phase III Studies

If a phase III clinical trial is conducted and a "significant" difference is not discerned, it is not uncommon for the trial to be classified as a negative study. How should such a study be interpreted? Recalling the terminology explained above, there is always the possibility that a false-negative error is being committed. Hopefully, the study was designed and conducted in such a fashion that an accurate measure of the probability, β, of committing this type of error is available and appropriate. As pointed out above, a frequent choice for β is 0.2. In such a case, once the results are known from the analysis there is a 1 in 5 chance that an undetected difference really existed. At this stage nothing can be done to alter the chance of committing such an error. However, in interpreting results one should be aware of the possibility of a false-negative error. (If fewer than the prescribed number of patients were entered the probability is even higher.)

Note that a negative study does not imply that a treatment difference does not exist. Rather, the implication is that a treatment difference of the magnitude initially considered desirable to detect does not exist. It may well be that a true therapeutic difference of a lesser magnitude exists but was undetectable owing to the original study objectives and required number of patients entered. For example, if a study had been designed to detect a 20% improvement in complete response rates from 20% to 40% with $\alpha = 0.05$ and $\beta = 0.02$ (one-sided), then 73 patients per regimen would have been required. Suppose that upon conducting the study and analyzing the data, the complete response rates were as shown in Table IX.

Assuming equal distribution of prognostic factors and the appropriateness of a straightforward treatment comparison of complete response rates, a significant difference is not found. This does not address the issue of whether or not a 10% difference in complete response rates exists, nor should it. To consider that difference would have required 249 patients per

TABLE IX. Hypothetical Tabulation of Response by Regimen

	Regimen		
Response category	A	B	Total
Complete response	15	23	38
Others[a]	60	52	112
Total	75	75	150

[a]Partial response, stable disease, and increasing disease.

regimen! Moreover, that decision should have been made in the design phase of the study. To let the results dictate the objectives is totally inappropriate. This example emphasizes the need for careful deliberation in the design phase of a clinical trial. In summary, a negative study does not proclaim treatment equivalence, but merely fails to confirm a therapeutic difference initially thought meaningful and possible to detect.

A phase III clinical trial that pronounces some statistically significant therapeutic difference is considered a positive study. In light of previous discussions a few points should be reiterated. The P value associated with the result is *not* the probability that the stated difference does not exist. It is the probability that *if* no such difference really existed, the experiment would produce results as different as observed. Secondly, "significant" results with associated P values between 0.03 and 0.05 should be considered marginal and taken with a grain of salt as repeated analyses have no doubt occurred. Lastly, one should avoid too great a dependence upon P values, as a possible consequence is the overemphasis on mathematical significance at the expense of medical importance.

In gynecologic studies there is sometimes a tendency to view survival as the only parameter of real importance. Improvements in response rates are minimized if overall survival is not appreciably improved. Again, one must be aware of the different nature of binary and time variables. Differences in response rates are likely to occur far earlier than differences in time variables, particularly survival. Differences in time variables are observable only after a substantial number of failures have occurred. Consequently, it is quite possible for a response difference to be seen and an accompanying significant difference in survival seen in a subsequent analysis after more follow-up data are available.

Caution must be used in interpreting graphs depicting treatment comparisons of time variables. Frequently investigators will be misled by the "tails" of survival or progression-free interval curves. It is not uncommon for curves displaying no significant treatment difference to be visibly distinct at 2 or 3 years. This does not represent a delayed treatment advantage; such fluctuations may be based on only a handful of patients and are subject to substantial change with the occurrence of as few as one new failure. Credence must be given to the early part of the curve, which is based on the majority of patients. Likewise, curves that do depict real treatment differences may cross in the tail. Here, the difference must not be discounted as such an event may also occur owing to one late-occurring failure. Figure 4 depicts the first situation. A comparison of progression-free interval for two

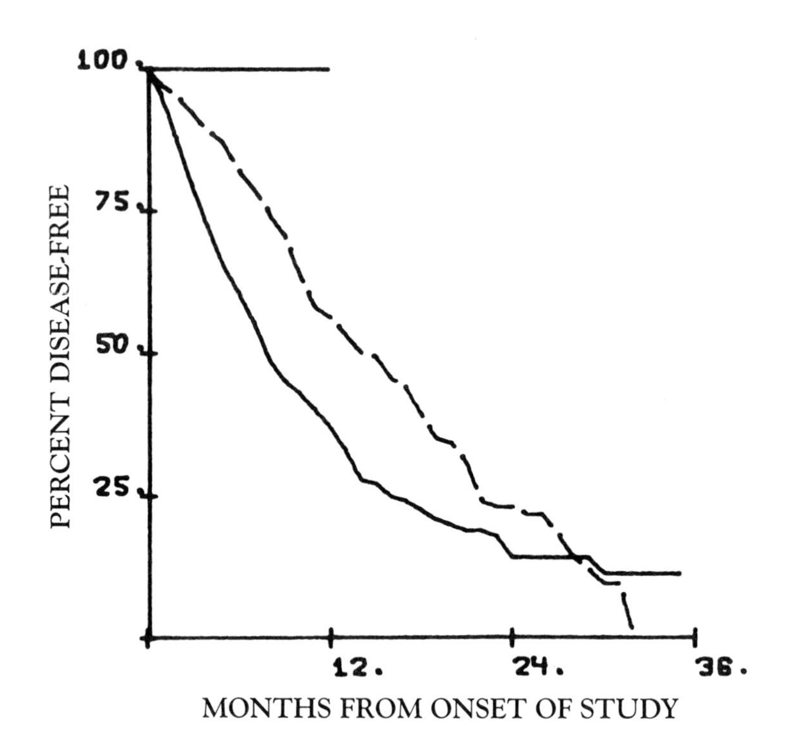

	Regimen	No. progression-free	No. failed	Total	Median
————————	I	84	119	203	8.1 months
— — — —	II	89	101	190	13.4 months

Fig. 4. Regimen II has highly significant ($P < 0.0001$) longer progression-free time interval than Regimen I.

groups of patients reveals that the two treatment arms are significantly different ($P < 0.0001$). Two late-occurring failures have caused the curves to cross. This is of no consequence; the overall life table is based upon 393 patients! Figure 5 displays a simulation of two regimens that are not significantly different. Median survival is 4.8 months for both curves and $P > 0.50$!

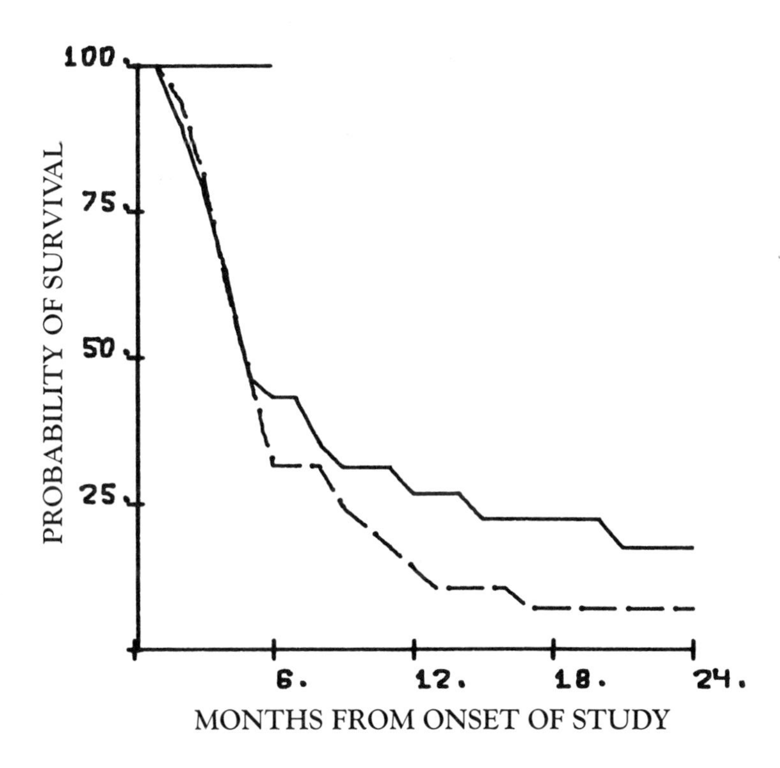

	Regimen	No. alive	No. dead	Total	Median
————————	I	9	22	31	4.8 months
— — — —	II	3	29	32	4.8 months

Fig. 5. There is no significant difference in survival between the two regimens ($P > 0.050$).

Collaboration in Interpretation

As in the other facets of clinical investigation, interpretation of the results should be a joint venture between the clinician and statistician. It would obviously be inappropriate for a statistician to attempt to analyze and interpret the data without detailed medical advice. However, the converse is equally true. The role of the statistician must not end with data analysis. As statistical methodology becomes more complex, expertise is required to verify that a correct interpretation is made. In this light, the area of clinical trials provides an excellent forum for the interchange between statistical and medical science in clinical investigation.

REFERENCES

Bonomi P, Bruckner H, Cohen C, Marshall R, Blessing J, Slayton R (1982): A randomized trial of three cisplatin regimens in squamous cell carcinoma of the cervix. Proc Am Soc Clin Oncol C425:110.

Breslow N (1970): A generalized Kruskal-Wallis test for comparing K samples subject to unequal patterns of censorship. Biometrika 57:579–594.

Bross IDJ (1974): The role of the statistician: Scientist or shoe clerk. Am Stat 28:126–127.

Brown BW (1980): The crossover experiment for clinical trials. Biometrics 36:69–70.

Byar DP (1980): Why data bases should not replace randomized clinical trials. Biometrics 36:337–342.

Casagrande JT, Pike MC, Smith PG (1978): The power function of the "exact" test for comparing two binomial distributions. Appl Stat 27:176–180.

Cochran WG, Cox GM (1957): "Experimental Designs," Ed 2. New York: John Wiley.

Cohen CJ, Bruckner HW, Deppe G, Blessing JA, Homesley H, Lee JH, Watring W (1983): A randomized study comparing multi-drug chemotherapeutic regimens in the treatment of advanced and recurrent endometrial carcinoma: A Gynecologic Oncology Group study. Am J Obstet Gynecol (in press).

Cox DR (1970): "The Analysis of Binary Data." London: Methuen & Co. Ltd; reprinted Chapman and Hall, Ltd. (1977).

Cox, DR (1972): Regression models and life tables (with discussion). J R Stat Soc B 34:187.

Cutler, SJ, Ederer F (1958): Maximum utilization of the life table method in analyzing survival. J Chron Dis 8:699–712.

Efron B (1978): Regression and ANOVA with zero-one data: Measure of residual variation. J Am Stat Assoc 73:113.

Fisher RA (1935): The logic of inductive inference. J R Stat Soc A 98:39–54.

Gehan EA (1961): The determination of the number of patients required in a preliminary and a follow-up trial of a new chemotherapeutic agent. J Chron Dis 13:346–353.

Gehan EA (1965): A generalized Wilcoxon test for comparing arbitrarily singly-censored samples. Biometrika 52:203–223.

Gehan EA, Freireich EJ (1974): Non-randomized controls in cancer clinical trials. N Engl J Med 290:198–203.

Gehan EA, Schneiderman MA (1982): Experimental design of clinical trials. In Holland JF, Frei E (eds): "Cancer Medicine," Ed 2. Philadelphia: Lea & Febiger, pp. 531–552.

George, SL, Desu MM (1974): Planning the size and duration of a clinical trial studying the time to some critical event. J Chron Dis 27:15–24.

Gordon RS (1978): Clinical trials. N Engl J Med 298:400–401.

Green SB (1982): Patient heterogeneity and the need for randomized clinical trials. Controlled Clin Trials 3:189–198.

Hammond D (1980): The training of clinical trials statisticians: A clinician's view. Biometrics 36:679–685.

Hannigan JF, Brown BW (1982): Adaptive randomization biased coin-design: Experience in a cooperative group clinical trial. Technical Report No. 74, Division of Biostatistics, Stanford University, Stanford, California.

Kaplan, EL, Meier P (1958): Nonparametric estimation from incomplete observations. J Am Stat Assoc 53:457.

Kruskal WH, Wallis WA (1952): Use of ranks in one-criterion variance analysis. J Am Stat Assoc 47:583–621.

Omura GA, Morrow CP, Blessing JA, Miller A, Buchsbaum HJ, Homesley HD, Leone L (1983): A randomized comparison of melphalan versus melphalan plus hexamethylmelamine versus adriamycin plus cyclophosphamide in ovarian carcinoma. Cancer 51:783–789.

Pearson K (1900): On the criterion that a given system of deviations from the probable in the case of a correlated system of variables is such that it can be reasonably supposed to have arisen from random sampling. Phil Mag Ser 5, 50:157.

Peto R, Pike MC, Armitage P, Breslow NE, Cox DR, Howard SV, Mantel N, McPherson K, Peto J, Smith PG (1976): Design and analysis of randomized clinical trials requiring prolonged observation of each patient. I. Introduction and design. Br J Cancer 34:585–612.

Peto R, Pike MC, Armitage P, Breslow NE, Cox DR, Howard SV, Mantel N, McPherson K, Peto J, Smith PG (1977): Design and analysis of randomized clinical trials requiring prolonged observation of each patient. II. Analysis and examples. Br J Cancer 35:1–27.

Schoenfeld, DA, Richter JR (1982): Nomograms for calculating the number of patients needed for a clinical trial with survival as an endpoint. Biometrics 38:163–170.

Simon R (1979): Restricted randomization designs in clinical trials. Biometrics 35:503–512.

Tannock I, Murphy K (1983): Reflections on medical oncology: An appeal for better clinical trials and improved reporting of their results. J Clin Oncol 1:66–70.

Thigpen T, Shingleton H, Homesley H, Lagasse L, Blessing JA (1979): Dis-dichlorodiammineplatinum (II) in the treatment of gynecologic malignancies: Phase II trials by the Gynecologic Oncology Group. Cancer Treat Rep 63:1549–1555.

Yates F (1934): Contingency tables involving small numbers and the chi-square test. J R Stat Soc Suppl 1:217–235.

Zelen M (1983): Guidelines for publishing papers on cancer clinical trials: Responsibilities of editors and authors. J Clin Oncol 1:164–169.

Chemotherapy of Vulvar and Vaginal Neoplasms

Edgardo L. Yordan, Jr., Philip D. Bonomi, and George D. Wilbanks

Section of Gynecologic Oncology (E.L.Y., G.D.W.) and Section of Medical Oncology (P.D.B.), Rush-Presbyterian-St. Luke's Medical Center, Chicago, Illinois 60612

Carcinoma of the vulva accounts for 3–5% of gynecologic malignancies, in most series, and its incidence may be on the rise. Carcinoma of the vagina is less frequently seen; a relative frequency figure of 2% of all female genital malignancies is accepted but likely represents a ceiling figure. Treatment of these tumors has traditionally revolved around diverse modalities of surgery and radiation therapy, depending on multiple aspects of tumor extension and location. The therapeutic role of chemotherapy in the management of either disease has remained almost exclusively a palliative concern. Chemotherapeutic experience, in general, has been limited in numbers and exposition and has been vague in definition. Of course, use of topical chemotherapy in the management of the premalignant or intraepithelial phases of both vulvar and vaginal neoplasia has attained a reasonably well-defined status over the past decade and has become an accepted modality of treatment. Not so with the invasive forms of disease. We may well be seeing, however, emerging trends in multimodal therapy that may eventuate in a strong role for chemotherapy in the primary management of vulvar and vaginal neoplasms.

CARCINOMA OF THE VULVA

The relative distribution of vulvar neoplasms by histologic type is as follows: squamous 86.2%, melanoma 4.8%, undifferentiated 3.9%, sarcoma 2.2%, basal cell 1.4%, adenocarcinoma 0.6%, bartholin gland 0.6%, bartholin duct (squamous) 0.4% [Plentl and Friedman, 1971]. The disease affects women during the postmenopausal years, but approximately 15% of

Chemotherapy of Gynecologic Cancer, pages 85–101

tumors will occur under the age of 40. As in the case of cervical neoplasia, it appears that invasive carcinoma may be preceded by a dysplastic form of disease that is referred to as a vulvar intraepithelial neoplasm (VIN); unlike cervical neoplasia, the process can be multifocal. Certainly the steps of progression from preinvasive disease to invasive carcinoma are less well defined for VIN than for CIN. Lesions can be found on any part of the vulva or perineum, but lesions on the labium majus and/or labium minus account for 70% of occurrence sites. Lesions are less frequently located on clitoris or perineum. The disease usually attracts attention to itself by symptoms of a lump or mass, pruritus, pain, bleeding, or dysuria.

Tumor growth tends to be indolent, and regional spread seems to be preceded by a mechanism of tumor microembolization to the inguinofemoral lymph nodes. Although spread to the pelvic lymph nodes or the aortolumbar lymph nodes may on occasion bypass the groin nodes, presumably by direct propagation through the clitoral or anal lymphatic routes, as a practical matter this is seldom seen in the clinical setting.

Stage grouping of vulvar carcinoma, as adopted by FIGO, involves the TNM system in which disease is defined by the status of tumor, lymph nodes, and metastatic presence (Table I). Prognosis correlates with size of lesion, histologic grade, and particularly with lymph node metastases. Inguinal nodes are pathologically involved in approximately one-third of the cases; pelvic nodes are involved in approximately 10% of the cases. The corrected 5-year survival for patients with squamous cell carcinoma of the vulva is 89.7% for stage I, 79.6% for stage II, 47.9% for stage III, and 15.2% for stage IV. The overall salvage for all stages is 66.3% [Morrow and Townsend, 1981].

Vulvar Intraepithelial Neoplasia (VIN)

The importance of VIN as a concept is underlined by the cancer prevention opportunities it presents and by the increasing incidence of the disease in premenopausal women. Observation of VIN over time carries an indeterminate risk of progression to invasive disease. Lesions are often keratinized and/or pigmented, facilitating gross clinical assessment. Furthermore, even subclinical lesions can be accentuated with dilute acetic acid for ease of colposcopic evaluation; characteristically, the lesions can be keratinized, irregularly surfaced, and with sharp borders and occasional punctation. Supravital nuclear staining with the use of toluidine blue is yet another diagnostic aid. But physical appearance can be highly variable and inconsistent, colposcopy tedious to the physician and uncomfortable to the patient, and toluidine blue notoriously unreliable. Difficulty tends to be

TABLE I. FIGO and TNM Classification for Clinical Stage Grouping of Vulvar Carcinoma

FIGO nomenclature	
Stage 0	Carcinoma in situ.
Stage I	Tumor confined to vulva, 2 cm or less in diameter. Nodes not clinically suspicious (not enlarged and mobile).
Stage II	Tumor confined to vulva, 2 cm in diameter. Nodes not clinically suspicious (not enlarged and mobile).
Stage III	Tumor of any size with 1) adjacent spread to urethra and/or vagina and/or perineum and/or anus; 2) nodes not fixed but clinically suspicious (enlarged, firm); 3) both.
Stage IV	Tumor of any size 1) infiltrating bladder and/or rectal mucosa, including upper urethral mucosa; 2) fixed to bone or other distant metastases; 3) both. Fixed or ulcerated nodes.
TNM nomenclature	
Primary tumor (T)	
Tis, T1, T2, T3, T4—see corresponding FIGO stages	
Nodal involvement (N)	
NX	Minimum requirements to assess regional nodes cannot be met.
NO	No involvement of regional nodes.
N1	Evidence of regional node involvement.
N3	Fixed or ulcerated nodes.
N4	Juxtaregional node involvement.
Distant metastasis (M)	
MX	Minimum requirements to assess presence of distant metastasis cannot be met.
MO	No (known) distant metastasis.
M1	Distant metastasis present; specify site.

compounded by the multifocal nature of the disease, especially in younger women. The technique, of course, is totally dependent on the acquired skills of an individual, since accurate evaluation relies on the physician's ability to colposcopically detect areas of potentially invasive disease. Liberal use of vulvar biopsies is advocated for diagnostic definition of disease and suitable follow-up.

Local excision of the lesion(s) or partial vulvectomy are considered the standard of treatment for VIN. When the lesions are confluent, or particularly widespread, or involving the perineum and/or perianal regions, a "skinning vulvectomy" with split-thickness skin grafting is indicated [Rutledge and Sinclair, 1968]. Cryotherapy is a more conservative alternative but is relatively inapplicable to cases with widespread disease and more applicable to selected cases with limited distribution of disease, since hyperkeratinization in VIN can often render the technique cumbersome and ineffective. Use of carbon dioxide laser is more versatile and less cumbersome for the widespread or multifocal lesions, and the discomfort to the patient is usually minimal. With both of these modalities, however, one forgoes the safety margin of pathologic backup to rule out potential and unsuspected invasive disease. Certainly the metachronously multifocal nature of the disease process can lead to a chronicity of recurrence; on the other hand, even the more comprehensive and definitive surgical modalities fail to provide absolute prophylaxis against recurrence.

A number of reports in the 1960s and 1970s, mostly from the dermatology and otolaryngology literature, introduced gynecologists to the possibilities of topical chemotherapy for treatment of intraepithelial neoplasia of the genital tract. There were obvious advantages seen in a modality that would be anatomically conservative while at the same time universally therapeutic by self-selecting and obliterating all dysplastic lesions in the area of topical application. These techniques have been widely adapted to the treatment of vulvar and vaginal intraepithelial neoplasia (VIN and VAIN) and multiple clinical trials have taken place. The most popular agent has been a cream with a 5% concentration of 5-fluorouracil in an aquafor base (Efudex), and there are several studies in the literature reporting on clinical experience. It is recommended that the cream be topically applied once or twice daily after cleansing the areas with nonmedicated soap. Duration of treatment has ranged between courses of 14 days and 50 days. One to four courses of treatment have been required to eradicate intraepithelial disease with intervals between courses ranging between 2 and 14 weeks and averaging 4–6 weeks. Carson et al. [1976] claim an element of selectivity in the incorporation of 5-fluorouracil into the metabolic pathways of VIN, such that areas of abnormal skin that may appear normal will undergo the same characteristic slough of the more obvious dysplastic lesions. Given the known multifocal nature of VIN, this selectivity may afford a further margin of reliability toward eradication of disease and, as such, may be a silent argument in favor of topical application to the overall vulvar perineal areas without undertaking any protective or occlusive measures for the benefit of "normal" skin. Other authors, on the other hand, do advocate occlusive bandages or use of barrier creams, such as zinc oxide, to protect nondiseased areas of perineum and upper thighs. Krupp and Bohm [1978] and Carson et al. [1976] describe a mild inflammatory reaction which is evident on the skin approximately 7–14 days into treatment, followed by eczematoid changes and histologic evidence of early skin erosion. Finally, there is escharification and slough of the diseased skin, usually 3–4 weeks into treatment, followed by subsequent healing. The process of skin healing appears to reach completion within 4–6 weeks following treatment.

Remission of VIN has been variously reported between 0% and 100% (Table II). Woodruff et al. [1975] report eight remissions in 13 patients,

TABLE II. 5-Fluorouracil Treatment of Vulvar Carcinoma In Situ

Reference	No. patients	Remission	
		No.	%
Woodruff et al., 1973	13	8	62
Carson et al., 1976	1	1	100
Krupp and Bohm, 1978	8	6	75
Forney et al., 1977	6	0	0
Lifshitz and Roberts, 1980	12	2	17
Caglar et al., 1981	3	0	0
Total	43	17	40

Carson et al. [1976] report one remission in one patient, Krupp and Bohm [1978] report six remissions in eight patients, Forney et al. [1977] report no remissions in six patients, Lifschitz and Roberts [1980] report two remissions in 12 patients, and Caglar et al. [1981] report no remissions in three patients. One arrives at an average remission rate of 40%; however, since in some of these studies clinical remission is imprecisely defined, one worries about the reliability of statements on remission of disease. Undoubtedly, the remission rate from topical 5-fluorouracil therapy for VIN is significant, but the medication is irritating in the extreme, and this tends to affect patient compliance. The often unimpressive results of therapy must be weighed together with the extreme discomfort caused by the intense inflammatory reaction to the vulvar and perineal skin, especially considering that there are other therapeutic alternatives which appear to be more effective and certainly less symptomatically objectionable to the patient. In summary, topical 5-fluorouracil cannot be considered a treatment of choice for VIN, although in select individuals it may have a therapeutic role to play.

More recently, there have been two reports on the use of topical bleomycin for VIN and recurrent vulvar Paget's disease. Roberts et al. [1980] report on seven patients treated with 5% bleomycin in an aquafor base, used twice daily for 21 days and averaging three courses of treatment. While all patients developed a symptomatic chemical vulvitis, there were no disease remissions. The authors concluded that the keratinization in the lesions was effectively preventing the drug from reaching the diseased layers of skin; therefore, intradermal injections of 1% bleomycin were then applied to the next ten patients in the series, in an attempt to bypass the keratinized layer of skin. They observed remissions in two of the ten patients, and no significant systemic toxicity was observed. Again, the results do not appear to justify the choice of this particular modality for the management of VIN.

Invasive Carcinoma of the Vulva

In the 1940s, Taussig and Way established the radical vulvectomy and bilateral inguinofemoral lymphadenectomy as the standard of primary treatment for carcinoma of the vulva. Radical surgery dramatically improved the overall survival, as compared to the less than radical forms of surgical therapy of the preceding era. In recent years, there has been a tendency to question the absolute necessity of radical surgery for all cases, and efforts have been directed at precisely defining those subsets of patients for whom more individualized and conservative methods might be appropriate without compromising survival results. In contradistinction, there are other subsets of patients, on the other end of the disease spectrum, in whom surgery alone, however radical, is insufficient to ensure long-term survival. The specter of recurrent disease in these advanced or anatomically defiant cases certainly begs for innovative approaches to the disease, and one suspects that therapeutic refinements in combination chemotherapy, as well as refinements in multimodal therapeutic approaches, will gradually pave the way to improved survival for the advanced stages of the disease.

Experience with chemotherapy in the management of vulvar carcinoma has been extremely limited, probably for three principal reasons. First, the activity of chemotherapeutic agents against squamous carcinoma has been and remains disappointing. Second, because the disease is relatively rare and the surgical cure rate is relatively high, the use of chemotherapy is seldom indicated as primary therapy. The general paucity of study cases is of a magnitude sufficient to challenge the resources of even the national study groups. This scarcity of clinical material is reflected in a medical literature replete with case reports and very small study series; of course, there is a conspicuous absence of controlled comparative studies, even within the national study groups. Third, chemotherapeutic efforts have been traditionally biased against patients with compromised performance status; although we may be starting to see vulvar carcinoma at relatively younger ages, it remains a disease of elderly women.

A literature review was undertaken by Deppe et al. [1979], summarizing chemotherapeutic experience in metastatic and/or recurrent squamous carcinoma of the vulva. An update of the experience in the literature for single-agent chemotherapy is depicted in Table III. This is a compendium of many small series; staging, performance status, drug dosage schedules, drug administration detail, definition of chemotherapeutic response, progression-free

TABLE III. Single Agent Chemotherapy in Vulvar Squamous Carcinoma

Agent	No. patients	Response No.	Response %	Reference
Adriamycin	6	4	67	Barlow et al., 1973; Deppe et al., 1977
Bleomycin	46	27	59	Barlow et al., 1973; Blum et al., 1973; Bull et al., 1972; Edsmyr, 1972; Encalada et al., 1973; Ichikawa, 1970; Schneider and Gebhartz, 1973; Sirisabya, 1974; Srivannaboon et al., 1973; Tojo et al., 1972; Trope et al., 1980; Yahia et al., 1978
Cyclophosphamide	2	0	0	Frick et al., 1965; Malkasian et al., 1968a
Cytembena	26	4	15	Dvorak, 1971
5-Fluorouracil	2	0	0	Masterson and Nelson, 1965
6-Mercaptopurine	1	0	0	Masterson and Nelson, 1965
Methotrexate	5	2	40	Chamoun et al., 1974; Gorgun et al., 1967; Haffner and Frick, 1970; Masterson and Nelson, 1965
Mitomycin C	1	0	0	Masterson and Nelson, 1965
Porfiromycin	1	0	0	Loo et al., 1967
Total	90	37	41	

interval, survival, and drug toxicity were not always defined with precision in these reports. Furthermore, the table seeks, however appropriately, to derive an estimate of drug activity by presenting regression of disease in aggregate. Chemotherapeutic agents reported include adriamycin, bleomycin, CCNU, methyl-CCNU, cyclophosphamide, cytembena, 5-fluorouracil, 6-mercaptopurine, methotrexate, mitomycin C, and porfiromycin.

The range of response seems very broad, but bleomycin, adriamycin, and methotrexate appear the three most active drugs. Among single-agent treatment reports, bleomycin appears to be the most extensively used drug, as well as the most effective; there have been 27 of 46 (59%) responses to the drug in aggregate. Responses were also demonstrated in two-thirds of the patients treated with adriamycin and in two-fifths of the patients treated with methotrexate, although the numbers were small. It is perhaps appropriate to state that the reporting of response rates in aggregate, considering that these are relatively rare clinical situations, may result in falsely optimistic representation, because of the tendency to report successful chemotherapeutic enterprise but to underreport the unsuccessful attempts. Furthermore, duration of response has been in general short-lived, although there have been some prolonged responses, particularly to adriamycin and bleomycin.

There have also been a number of reports on treatment with combination chemotherapy, but in this area the reported experience has been exceedingly limited. Deppe et al. [1979] summarized seven reports; the experience with combination chemotherapy is updated in Table IV. This is for the most part a compendium of case reports and, by and large, an expression of therapeutic disappointment. Perhaps the one exception is a recent small series by Trope et al. [1980], wherein five responses are reported out of nine patients treated with a combination of bleomycin and mitomycin C. There were four partial responses and one complete response, but the maximum follow-up was only 7 months. They reported, in addition, objective responses in five of 11 patients treated with single-agent bleomycin; there were three short-lived partial responses and two complete responses reported at 4 and 24 months respectively. While other reports of response are essentially anecdotal, it does appear that inclusion of bleomycin in the drug combination may be a common theme among the successful attempts. More recently, Kalra et al. [1981] reported dramatic shrinkage of a vulvar lesion following treatment with a combination of mitomycin C, 15 mg/M^2 day 1 and 5-FU, 750 mg/M^2 day 1–5 by continuous IV infusion, but regression was only observed following subsequent external irradiation to a total of 3,000 rads over 3 weeks. One patient was recently treated at our institution for squamous carcinoma of the vulva recurrent to the groin following radical excision, bilateral groin lymphadenectomy, and postoperative pelvic irradia-

TABLE IV. Combination Chemotherapy in Vulvar Squamous Carcinoma

Agents	No. patients	Response	Reference
Bleomycin, methotrexate	1	1	Mosher et al., 1972
Adriamycin, cis-platinum	1	0	Vogl et al., 1976
Methotrexate, hydroxyurea, vincristine	2	0	Morrow et al., 1973
6-Mercaptopurine, thiotepa, D-phenylalanine mustard	2	0	Frick et al., 1965
Cyclophosphamide, 5-fluorouracil, actinomycin D, cyotosine arabinoside, methotrexate, bleomycin, vincristine	1	1	Forney et al., 1975
Mitomycin C, bleomycin	9	5	Trope et al., 1980
Mitomycin C, 5-fluorouracil	1	1	Kalra et al., 1981
Cis-platinum, 5-fluorouracil	1	1	Yordan, unpublished data
Total	18	9	

tion because of two positive inguinal lymph nodes. She received 50 mg/M^2 cis-platinum day 1, followed by 500 mg/M^2 5-fluorouracil day 1–5 by continuous IV infusion. She received three monthly courses and experienced a partial response, but disease progressed promptly after her third course.

In recent years, the literature on squamous carcinomas of the oropharyngeal tract has shown a growing enthusiasm for the use of chemotherapy combinations that include cis-platinum. This has promoted in some centers an interest in platinum-containing combinations for the treatment of advanced or recurrent vulvar (and vaginal) carcinomas. The role of cis-platinum alone, however, is as yet undefined. The Gynecologic Oncology Group has been investigating the use of cis-platinum alone in advanced or recurrent gynecologic malignancies as part of a phase II drug study program. An overall response rate of 38% was observed in 34 patients with carcinoma of the cervix. For vulvar carcinoma, 17 cases have been treated with cis-platinum, and three cases have been treated with VP-16 to date; the response and survival data for cis-platinum should soon be available. It is possible that cis-platinum will play a significant role in vulvar carcinoma. The combination cis-platinum and 5-fluorouracil, as induction chemotherapy, appears promising at this time.

Vulvar sarcoma is a rare entity, indeed. DiSaia et al. [1971] report on twelve such cases. The use of vincristine, actinomycin D, and cyclophosphamide (VAC) was found to have minimal local effect among six patients treated; on the other hand, pulmonary metastases on two other patients showed significant regression. Vulvar melanoma is a similarly rare disease. No reports were identified showing significant chemotherapeutic activity for recurrent melanoma. As more active drugs are identified, it is possible that a role for adjunctive chemotherapy, or chemotherapy as part of a multimodal approach, may evolve in the treatment of these highly virulent diseases, but definition of such a role is likely to require the joint efforts of a cooperative study group, because of the relative rarity of these diseases.

Unfortunately, the data available on the chemotherapy of vulvar malignancies are quite limited. With increased sophistication in surgical rehabilitation of these patients, in multimodal approaches to treatment, in administration of single-agent and combination chemotherapy, and in the medical management of intercurrent diseases in this elderly group of patients, a more aggressive role for the chemotherapy of vulvar carcinoma may be in the process of emergence, as we seek to establish what is feasible, appropriate, safe, and most importantly, worthwhile.

CARCINOMA OF THE VAGINA

The relative distribution of vaginal neoplasms by histologic type is as follows: squamous 93.5%, adenocarcinoma 4.2%, sarcomas 1.6%, and other rare types (DES-related adenocarcinomas, botryoid tumors, melanomas, endodermal sinus tumors, etc.) making up the remaining 0.6% [Plentl and Friedman, 1971]. The disease characteristically develops in the postmenopausal years, and there is a well-known association with prior carcinoma of the cervix. Indeed, vaginal carcinomas have much in common, epidemiologically as well as pathogenetically, with cervical carcinomas. Evaluation of vaginal neoplasms, as a practical matter, often requires exercise of critical clinical judgment in the distinction between primary neoplastic disease and metastatic disease; vaginal metastases usually arise from tumors of uterine cervix or corpus.

The vagina is a thin-walled structure with an anastomosing lymphatic network that drains the entire length of the vaginal tube. In general, the upper two-thirds of the vagina drain directly into the pelvic lymph nodes, and the lower one-third drains into the inguinal lymph nodes; however, the pattern of drainage is complex. Primary squamous carcinomas arise in the mucosa and invasion is thought to be preceded by vaginal intraepithelial neoplasia (VAIN), in a manner similar to that for cervical and vulvar neoplasia; unlike CIN, VAIN is often a multifocal process.

Prognosis correlates with the stage of disease, the size of the lesion, and the site of the lesion. The most common tumor location is the upper third of the vagina, particularly the posterior wall, with the anterior lower third of the vagina being the second most common site. A significant number of these patients have had prior hysterectomy and/or pelvic irradiation. These circumstances of clinical history bear on treatment planning, whether surgical or radiotherapeutic; furthermore, they bear on prognosis, since they may impose some sobering limitations on the therapeutic alternatives available to the patient. In vaginal malignancies, the FIGO stage grouping is most widely accepted, and the TNM nomenclature is modeled after the FIGO system (Table V). By convention, when cervix, vulva, and urethra are involved, these tumors are designated cervical, vulvar, and urethral malignancies respectively. The corrected 5-year survival for patients with vaginal carcinoma is 90% for stage I, 56% for stage II, 36% for stage III, and 3% for stage IV [Morrow and Townsend, 1981].

Vaginal Intraepithelial Neoplasia (VAIN)

A significant number of women with VAIN have had CIN in the past. Often the presence of dysplasia is heralded by abnormal cytology. Evalua-

TABLE V. FIGO and TNM Classification for Clinical Stage Grouping of Vaginal Carcinoma

FIGO nomenclature	
Stage 0	Intraepithelial carcinoma, carcinoma in situ.
Stage I	Carcinoma limited to vaginal wall.
Stage II	Carcinoma has involved the subvaginal tissues but has not extended to pelvic wall.
Stage III	Carcinoma has extended to pelvic wall.
Stage IV	Carcinoma has extended beyond true pelvis or has involved bladder or rectal mucosa. Bullous edema, as such, does not permit allotment to Stage IV.
	Stage IVa—Spread of growth to adjacent organs.
	Stage IVb—Spread to distant organs.
TNM nomenclature	
Primary tumor (T)	
Tis, T1, T2, T3, T4—see corresponding FIGO stages	
Nodal involvement (N)	
NX	Minimum requirements to assess regional nodes cannot be met.
NO	No involvement of regional nodes.
N1	Evidence of regional node involvement.
Distant metastasis (M)	
MX	Minimum requirements to assess presence of distant metastasis cannot be met.
MO	No (known) distant metastasis.
M1	Distant metastasis present; specify site.

tion is best accomplished by colposcopy and colposcopically directed biopsies, although vaginal colposcopy requires considerable skill and experience. These lesions have a well-defined and characteristic appearance that is facilitated by the application of dilute acetic acid and/or Lugol's solution. The majority of lesions are visualized in the upper third of the vagina and are often multifocal.

Partial colpectomy has been the traditional approach to treatment, sometimes at the expense of markedly shortening the vagina, but the multifocal nature of the disease will often render the surgical approach insufficient. Similarly, radiation therapy is effective but can result in vaginal dysfunction. Carbon dioxide laser therapy is a highly versatile modality, particularly for lesions that are limited in size or multifocal, but one that by necessity relies on technical skills that can be difficult to attain and retain. Not infrequently, the patient has a history of previous irradiation for cervical carcinoma. Not only is diagnostic evaluation of VAIN rendered considerably more difficult, but any surgical approach, even a simple biopsy, must be weighed against the risk of precipitating a fistula.

The ideal treatment should minimize morbidity and dysfunction while addressing the multifocal nature of the disease. Use of 5% 5-fluorouracil

(Efudex) has been supported by a number of reports in the literature claiming effectiveness (Table VI). The medication is applied intravaginally by applicator, on a tampon, or with a gloved finger; application twice daily for 5–14 days has been described, allowing a suitable time period for healing, and patients have required 1–3 courses to achieve remission. While the medication causes widespread sloughing of diseased mucosa, the general inflammatory effect is far better tolerated when Efudex is used for VAIN than when used for VIN. Indeed, with intravaginal use, most of the symptoms arise from the drug's effect on vulvar epithelium and can be minimized by measures preventing external spillage of drug. In an attempt to protect vulvar skin as much as possible, bedtime application and the use of a barrier ointment, such as zinc oxide, on the vulvar epithelium are recommended. There does not appear to be detectable systemic toxicity or significant compromise of vaginal function resulting from the use of topical 5-fluorouracil in VAIN.

This topical agent appears at least 80% effective in eradicating VAIN and has become the preferred treatment for this condition, when there has been prior radiation, reserving surgery and carbon dioxide laser treatment for cases where Efudex has failed or where the dysplastic lesion has recurred despite an earlier remission (Table VI). Woodruff et al. [1975] caution that the hyperkeratotic lesions may be more resistant to eradication by Efudex. While the use of topical 5FU cannot be enthusiastically recommended for the treatment of VIN, the same agent appears satisfactorily effective and minimally morbid when used for VAIN. Furthermore, since routine Pap smears of the vagina are more reliable than vulvar smears in screening for the presence of dysplasia, remission of VAIN following the use of topical 5-fluorouracil can be defined with greater confidence than remission in VIN.

Invasive Carcinoma of the Vagina

The preferred modalities for management of vaginal carcinoma, depending on extent of disease, are radiation therapy and surgery. Often the

TABLE VI. 5-Fluorouracil Treatment of Vaginal Carcinoma In Situ

		Remission		
Reference	No. patients	No.	%	Recurrence
Woodruff et al., 1975	9	8	88	
Ballon et al., 1979	12	12	100	3
Daly and Ellis, 1980	17	17	100	0
Petrilli et al., 1980	15	12	80	
Caglar et al., 1981	27	27	100	3
Total	80	76	95	6 (9%)

performance scale will dictate choice of irradiation over surgery as treatment for this generally elderly group of patients; certainly, irradiation has traditionally been the treatment of choice, although there are data to suggest that, when medically feasible, surgery may be at least as effective for the early lesions [Herbst et al., 1972]. Of course, patients with early lesions constitute precisely that clinical subset where anatomic considerations similarly favor treatment by a combination of external irradiation and intracavitary brachytherapy. Considering the anatomic handicap of radiation therapy in the clinical situation of carcinoma in the upper vagina and a surgically absent uterus, recent applications of brachytherapy by interstitial template seem promising. Furthermore, those cases that are anatomically inappropriate for radiation therapy may well benefit from a multimodal approach, combining chemotherapy with radiation therapy.

The effectiveness of chemotherapy in vaginal carcinoma is poorly documented in the literature, but the general experience has been disappointing. Malkasian et al. [1968] reported two responses out of five patients treated with 5-fluorouracil 15 mg/kg/day, day 1–5, repeated monthly; however, responses were very brief. Piver et al. [1980] reported on two patients with vaginal carcinoma, among a group of 34 patients with carcinoma of the cervix, all of whom received cyclophosphamide, adriamycin, and 5-fluorouracil; the overall response rate was very low and the complications rate high. Piver's group [1978] also reported on seven patients with vaginal carcinoma receiving diverse adriamycin-containing combinations; there were two responses, one complete response to adriamycin 90 mg/M^2 and one partial response to cyclophosphamide 200 mg/M^2 day 1–5, adriamycin 60 mg/M^2 day 1, and 5-fluorouracil 200 mg/M^2 day 1–5. The former patient recurred after adriamycin was stopped at 550 mg/m^2. Omura et al. [1978] reported on three patients with vaginal carcinoma receiving methyl-CCNU and four patients receiving CCNU. There were no objective responses.

Emerging anecdotal evidence seems to favor use of cis-platinum or platinum-containing combinations, but there are no literature reports as yet. Twenty-three patients with vaginal carcinoma have been treated with cis-platinum alone in a GOG phase II study, and three have been treated with VP-16 alone. A response rate to cis-platinum will be determined in the near future. At our institution the current approach for advanced vaginal carcinoma is to precede brachytherapy by a combined approach using hyperfractionated external irradiation as well as chemotherapy, on alternating weeks, with cis-platinum 50 mg/M^2 day 1 and 5-fluorouracil 500 mg/M^2 day 1–5 by continuous IV infusion.

In studying 37 cases of recurrent DES-related clear cell adenocarcinomas of the cervix and vagina, Robboy et al. [1974] concluded that, in isolated instances, 5-fluorouracil and *Vinca* alkaloids were somewhat effective, although responses were brief; however, specific data were not isolated for the vaginal carcinoma group in particular. Fowler et al. [1979] reported on a patient receiving melphalan for clear cell adenocarcinoma of the vagina recurrent to lung and having no evidence of pelvic recurrence. Response was complete but the patient succumbed 2 years later to brain metastases. The suggestion is made that perhaps chemotherapy may be of adjunctive value as part of the primary treatment to the aggressive variants of disease.

Vaginal sarcomas are most commonly seen in the form of embryonal rhabdomyosarcoma in children, the so-called sarcoma botryoides. The traditional therapeutic approach has been that of exenterative surgery on these young patients; for years it provided the only hope of cure. Several reports in the early 1970s supported a combined modality approach using radical surgery, radiation therapy, and chemotherapy. In view of the marked success of multimodal therapy, more recent studies have questioned the need for routine radical surgery and instead have promoted the use of radical surgery selectively, only in those circumstances where chemotherapy and radiation therapy have failed to control disease. Dritschilo et al. [1978] found that radiation therapy in combination with nonradical surgery provided comparable local control of disease as well as comparable survival. There are, of course, long-term complications of irradiation to consider in children, and several groups are currently focusing their multimodal approach at minimizing, based on pretreatment with chemotherapy, the morbidity inherent in radical surgery and irradiation, while sustaining optimal survival figures. Specifically, the current approach of the Intergroup Rhabdomyosarcoma Study Protocol is predicated on initial chemotherapy with vincristine, actinomycin D, and cyclophosphamide, followed sequentially by radiation and then by surgery if disease remains uncontrolled. Initial data suggest that approximately one-half require low-dose irradiation and one-fourth require surgery. Survival statistics support the treatment rationale. It is possible that a trend toward multimodal therapy may similarly emerge in the treatment of the less rare variants of vaginal malignancy, such as the squamous carcinomas, simply because of the growing recognition that the traditional modalities of surgery and radiation therapy are so often handicapped by the extent of distribution of tumor or by previous cancer treatment.

REFERENCES

Ballon SC, Roberts JA, Lagasse LD (1979): Topical 5-fluorouracil in the treatment of intraepithelial neoplasia of the vagina. Obstet Gynecol 54:163.

Barlow JJ, Piver MS, Chuang JT, Cortes EP, Ohnuma T, Holland JF (1973): Adriamycin and bleomycin, alone and in combination, in gynecologic cancers. Cancer 32:735.

Blum RH, Carter SK, Agre K (1973): A clinical review of bleomycin—A new antineoplastic agent. Cancer 31:903.

Boronow RC (1973): Therapeutic alternative to primary exenteration for advanced vulvovaginal cancers. Gynecol Oncol 1:233.

Bull CA, Biggs JC, Newton NC, DeWilde FW, Chew KM (1972): Bleomycin in squamous cell carcinoma. Med J Aust 2:702.

Caglar H, Hertzog RW, Hreshchyshyn MM (1981): Treatment of vaginal intraepithelial neoplasia. Obstet Gynecol 58:580.

Carson TE, Hoskins WJ, Wurzel JF (1976): Topical 5-fluorouracil treatment of carcinoma in situ of the vulva. Obstet Gynecol 47:59(s).

Chamoun CD, Downing V, Huseby RA (1974): Vulvar carcinoma treated successfully. Rocky Mt Med J 71:89.

Daly JW, Ellis GF (1980): Treatment of vaginal dysplasia and carcinoma-in-situ with topical 5-fluorouracil. Obstet Gynecol 55:350.

Deppe G, Bruckner HW, Cohen CJ (1977): Adriamycin treatment of advanced vulvar carcinoma. Obstet Gynecol 50:13(s).

Deppe G, Cohen CJ, Bruckner HW (1979): Chemotherapy of squamous cell carcinoma of the vulva: A review. Gynecol Oncol 7:345.

DiSaia PJ, Rutledge F, Smith JP (1971): Sarcoma of the vulva: A report of 12 patients. Obstet Gynecol 38:180.

Dritschilo A, Weichselbaum R, Cassady JR, Jaffe N, Paed D (1978): The role of radiation therapy in the treatment of soft tissue sarcomas of childhood. Cancer 42:1192.

Dvorak O (1971): Cytembena treatment of advanced gynecologic carcinomas. Neoplasma 18:461.

Edsmyr F (1972): Bleomycin in the treatment of malignant diseases. In Proceedings of the International Symposium, London, England, November 1972, pp 95–103.

Encalada J, Bigalli A, Fernandez CA, Paulson G (1973) Clinical study of treatment with bleomycin in malignant tumors. Acta Folha Med 67:25.

Forney JP, Morrow CP, DiSaia PJ (1975): Seven-drug polychemotherapy in the treatment of advanced and recurrent squamous carcinoma of the female genital tract. Am J Obstet Gynecol 123:748.

Forney JP, Morrow CP, Townsend DE, DiSaia PJ (1977): Management of carcinoma-in-situ of the vulva. Obstet Gynecol 127:801.

Foster DC, Woodruff JD (1981): The use of dinitrochlorobenzene in the treatment of vulvar carcinoma-in-situ. Gynecol Oncol 11:330.

Fowler WC, Brantley JC III, Edelman DA (1979): Clear cell adenocarcinoma of the genital tract. South Med J 72:15.

Frick HC II, Atchoo N, Adamsons K Jr, Taylor HC Jr (1965): The efficacy of chemotherapeutic agents in the management of disseminated gynecologic cancer—A review of 206 cases. Am J Obstet Gynecol 93:1112.

Ghavimi F, Exelby PR, D'Angio GJ (1973): Combination therapy of urogenital embryonal rhabdomyosarcoma in children. Cancer 32:1178.

Gorgun B, Goplerud DR, Watne AL (1967): Intra-arterial chemotherapy in advanced pelvic tumors. Arch Surg 94:251.

Guthrie D (1978): The use of cytotoxic chemotherapy in conjunction with gynaecologic surgery. Clin Obstet Gynaecol 5:709.

Haffner WHJ, Frick HC II (1970): Intermittent intravenous methotrexate in the treatment of advanced epidermoid carcinoma of the cervix and vulvo-vagina. Cancer 24:812.

Hays DM, Ortega J (1977): Primary chemotherapy in the management of pelvic rhabdomyosarcoma in infancy and early childhood. In Salmon SE, Jones SE (eds): "Adjuvant Therapy of Cancer." Amsterdam: Elsevier/North Holland Biomedical Press.

Herbst AL, Kurman RJ, Scully RE, Poskanzer DC (1972): Clear-cell adenocarcinoma of the genital tract in young females: Registry report. N Engl J Med 287:1259.

Hilgers RD (1975): Pelvic exenteration for vaginal embryonal rhabdomyosarcoma: A review. Obstet Gynecol 45:175.

Ichikawa T (1970): Discovery of clinical effect of bleomycin against squamous cell carcinoma and further development of its research. Asian Med J 13:210.

Jaffe N, Filler RM, Farber S (1973): Rhabdomyosarcoma in children: Improved outlook with a multidisciplinary approach. Am J Surg 125:482.

Kalra JK, Grossman AM, Krumholz BA, Chen S, Tinker MA, Flores GT, Molho L, Cortes EF (1981): Preoperative chemoradiotherapy for carcinoma of the vulva. Gynecol Oncol 12:256.

Krupp PJ, Bohm JW (1978): 5-Fluorouracil topical treatment of in situ vulvar cancer. Obstet Gynecol 51:702.

Lifshitz S, Roberts JA (1980): Treatment of carcinoma-in-situ of the vulva with topical 5-fluorouracil. Obstet Gynecol 56:242.

Loo RV, Vaitkevicius VK, Reed ML (1967): Phase I trial of porfiromycin (NSC-56410). Cancer Chemotherapy Rep 51:497.

Malkasian GD Jr, Decker DG, Mussey E, Johnson CE (1968a): Chemotherapy of squamous cell carcinoma of the cervix, vagina, and vulva. Clin Obstet Gynecol 11:367.

Malkasian GD Jr, Decker DG, Mussey E, Johnson CE (1968b): Observations on gynecologic malignancy treated with 5-fluorouracil. Am J Obstet Gynecol 100:1012.

Masterson JG, Nelson JH (1965): The role of chemotherapy in the treatment of gynecologic malignancy. Am J Obstet Gynecol 93:1102.

Middleton AW Jr, Elman AJ, Stewart JR, O'Brien RT, Johnson DG (1981): Combined modality therapy with conservation of organ function in childhood genitourinary rhabdomyosarcoma. Urology 18:42.

Morrow CP, Townsend DE (1981): "Synopsis of Gynecologic Oncology." New York: John Wiley & Sons.

Morrow CP, Creasman WT, DiSaia PJ, Curry SL, DePetrillo AD (1973): Methotrexate, hydroxyurea, and vincristine: Combination chemotherapy in squamous carcinoma of the female genitalia. Gynecol Oncol 1:314.

Mosher MB, Deconti RC, Bertino JR (1972): Bleomycin therapy in advanced Hodgkin's disease and epidermoid cancers. Cancer 30:56.

Omura GA, Shingleton HM, Creasman WT, Blessing JA, Boronow RC (1978): Chemotherapy of gynecologic cancer with nitrosoureas: A randomized trial of CCNU and methyl CCNU in cancers of the cervix, corpus, vagina, and vulva. Cancer Treat Rep 62:833.

Ortega JA (1979): A therapeutic approach to childhood pelvic rhabdomyosarcoma without pelvic exenteration. J Pediatr 94:205.

Petrilli ES, Townsend DE, Morrow CP, Nakao CY (1980): Vaginal intraepithelial neoplasia: Biologic aspects and treatment with topical 5-fluorouracil and the carbon dioxide laser. Am J Obstet Gynecol 138:321.

Piver MS, Barlow JJ, Wang JJ, Shah NK (1973): Combined radical surgery, radiation therapy, and chemotherapy in infants with vulvovaginal embryonal rhabdomyosarcoma. Obstet Gynecol 42:522.

Piver MS, Barlow JJ, Xynos FP (1978): Adriamycin alone or in combination in 100 patients with carcinoma of the cervix or vagina. Am J Obstet Gynecol 131:311.

Piver MS, Barlow JJ, Dunbar J (1980): Doxorubicin, cyclophosphamide, and 5-fluorouracil in patients with carcinoma of the cervix or vagina. Cancer Treat Rep 64:549.

Plentl AA, Friedman EA (1971): "Lymphatic System of the Female Genitalia." Philadelphia: WB Saunders.

Rivard G, Ortega J (1975): Intensive chemotherapy as primary treatment for rhabdomyosarcoma of the pelvis. Cancer 36:1593.

Robboy SJ, Herbst AL, Scully RE (1974): Clear cell adenocarcinoma of the vagina and cervix in young females: Analysis of 37 tumors that persisted or recurred after primary therapy. Cancer 34:606.

Roberts JA, Watring WG, Lagasse LD (1980): Treatment of vulvar intraepithelial neoplasia (VIN) with local bleomycin. Cancer Clin Trials 3:354.

Rutledge F, Sinclair M (1968): Treatment of intraepithelial carcinoma of the vulva by skin excision and graft. Am J Obstet Gynecol 102:806.

Schneider J, Gebhartz H (1973): Therapy of squamous epithelial carcinoma with bleomycin. Verh Dtsch Ges Inn Med 78:163.

Sirisabya N (1974): Clinical trials of bleomycin on female genital cancer: A preliminary report. J Med Assoc Thai 56:101.

Smith JP, Rutledge F, Delclos L, Sutow W (1975): Combined irradiation and chemotherapy for sarcomas of the pelvis in females. Am J Roentgenol Radium Ther Nucl Med 123:571.

Soule EH, Newton W Jr, Moon TE, Tefft M (1978): Extraskeletal Ewing's sarcoma: A preliminary review of 26 cases encountered in the Intergroup rhabdomyosarcoma study. Cancer 42:259.

Srivannaboon S, Boonyanit S, Vatananusara C, Sophak P (1973): A clinical trial of bleomycin on carcinoma of the vulva: A preliminary report. J Med Assoc Thai 56:101.

Taussig FJ (1935): Primary cancer of the vulva, vagina, and female urethra: 5-year results. Surg Gynecol Obstet 60:477.

Taussig FJ (1940): Cancer of the vulva. Am J Obstet Gynecol 40:764.

Tojo S, Matsuura Y, Oku T (1972): Therapeutic effects of bleomycin on vulvar carcinoma. Adv Obstet Gynecol 24:236.

Trope C, Johnsson JE, Larsson G, Simonsen E (1980): Bleomycin alone or combined with mitomycin C in treatment of advanced or recurrent squamous cell carcinoma of the vulva. Cancer Treat Rep 64:639.

Usherwood M (1975): Management of vaginal carcinoma after hysterectomy. Am J Obstet Gynecol 122:352.

Vogl S, Ohnuma T, Perloff M, Holland JF (1976): Combination chemotherapy with adriamycin and cis-diaminedichloroplatinum in patients with neoplastic diseases. Cancer 38:21.

Watring WG, Roberts JA, Lagasse LD, Berman ML, Ballon SC, Moore JG, Schlesinger RE (1978): Treatment of recurrent Paget's disease of the vulva with topical bleomycin. Cancer 41:10.

Way S (1948): Primary carcinoma of the vagina. J Obstet Gynaecol Brit Emp 55:739.

Way S (1978): The surgery of vulvar carcinoma: An appraisal. Clin Obstet Gynaecol 5:623.

Woodruff JD, Julian C, Puray T (1973): The contemporary challenge of carcinoma-in-situ of the vulva. Am J Obstet Gynecol 115:677.

Woodruff JD, Parmley TH, Julian CG (1975): Topical 5-fluorouracil in the treatment of vaginal carcinoma-in-situ. Gynecol Oncol 3:124.

Yahia C, Fuller AF, Cloud LP (1978): Successful long-term palliation of stage IV vulvar carcinoma with operation and bleomycin sulfate. Am J Obstet Gynecol 130:360.

Chemotherapy of Cervical Carcinoma

Philip D. Bonomi and Edgardo L. Yordan, Jr.

Section of Medical Oncology, Department of Internal Medicine (P.D.B.) and Section of Gynecologic Oncology (E.L.Y.), Rush-Presbyterian-St. Luke's Medical Center, Chicago, Illinois 60612

Treatment of women with recurrent or metastatic carcinoma of the cervix is a difficult problem. Results obtained with a variety of chemotherapeutic agents indicate that cervical cancer is only moderately sensitive to chemotherapy [Wasserman and Carter, 1977]. Inherent insensitivity of the tumor is probably the primary reason for the relatively low response rates that have been observed. However, other factors that may contribute to the low level of responsiveness include the fact that many of these women have received prior pelvic irradiation. It is possible that a tumor that recurs or persists in an irradiated field consists of more resistant cells. Also, previous radiation might result in decreased tumor vascularity and hence decreased drug levels in the tumor. Finally, in many patients, the amount of drug that can be given will be compromised by increased myelosuppression or increased risk of mucositis associated with prior radiation.

Similarly, the inherent nature of the disease may preclude administration of full doses of chemotherapy. Ureteral obstruction resulting in impaired renal function and the development of pelvic necrosis which is frequently accompanied by smoldering infection may limit the choice and dose of drugs that can be given.

Assessment of tumor response presents another problem in treating this group of patients with chemotherapy. Computerized axial tomography has improved the ability to measure pelvic masses in some patients. However, many pelvic recurrences infiltrate surrounding structures or form sheets of tumor. These types of lesions remain difficult to measure, despite the availability of CAT scans.

Chemotherapy of Gynecologic Cancer, pages 103–124

The previously described considerations give an indication of the difficulty of doing clinical trials with chemotherapy in this group of patients. The situation has been complicated by the variation in response rates observed by different investigators. These inconsistencies, which are particularly apparent for some of the combination regimens, probably reflect differences in prognostic factors in the various series of patients as well as differences in methodology and criteria of tumor response. However, prognostic factors for response to chemotherapy have not been clearly defined for cervical cancer. For instance, performance status, which has been shown to have major importance in chemotherapy trials in other solid tumors [Zelen, 1973], is frequently not described in cervical cancer trials. Other possible prognostic factors include site of disease (pelvic vs. extrapelvic), previous radiation therapy, number of sites of disease, size of pelvic mass, and disease-free interval, initial stage and size of tumor, and grade of differentiation.

Despite the previously described problems, response to chemotherapy provides palliation of symptoms. [Hreshchyshyn and Holland, 1962; Smith et al., 1967]. Also, response to chemotherapy appears to prolong survival with median survival for responders being approximately 7–10 months compared to 3–5 months for nonresponders. [Hreshchyshyn and Holland, 1962; Smith et al., 1967; Baker et al., 1978; Trope et al., 1980, 1983; Bonomi et al., 1982].

The histology of most cervical tumors is squamous cell carcinoma, and therefore most of this chapter will deal with chemotherapeutic trials for this histologic type. Nonsquamous cell tumors including adenocarcinoma and neuroendocrine small cell carcinoma of the cervix will be discussed briefly.

SINGLE AGENTS

Drugs that have activity in squamous cell carcinoma of the cervix [Wasserman and Carter, 1977; Bonomi et al., 1982; Piver et al., 1978; Wallace et al., 1978; Malkasian et al., 1977, Thigpen et al., 1981] are listed in Table I. The presumed mechanism of action, pharmacology, and toxicity for each of these agents is discussed briefly.

Alkylating Agents

The nitrogen mustard–derived alkylating agents including cyclophosphamide, melphalan, and chlorambucil have shown activity in squamous cell carcinoma of the cervix. [Wasserman and Carter, 1977]. The antineoplastic activity of these drugs appears to result from alkylation of DNA with subsequent interstrand and intrastrand crosslinking of DNA [Colvin, 1982].

TABLE I. Active Single Agents

Drug	Responses/evaluable patients	Response rate (%)	References
Cisplatin (100 mg/m^2)	38/138	27	Bonomi et al., 1982
Chlorambucil	11/44	25	Wasserman and Carter, 1977
Cisplatin (50 mg/m^2)	28/122	23	Bonomi et al., 1982
Vincristine	10/44	23	Wasserman and Carter, 1977
Hexamethylmelamine	11/49	22	Wasserman and Carter, 1977
Porfiromycin	17/78	22	Wasserman and Carter, 1977
Mitomycin	4/18	22	Wasserman and Carter, 1977
Melphalan	4/20	20	Wasserman and Carter, 1977
Dianhydrogalactitol	7/36	19	Thigpen et al., 1981
ICRF 159	5/28	18	Thigpen et al., 1981
Baker's Antifol	5/32	16	Thigpen et al., 1981
Methotrexate	12/77	16	Wasserman and Carter, 1977
Cyclophosphamide	29/188	15	Wasserman and Carter, 1977
Methyl CCNU	4/32	13	Wasserman and Carter, 1977
Bleomycin	17/172	10	Wasserman and Carter, 1977
Doxorubicin	9/88	10	Piver et al., 1978; Wallace et al., 1978
5-Fluorouracil	208	9	Malkasian et al., 1977

Myelosuppression, the dose-limiting toxicity of this group of drugs, is troublesome because the majority of these patients have compromised bone marrow function from previous pelvic radiation. Cyclophosphamide is unique among the nitrogen mustard derivatives because it may induce hemorrhagic cystitis. Patients should be hydrated adequately prior to and during cyclophosphamide therapy.

None of these drugs has been shown to be clearly superior, in terms of antitumor effect [Wasserman and Carter, 1977] but cyclophosphamide has been most widely used in combination regimens probably because its myelosuppression tends to be less prolonged than other alkylating agents and because it was tested more extensively as a single agent [Wasserman and Carter, 1977; Solidoro et al., 1966]. Cyclophosphamide is metabolized by hepatic microsomal enzymes, and the metabolites, particularly 4-hydroxycyclophosphamide, appear to account for the antitumor effect [Colvin, 1982]. Metabolites of the drug are excreted primarily in the urine [Colvin, 1982].

Methyl CCNU, one of the nitrosourea derivatives which are another class of alkylating agents, has shown activity in a relatively small group of patients [Wasserman and Carter, 1977]. The major drawback of this class of drugs is myelosuppression, which is delayed and may be severe and prolonged [Katz and Glick, 1979].

Hexamethylmelamine

While some investigators have observed activity with hexamethylmelamine [Wasserman and Carter, 1977], others have not confirmed their findings [Freedman et al., 1980]. This drug was originally thought to exert its antitumor effect by alkylation of DNA, but more recent data suggest that it may act as an antimetabolite [Legha et al., 1976]. Hexamethylmelamine produces mild myelosuppression, but may cause considerable nausea and vomiting. Prolonged use may result in peripheral neuropathy [Legha et al., 1976], and combination with other neurotoxic drugs might result in an increased frequency of neurologic side effects. This drug has not been used in combination regimens in cancer of the cervix.

5-Fluorouracil

The fluorinated pyrimidine 5-fluorouracil (5FU) has produced a regression rate of 9% in cervical cancer [Malkasian et al., 1977]. Fluorine replaces a hydrogen atom in the 5 position of the pyrimidine ring which results in inhibition of the enzyme thymidylate synthetase. This enzyme inhibits the conversion of uridine to thymidine, which is necessary for DNA synthesis [Chabner, 1982a]. Originally the antitumor effect of 5FU was believed to be due solely to inhibition of this enzyme. However, 5-fluorouracil is incorporated into ribosomal RNA resulting in abnormalities in protein synthesis, which may account at least partially for the antineoplastic effect [Chabner, 1982a]. Myelosuppression and mucositis are the dose-limiting side effects of 5FU. Administering the drug by continuous intravenous infusion as opposed to bolus intravenous infusion reduces the myelosuppression considerably [Fraile et al., 1980]. We are currently evaluating cisplatin plus 5FU given by continuous infusion in squamous cell carcinoma of the cervix. The drug is eliminated predominantly by metabolism rather than by urinary or biliary excretion [Chabner, 1982a].

Vincristine

Hreshchyshyn [1963] reported a 31% response rate with vincristine. This drug is a *Vinca* alkaloid which disrupts the mitotic spindle resulting in transient metaphase arrest at low doses. Cell death occurs at higher doses. [Bender and Chabner, 1982]. The dose-limiting toxicity is peripheral neuropathy which may result in weakness and severe paresthesias. The drug produces virtually no myelosuppression. Biliary excretion is the primary mode of drug elimination [Bender and Chabner, 1982].

Methotrexate

The review conducted by Wasserman and Carter [1982] showed that the antifolate, methotrexate, produced a cumulative response rate of 16% in 77 patients. This drug inhibits the enzyme dihydrofolate reductase which is necessary for the transfer of the single carbon moiety in the synthesis of thymine [Chabner, 1982b]. Inhibition of this enzyme results in the inhibition of DNA synthesis which is presumed to be the basis for methotrexate antitumor effect. The major toxicities of methotrexate are myelosuppression and mucositis. The use of folinic acid (rescue factor, citrovorum) which is tetrahydrofolate ameliorates the toxicities enabling administration of much higher doses of methotrexate [Chabner, 1982b]. High-dose methotrexate combined with vincristine has been tried in treating cervical carcinomas producing a response rate of 17% in 31 patients [Hakes et al., 1979]. From these results it appears that there is no advantange for using high-dose methotrexate in patients with cancer of the cervix.

Methotrexate is excreted primarily by the kidneys. Increased myelosuppression and mucositis are observed in patients with decreased renal function. In addition, methotrexate, particularly at higher doses, may be nephrotoxic, resulting in further decrease in renal function in patients who initially have impaired kidneys. [Chabner, 1982b].

Doxorubicin

Doxorubicin, an antitumor antibiotic, has produced a 10% response rate in squamous cell cancer of the cervix [Piver et al., 1978; Wallace et al., 1978]. This drug is an intercalating agent which produces damage to DNA strands resulting in inhibition of DNA and RNA synthesis leading to cell death [Myers, 1982]. Dose-limiting toxicities include myelosuppression, mucositis, and cardiac toxicity.

The cardiac injury involves mitochondrial injury presumably from interaction of doxorubicin-derived free radicals and lipids in the mitochondrial membrane. The mitochondrial injury is believed to result in degeneration of cardiac myofibrils leading to cardiomyopathy which is fatal in as high as 50% of cases. [Lefrak et al., 1973].

The frequency of cardiomyopathy is directly related to the cumulative dose. Below doses of 550 mg/m^2 the frequency of heart failure was 0.27% and above 550 mg/m^2 it increases to as high as 30% [Lefrak et al., 1973]. Previous heart failure, hypertension, and previous mediastinal irradiation are risk factors which predispose to the development of clinically significant cardiomyopathy [Lefrak et al., 1973]. Endomyocardial biopsy reveals abnormalities in cardiac myofibrils which increase with increasing doses of the drug [Bristow et al., 1978]. Radionuclide cardiac (MUGA) scans have been shown to have predictive values in detecting patients who have a high risk of developing clinically significant cardiomyopathy [Alexander et al., 1979]. Most clinicians limit the dose of doxorubicin to 550 mg/m^2 in patients who have not received prior mediastinal radiation, and 400 mg/m^2 in patients who have received mediastinal radiation.

Mitomycin

Regression of cervical cancer has been observed with the antitumor antibiotic mitomycin [Wasserman and Carter, 1977] and the closely related compound Porfiromycin. This drug binds covalently to DNA and its antitumor action is presumed to be similar to that of alkylating agents [Glaubiger and Rama, 1982]. Myelosuppression which may be severe and prolonged is the dose-limiting toxicity. Pulmonary toxicity in the form of interstitial pneumonitis has been observed in three patients with this compound [Orwell et al., 1978]. Treatment with corticosteroids resulted in improvement in each case [Orwell et al., 1978].

Bleomycin

Bleomycin, an antitumor antibiotic isolated by the Japanese, is active in cervical cancer [Wasserman and Carter, 1977]. This agent binds to DNA, resulting in breaks in the DNA strands and subsequent cell death [Bennett and Reich, 1979]. Mucositis and interstitial pulmonary fibrosis are the dose-limiting side effects [Bennett and Reich, 1979]. The risk of pulmonary toxicity increases with increasing cumulative dose and with increasing age [Bennett and Reich, 1979; Blum, 1973]. Bleomycin is generally discontinued at a total dose of 400–450 mg. Excretion of the drug is predominantly renal, and there is evidence that impaired renal function results in an increased toxicity and that the frequency of drug administration should be reduced in patients with renal impairment [Petrilli et al., 1982].

Bleomycin has been used in a variety of doses and schedules. There is evidence that continuous infusion of bleomycin may be more effective in squamous cell carcinoma of the cervix. In a nonrandomized trial Krakoff et al. [1977] observed ten responses in 32 patients (30% response rate) who received a continuous infusion of bleomycin compared to a previous trial in which no responses occurred in patients given bolus injection of the drug [Yagoda et al., 1972]. Although this approach has not been evaluated in a randomized study, Baker et al. [1980] evaluated bleomycin by bolus injection versus continuous infusion in sequential studies in which bleomycin was combined with mitomycin and vincristine. The response rate for the continuous infusion regimen was 39% compared to 60% for the bolus regimen.

Cisplatin

Cisdiamminedichloroplatin (cisplatin) is the most extensively studied single agent in squamous cell cancer of the cervix. Thigpen et al. [1979] were the first to report activity for cisplatin. At a moderate dose (50 mg/m^2 every 3 weeks), they observed 11 partial remissions in 25 patients. Based on these data, the Gynecologic Oncology Group initiated a study to evaluate the dose-response relationship for cisplatin. In this trial, women with recurrent or metastatic squamous cell cancer were randomized to cisplatin 50 mg/m^2, 100 mg/m^2, or to 20 mg/m^2 daily for 5 consecutive days [Bonomi et al., 1982]. Each regimen was repeated every 3 weeks and treatment was discontinued at a cumulative dose of 400 mg/m^2. The response rates were virtually identical, ranging from 23% to 27%. Similarly, there was no difference in complete remission (10%) time to progression (4 months), or in median survival (7 months). In summary, the GOG study has shown no advantage of 100 mg/m^2 over 50 mg/m^2 of cisplatin.

The mechanism of action of cisplatin appears to be similar to alkylating agents. The dose-limiting toxicity and mode of excretion of cisplatin are renal [Zwelling and Kohn, 1982]. At moderate doses (50 mg/m^2) it appears that hydration alone is adequate protection for the kidney [Bonomi et al., 1982]. However, at higher doses (3 mg/kg) it appears that diuretics are required along with hydration [Cvitkovic, 1977; Hayes, 1977]. In the GOG study patients receiving 50 mg/m^2 or 20 mg/m^2 daily for 5 days received hydration only, whereas patients receiving 100 mg/m^2 as a single infusion received mannitol, furosemide, and hydration. The administration of diuretics and fluid for the single dose 100 mg/m^2 regimen required hospitalization. Nephrotoxicity was not a significant problem in the GOG trial. BUN $\geqslant$ 40 mg/dl and/or creatinine $\geqslant$ 2.0 mg/dl were observed in 5% of patients receiving 50 mg/m^2 with hydration only, 10% of patients receiving 20 mg/m^2 daily for 5 days with hydration only, and 10% of patients receiving diuretics and hydration with 100 mg/m^2 as a single dose [Bonomi et al., 1982].

Nausea and vomiting are major problems associated with cisplatin treatment. Standard antiemetics are frequently ineffective for cisplatin-induced nausea and vomiting, which may persist for days. Metoclopramide appears capable of reducing this side effect in some patients [Gralla et al., 1981]. Although auditory toxicity, peripheral neuropathy, and anaphylactic reactions may occur with cisplatin [Zwelling and Kohn, 1982], these were reported infrequently in the GOG study [Bonomi et al., 1982].

Dianhydrogalactitol and ICRF 159

The GOG has been conducting phase II trials of new agents in cervical cancer. Two agents have shown activity in these trials. Dianhydrogalactitol produces a 19% response rate, and ICRF 159 produced an 18% response rate [Thigpen et al., 1981]. The presumed mechanism of action for both of these agents is alkylation of DNA. Myelosuppression is the dose-limiting toxicity for each drug.

COMBINATION CHEMOTHERAPY

Although a variety of combination regimens have been tried in cervical cancer, most of these trials have involved small groups of patients. Only two randomized prospective studies of combination chemotherapy have been reported [Wallace et al., 1978; Omura et al., 1981].

As mentioned earlier, results using the same combination regimen have varied considerably. These inconsistencies probably reflect differences in prognostic factors in different patient populations as well as the wide confidence limits which are associated with results obtained from small groups of patients.

Doxorubicin Combinations

Doxorubicin-containing regimens that have been tried in cervical cancer are listed in Tables II and III. Wallace et al. [1978] conducted a randomized trial of doxorubicin versus doxorubicin and vincristine versus doxorubicin and cyclophosphamide. Comparison of the combination regimens against doxorubicin alone showed no difference in time to progression, response rates, or survival durations. Others have reported similar results for doxorubicin and cyclophosphamide [Alberts and Ignoffo, 1978; Hanjani and Bonnell, 1980] and Piver et al. [1980] have observed virtually the same results for doxorubicin, 5FU, and cyclophosphamide.

TABLE II. Doxorubicin-Containing Regimens

Drugs	Dose/schedule	Evaluable patients	Response rate (%)	Median duration of response (months)	References
Doxorubicin Cyclophosphamide Vincristine 5-Fluorouracil	45 mg/m^2 d 1[a] 100 mg/m^2 d 1–14 1.4 mg/m^2 d 1 and 8 500 mg/m^2 d 1 and 8	31	58	5	Chan et al., 1982
Doxorubicin Methyl CCNU	45–60 mg/m^2 d 1 and 22 q. 42 d 175 mg/m^2 d 1 q. 42 d	31	45	CR-7 PR-4	Day et al., 1978
Doxorubicin Cyclophosphamide	50 mg/m^2 q. 21 d 500 mg/m^2 q. 21 d	39	18	—	Wallace et al., 1978
Doxorubicin Cyclophosphamide	50 mg/m^2 q. 21 d 500 mg/m^2 q. 21 d	20	20	4	Hanjani and Bonnell, 1980
Doxorubicin Vincristine	60 mg/m^2 q. 21 d 1.5 mg/m^2 q. 21 d	54	17	—	Wallace et al., 1978
Doxorubicin Cyclophosphamide 5-Fluorouracil	60 mg/m^2 d 1[b] 200 mg/m^2 d 1–5 200 mg/m^2 d 1–5	36	16	4	Piver et al., 1980
Doxorubicin Vincristine 5-Fluorouracil	50 mg/m^2 d 1 1.4 mg/m^2 d 1 and 8 500 mg/m^2 d 1 and 8	31	10	6	Omura et al., 1981
Doxorubicin Cyclophosphamide	40 mg/m^2 q. 21 d 200 mg/m^2 d 3–6, q. 21 d	10	10	—	Alberts and Ignoffo, 1978
Doxorubicin Bleomycin	20 mg/m^2 d 1–3 15 mg/m^2 d 1–5 q. 21 d	16	6	—	Piver et al., 1978
Doxorubicin Bleomycin	30–60 mg/m^2 q. 21 d 10 mg/m^2 weekly	11	0	—	Greenberg et al., 1977

[a]This regimen was repeated every 28 days.
[b]This regimen was repeated every 21 days.

TABLE III. Doxorubicin-Methotrexate Trials

Drugs	Doses/ Schedules	Evaluable patients	Response rate (%)	Median duration (months)	References
Doxorubicin Methotrexate	50 mg/m^2 q. 21 d 20 mg/m^2 d 1 and 8 q. 21 d	23	65	—	Guthrie and Way, 1978
Doxorubicin Methotrexate	50 mg/m^2 q. 21 d 20 mg/m^2 d 1 and 8 q. 21 d	24	29	—	Papavasilou et al., 1978
Doxorubicin Methotrexate	50 mg/m^2 q. 21 d 45 mg/m^2 d 8 q. 21 d	24	21	5	Trope et al., 1980
Doxorubicin Methotrexate Leucovorum	30 mg/m^2 d 1 and 2 500 mg/m^2 d 1 10 mg/m^2 q. 6 h × 12	15	0	—	Piver et al., 1978

In another randomized trial Omura et al. [1981] reported a 10% response rate for the combination of doxorubicin, vincristine, and 5FU, and a 7% response rate for cyclophosphamide. Similarly, disappointing results have been obtained with the combination of doxorubicin and bleomycin [Piver et al., 1978; Greenberg et al., 1977]. In 31 patients Chan et al. [1982] observed a 58% response rate for the regimen which consisted of doxorubicin, cyclophosphamide, 5-fluorouracil, and vincristine. Median survival for responders was 10 months as opposed to 3 months for nonresponders. Additional trials with this regimen have not been reported.

Doxorubicin-Methotrexate Trials

Results of doxorubicin-methotrexate trials are summarized in Table III. Guthrie and Way [1978] were the first investigators to combine doxorubicin with methotrexate. They observed a response rate of 67%. Subsequently, Trope et al. [1980], Papavasiliou et al. [1978], and Piver et al. [1978] have observed response rates of 21%, 29% and 0% respectively. In addition, two of these groups of investigators [Trope et al., 1980, Papavasiliou et al., 1978] observed considerable myelosuppression from this regimen. The response rate for doxorubicin alone observed in the GOG trial [Wallace et al., 1978] was similar to the response rate for doxorubicin combined with methotrexate observed by Trope et al. [1980] and Papavasilliou et al. [1978].

A 45% response rate for doxorubicin combined with methyl CCNU has been reported by Day et al. [1978]. Subsequent trials with this combination have not been described.

Bleomycin-Mitomycin Regimens

The regimen of mitomycin and bleomycin has been evaluated by several different groups (see Table IV). Miyamoto et al. [1978] were the originators of this regimen, which includes bleomycin 5 mg infused intravenously over 3–4 h daily for 7 consecutive days and mitomycin 10 mg intravenously on day 8. They utilized this schedule hoping to capitalize on theoretical considerations which suggested that multiple small doses of bleomycin would result in increased effectiveness and decreased toxicity. In 1978 they reported 14 responses in 15 patients with 12 complete remissions. Subsequent trials by other investigators have shown response rates of 16% [Leichman et al., 1980], 22% [Petrilli et al., 1980; Greenberg et al., 1982], 36% [Trope et al., 1983], and 40% [Krebs et al., 1980].

Miyamoto series included only 3/15 [Miyomoto et al., 1978] patients with pelvic and abdominal masses, while 19/20 in the series of Krebs et al. [1980] and 23/33 in the series of Trope et al. [1983] had disease in these sites. Perhaps these differences in distribution of disease sites account for the differences in response rates. However, response rate related to site of disease is an unsettled issue. In small groups of patients some investigators [Piver et al., 1978] have observed higher response rates in extrapelvic and nonirradiated disease sites, while others [Wallace et al., 1978] have observed no significant differences.

Differences in PS may account for the different response rates. None of these investigators described the performance status of their patients [Miyamoto et al., 1978; Leichman et al., 1981; Petrilli et al., 1980; Greenberg et

TABLE IV. Mitomycin-Bleomycin Trials

References	Evaluable patients	Response rate (%)	Median response duration (months)
Miyamota et al., 1978	15	93	5
Krebs et al., 1980	20	40	3
Trope et al., 1983	33	36	CR-12, PR-6
Greenberg et al., 1982	18	18	3
Petrilli et al., 1980	9	18	—
Leichman et al., 1980	19	16	3

Drug doses and schedule: bleomycin 5 mg daily on days 1–7; mitomycin 10 mg on day 8. Treatment was repeated every 14 days.

al., 1982; Krebs et al., 1980]. Although this variable has not been evaluated in cancer of the cervix, it has been shown to be an important prognostic variable and predictor of response to in other types of tumors [Zelen, 1973].

Bleomycin-Mitomycin-Vincristine Trials

Baker et al. have evaluated mitomycin C and bleomycin combined with vincristine in cervical cancer [Baker et al., 1976, 1978] (Table V). They included vincristine because of evidence that giving this drug 6–12 h before bleomycin produced higher response rate in miscellaneous squamous cell carcinomas. The schedule employed was mitomycin C 20 mg/m^2 every 6 weeks and vincristine 0.5 mg/m^2 6 h before bleomycin 6 mg/m^2. Vincristine and bleomycin were given trial biweekly weeks for 12 weeks, and subsequent doses of mitomycin were reduced. Initally they reported a 48% response

TABLE V. Mitomycin-Bleomycin-Vincristine Trials

Schedule	Evaluable patients	Response rate (%)	Median response duration (months)
Regimen I			
Vincristine 0.5 mg/m^2 twice weekly for 24 doses			
Bleomycin 6 mg/m^2 weekly for 12 doses	50	60	2
Mitomycin 20 mg/m^2 on day 1 every 6 weeks			
Regimen II			
Vincristine 0.5 mg/m^2 on days 1 and 4[a]			
Bleomycin 30 U daily as a continuous IV infusion days 1–4	41	39	4
Mitomycin 20 mg/m^2 on day 2			
Regimen III			
Vincristine 0.5 mg/m^2 weekly for 24 doses			
Bleomycin 6 U/m^2 weekly for 24 doses	24	25	3
Mitomycin 20 mg/m^2 on day 1 every 6 weeks			

[a]Repeated every 6 weeks.
From Baker et al., 1978.

rate in 27 patients [Baker et al., 1976]. In subsequent trials bleomycin and vincristine were given once weekly, producing a 25% response rate, and bleomycin was given as a continuous infusion producing a 39% response rate [Baker et al., 1978]. Further experience with the twice-weekly vincristine-bleomycin schedules revealed a 60% response rate in 50 patients, suggesting that this schedule was superior. However, these regimens were not compared in a prospective randomized trial.

These results have led the Southwestern Oncology Group to initiate a randomized trial of cisplatin versus mitomycin and cisplatin, versus mitomycin, vincristine, bleomycin, and cisplatin.

Methotrexate Combination Regimens

There have been two trials of bleomycin combined with standard dose methotrexate given orally [Conroy et al., 1976; Benham et al., 1981] (Table VI). Vincristine was also included in one of these regimens [Conroy et al., 1976]. There were 12 responses in 20 patients with 2-day drug regimen [Benham et al., 1981] and eight responses in 17 patients with the three-drug regimen [Conroy et al., 1976]. Despite the relatively high response rates,

TABLE VI. Methotrexate Trials

Drugs	Doses/schedules	Evaluable patients	Response rate (%)	Median duration (months)	References
Methotrexate Bleomycin	10 mg/m^2 q. 4 d 10 mg/m^2 q. 7 d	20	60	7.5	Benham et al., 1981
Methotrexate Bleomycin Vincristine Cyclophosphamide 5-Fluorouracil Actinomycin D Cytosinearabinoside Leucovorum	100 mg/m^2 cont IV 30 U 1 mg/m^2 600 mg/m^2 500 mg/m^2 0.25 mg/m^2 100 mg q. 6 h × 6 d 15 mg q. 6 h × 5 doses	18	50	5	Forney et al.,[a] 1975
Methotrexate Bleomycin Vincristine	10 mg/m^2 P.O. q. 7 d 15 mg IM q. 7 d 1.5 mg/m^2 q. 14 d	17	47	2.5	Conroy et al., 1976
Methotrexate Vincristine	250 mg/m^2 to 10 g/m^2 q. 21 d 1.4 mg/m^2 q. 21 d	31	17	3	Hakes et al., 1979

[a]This regimen was given every 28 days.

duration of response and survival were similar to cisplatin alone [Bonomi et al., 1982].

Two groups of investigators [Hakes et al., 1979; Forney et al., 1975] have utilized high-dose methotrexate and citrovorum in combination regimens. Hakes et al. [1979] gave vincristine with doses of methotrexate as high as 10 g/m^2 and observed a 17% response rate. Forney et al. [1975] administered a relatively small dose of methotrexate with six drugs over a 24 h period. Although nine of 18 patients responded, this regimen appears to offer no advantage over less complicated regimens.

Cisplatin Combination Regimens

Vogl and his colleagues [1979, 1980, 1982] have conducted a series of phase II trials of cisplatin-containing combination regimens in cervical cancer. Recently Surwit et al. [1983] and Fine et al. [1983] have reported additional results with cisplatin combination regimens (see Table VII). In their first trial Vogl et al. [1979] combined cisplatin with methotrexate and bleomycin. Eight of nine patients had partial remissions with a median duration of 4 months. The median duration of response is similar to cisplatin alone. Myelosuppression and mucositis were moderately severe, and trial of this regimen was discontinued.

Next, Vogl et al. [1980] combined mitomycin with bleomycin, cisplatin, and vincristine. Ten of 16 patients had objective remissions with a median duration of 4 months. Using the same drugs with a slightly different schedule (see Table VI), Surwit et al. [1983] observed eight responses in 17 patients. Four of these remissions were complete with durations of 5, 20, 37, and 46 months.

Fine et al. [1983] have combined doxorubicin and methotrexate with a cisplatin. In 48 patients the regimen produced a 38% response rate with a median response duration of 5 months. Combining dianhydrogalactitol with cisplatin [Vogl et al., 1982] produced a 39% response rate with a median duration of 5 months, which is virtually the same as cisplatin alone. Myelosuppression was severe.

In summary, although response rates for some combination regimens [Baker, 1980; Chan et al., 1982; Trope et al., 1983; Vogl et al., 1979; Fine et al., 1983] are higher than for cisplatin alone [Bonomi et al., 1982], comparison of the median duration of response and median survival for trials of combination regimens versus results from a trial for cisplatin alone show virtually no difference. Also, in two randomized prospective studies which compared combination regimens to single agents there was no significant difference in median survival and response duration or in response rate

TABLE VII. Cisplatin Regimens

Doses/schedule	Evaluable patients	Response rate (%)	Median duration (months)	References
Regimen I[a]				
Cisplatin 50 mg/m^2 d 4 Methotrexate 40 mg/m^2 d 1 and 15 Bleomycin 10 U d 1, 8, 15	9	90	4	Vogl et al., 1979
Regimen II[b]				
Cisplatin 50 mg/m^2 d 1 and 22[a] Bleomycin 10 U weekly Vincristine 1 mg/m^2 d 1, 8, 22, 29 Mitomycin 10 mg/m^2 d 1	13	77	4	Vogl et al., 1980
Regimen III[b]				
Cisplatin 50 mg/m^2 d 1 and 22 Mitomycin 10 mg/m^2 d 1 Vincristine 0.5 mg/m^2 d 1 and 4 Bleomycin 30 U cont IV daily d 1 and 4	17	47	—	Surwit et al., 1983
Cisplatin 50 mg/m^2 q. 21 d Methotrexate 40 mg/m^2 q. 21 d Doxorubicin 50 mg/m^2 q. 21 d	48	38	5	Fine et al., 1983
Cisplatin 50 mg/m^2 q. 21 d Dianhydrogalactitol 15 mg/m^2 q. 21 d	18	40	5	Vogl et al., 1982

[a]This regimen was repeated every 21 days.
[b]This regimen was repeated every 42 days.

[Wallace et al., 1978; Omura et al., 1981]. Cisplatin was not included in these trials [Wallace et al., 1978; Omura et al., 1981].

Identification of prognostic factors is important in order to have a means of comparing results obtained with various combination regimens, but more important is the development of randomized prospective trials comparing combination regimens and single agents.

Intra-Arterial Chemotherapy

Cervical cancer has been treated by arterial infusion of chemotherapy via a catheter placed at the level of the aortic bifurcation or in the common iliac arteries. Nitrogen mustard [Kramer et al., 1952; Bolman et al., 1956], methotrexate [Sullivan et al., 1960; Bateman et al., 1966; Averette et al., 1976], 5-fluorouracil [Rutledge, 1976], bleomycin [Morrow et al., 1977], and cisplatin [Carlson et al., 1981] have been infused intra-arterially in single-agent trials. In addition, the following combination regimens have been evaluated as intra-arterial infusions: vincristine-methotrexate [Averette et al., 1976], 5FU-methotrexate, alkylating agent [Cavanaugh et al., 1975], and bleomycin-vincristine-mitomycin [Swenerton et al., 1979]. Although some long-term remissions have been observed, intra-arterial chemotherapy has shown no apparent increase in tumor regression over peripheral venous infusion. [Morrow et al., 1977; Carlson et al., 1981; Swenerton et al., 1979]. In addition, there was no difference in systemic toxicity between these two methods of treatment [Morrow et al., 1977; Swenerton et al., 1979].

Local Application of Chemotherapy

Masuda et al. [1981] have utilized vaginal suppositories of either bleomycin or 5-fluorouracil in treating stages O and IA squamous cell carcinoma. Subsequent hysterectomy revealed no residual tumor in 17 of 33 women with stage O lesions and in nine of 42 women with stage IA lesions. This method of using chemotherapy is being evaluated with the possibility that young women with early cervical cancer might have the opportunity for childbirth.

Hormonal Therapy

Recent reports of the presence of estrogen and progesterone receptors [Hahnel et al., 1979; Farley et al., 1982; Ford et al., 1983] in cancer of the cervix raise the question of whether some cervical cancers might regress with hormonal therapy. Progestational agents have been tried in a small number of women with cervical cancer [Smith et al., 1967; Malkasian et al., 1977], and no objective responses were observed. However, in one report vaginal bleeding stopped in three of four women treated with medroxy-progesterone [Smith et al., 1967].

Radiation Sensitizers

The use of chemical agents to potentiate the effect of radiation therapy in locally advanced carcinoma of the cervix was evaluated in a double-blind study comparing hydroxyurea and placebo [Piver et al., 1977]. In this randomized trial, women with stage IIB cancer of the cervix received pelvic radiation. Hydroxyurea 80 mg/kg every third day was given to 22 patients and a placebo was given on the same schedule to 37 patients. Either the placebo or hydroxyurea was continued for 12 weeks. At 2 years 74% of the hydroxyurea-treated group and 43% of the placebo-treated group are alive and free of disease ($P = 0.01$). In stage IIIB cervical cancer there was a trend for higher disease-free survival in women treated with the sensitizer, but this difference was not statistically significant.

Currently the radiation sensitizers misonidazole and hydroxyurea are being compared in women receiving pelvic radiation for stages IIB–IVA squamous cell carcinoma of the cervix with negative para-aortic nodes.

Adjuvant Chemotherapy

Although no randomized trials of adjuvant chemotherapy in cervical cancer have been reported, the Gynecologic Oncology Group is currently conducting a randomized adjuvant trial in women with metastases to para-aortic lymph nodes. Histologic confirmation of lymph node metastases is required in this study. All patients receive hydroxyurea 80 mg/kg twice weekly and radiation which includes the pelvis and para-aortic areas. After completion of radiation, the women are randomized to either treatment with six cycles of cisplatin at 50 mg/m^2 every 3 weeks or to no additional treatment.

Merwe et al. [1983] have repeated preliminary data from a nonrandomized trial of neoadjuvant chemotherapy in stage IIIB cancer of the cervix. They gave cisplatin, bleomycin, and methotrexate prior to pelvic radiation. After receiving two courses of this regimen, partial remissions occurred in 11 of 22 women.

Preliminary data using another new approach in locally advanced cervical cancer have been presented by Kalra et al. [1983]. These investigators have given simultaneous 5-fluorouracil, mitomycin C, and pelvic radiation to ten women with advanced cervical cancer. Six complete remissions and two partial remissions were observed.

Nonsquamous Cell Carcinoma

In women with nonsquamous cell cancer of the cervix responses have been observed in 2/13 patients treated with cisplatin 50 mg/m^2 every 21 days and in 2/14 patients treated with piperazinedione 9 mg/m^2 every 3 weeks. [Thigpen et al., 1981]. The histology in most of these cases was adenocarcinoma.

Small Cell Carcinoma of the Cervix

Small cell carcinoma has been classified as a type of squamous cell carcinoma [Reagan et al., 1957]. Some investigators have emphasized the aggressive nature of these tumors and have compared them to small cell cancer of the lung, which is a neuroendocrine carcinoma. Since then, several reports [Jones et al., 1976; Pazdur et al., 1981] have shown that some small cell carcinomas of the cervix demonstrate neuroendocrine features. Complete remission of bulky tumor was observed in one of four patients treated with doxorubicin and cyclophosphamide [Pazdur et al., 1981].

The regimen of cyclophosphamide, doxorubicin, and vincristine, which is active in small cell bronchogenic carcinoma, is being evaluated in patients with recurrent or metastatic small cell carcinoma of the cervix in a Gynecologic Oncology Group protocol.

REFERENCES

Alberts DS, Ignoffo R (1978): Adriamycin-cyclophosphamide treatment of squamous cell carcinoma of the cervix. Cancer Treat Rep 62:143–144.

Alexander J, Dainak N, Berger HJ, Goldman L, Johnstone D, Reduto L, Duffy T, Schwartz P, Gottschalk A, Zaret B (1979): Serial assessment of doxorubicin cardiotoxicity with quantitative radionuclide angiography. N Engl J Med 300:278–283.

Averette HE, Weinstein GD, Ford JH, Girtanner RE, Hoskins WJ, Ramos R (1976): Cell kinetics and programmed chemotherapy for gynecologic cancer. Am J Obstet Gynecol 124:912–923.

Baker LH, Opipari MI, Izbicki RM (1976): Phase II study of mitomycin C, vincristine, and bleomycin in advanced squamous cell carcinoma of the uterine cervix. Cancer 38:2222–2224.

Baker LH, Opipari MI, Wilson H, Bottomley R, Coltman CA Jr (1978): Mitomycin, vincristine, and bleomycin for advanced cervical cancer. Obstet Gynecol 52:146–150.

Bateman JR, Hazen JG, Stolinsky DC, Steinfeld JL (1966): Advanced carcinoma of the cervix treated by intra-arterial methotrexate. Am J Obstet Gynecol 96:181–187.

Bender RA, Chabner BA (1982): Tubulin binding agents in pharmacologic principles of cancer treatment. In Chabner BA (ed): "Pharmacologic Principles of Cancer Treatment." Philadelphia: WB Saunders, pp 256–262.

Benham K, Lewis GC, Lee JH, Looka MH (1981): Treatment of cervical carcinoma with methotrexate, bleomycin and vincristine. Cancer Clin Trials 4:75–79.

Bennett JM, Reich SD (1979): Bleomycin. Ann Intern Med 90:945–948.
Blum RH, Carter SK, Agre K (1973) A clinical review of bleomycin—a new antineoplastic agent. Cancer 31:903–914.
Bolman RE, Holzapfel JH, Barnes AC (1956): Intra-arterial nitrogen mustard in advanced pelvic malignancies. Am J Obstet Gynecol 72:1319–1325.
Bonomi P, Bruckner H, Cohen C, Marshall R, Blessing J, Slayton R (1982): A randomized trial of three cisplatin regimens in squamous cell carcinoma of the cervix. Proc Am Soc Clin Oncol 18:110.
Bristow MR, Mason JW, Billingham ME (1978): Adriamycin cardiomyopathy: Evaluation by phonography, endomyocardial biopsy, and cardiac catheterization. Ann Intern Med 88:168.
Carlson JA Jr, Freedman RS, Wallace S, Chuang VP, Wharton TJ, Rutledge FN (1981): Intra-arterial cis-platinum in the management of squamous cell carcinoma of the uterine cervix. Gynecol Oncol 12:92–98.
Cavanaugh D, Hovadhanakul P, Comasm R (1975): Regional chemotherapy: A comparison of pelvic perfusion and intra-arterial infusion in patients with advanced gynecologic cancer. Am J Obstet Gynecol 123:435–440.
Chabner BA (1982a): Pyrimidine antagonists in pharmacologic principles of cancer treatment. In Chabner BA (ed): "Pharmacologic Principles of Cancer Treatment." Philadelphia: WB Saunders, pp 183–212.
Chabner BA (1982b): Methotrexate: Pharmacologic principles of cancer treatment. In Chabner BA (ed): "Pharmacologic Principles of Cancer Treatment." Philadelphia: WB Saunders, pp 229–255.
Chan WK, Aroney RS, Levi JA, Tattersall HA, Fox RM, Woods RL (1982): Four-drug combination chemotherapy for advanced cervical carcinoma. Cancer 49:2437–2440.
Colvin M (1982) The alkylating agents in pharmacologic principles of cancer treatment. In Chabner BA (ed): "Pharmacologic Principles of Cancer Treatment." Philadelphia: WB Saunders, 276–309.
Conroy JF, Lewis GC, Brady LW, Brodsky I, Kahn SB, Ross D, Nuss R (1976): Low dose bleomycin and methotrexate in cervical cancer. Cancer 37:660–664.
Cvitkovic E, Spaulding J, Bethune V, Martin J, Whitmore WF (1977): Improvement of cis-dichlorodiammineplatinum (NSC 119875): Therapeutic index in an animal model. Cancer 39:1357–1361.
Day TG Jr, Wharton JT, Gottlieb JA, Rutledge FN (1978). Am J Obstet Gynecol 132:545–548.
Farley AL, O'Brien T, Moyer D, Taylor CR (1982): The detection of estrogen receptors in gynecologic tumors using immunoperoxidase and the dixtran-coated charcoal assay. Cancer 49:2153–2160.
Fine S, Sturgeon JFB, Gospodorwicz MK, Dembo AJ, Bean HA, Bush RS, Beale FA, Pringle JF, Thomas GM, Herman TG, Rowlings G (1983): Treatment of advanced carcinoma of the cervix with methotrexate, adriamycin, cisplatin. Proc Am Soc Clin Oncol 2:154.
Ford LC, Berek JS, Lagasse LD, Hacker NF, Heins YL, DeLange RJ (1983): Estrogen and progesterone receptor sites in malignancies of the uterine cervix, vagina, vulva. Gynecol Oncol 15:27–31.
Forney JP, Morrow CP, DiSaia PJ, Futoran RJ (1975): Seven drug polychemotherapy in the treatment of advanced and recurrent squamous cell carcinoma of the female genital tract. Am J Obstet Gynecol 123:748–752.
Fraile RJ, Baker LH, Buroker TR (1980): Pharmacokinetics of 5-fluorouracil administered orally, by rapid intravenous and by slow infusion. Cancer Res 40:2223–2228.

Freedman RS, Herson J, Wharton JT, Rutledge FN (1980): Single agent chemotherapy for recurrent carcinoma of the cervix. Cancer Clin Trials 3:345–350.

Glaubiger D, Rama A (1982): Antitumor antibiotics in pharmacologic principles of cancer treatment. In Chabner BA (ed): "Pharmacologic Principles of Cancer Treatment." Philadelphia: WB Saunders, pp 402–415.

Gralla, RJ, Itri LM, Pisko SE, Squillante AE, Kelsen DP, Braun DW Jr, Bordin LA, Braun TJ, Young CW (1981): Antiemetic efficacy of high dose metoclopramide: Randomized trials with placebo and prochlorperazine in patients with chemotherapy-induced nausea and vomiting. N Engl J Med 305:905–909.

Greenberg BR, Kardinal CG, Pajakt F, Bateman JR (1977): Adriamycin versus adriamycin and bleomycin in advanced epidermoid carcinoma of the cervix. Cancer Treat Rep 61:1383–1384.

Greenberg BR, Hannigan J Jr, Gerretson L, Turbow MM, Friedman MA, Hendrickson CA, Glassberg A, Carter SK (1982): Sequential combination of bleomycin and mitomycin in advanced cervical cancer—an American experience: A Northern California Oncology Group Study. Cancer Treat Rep 66:163–165.

Guthrie D, Way S (1978): The use of adriamycin and methotrexate in carcinoma of the cervix. Obstet Gynecol 52:349–354.

Hahnel R, Martin JD, Masters AM, Ratijczak T, Twaddle T (1979): Estrogen receptors and blood hormone levels in cervical carcinoma and other gynecologic malignancies. Gynecol Oncol 8:226–233.

Hakes T, Majomosama N, Magill G, Ochoa M (1979): Cervix cancer: Treatment with combination vincristine and high doses of methotrexate. Cancer 43:459–469.

Hanjani P, Bonnel S (1980): Treatment of advanced and recurrent squamous cell carcinoma of the cervix with combination doxorubicin and cyclophosphamide. Cancer Treat Rep 64:1363–1365.

Hayes DM, Cvitkovic E, Golbey RB, Scheiner E, Nelson L, Krakoff IH (1977): High dose cis-platinum diammine dichloride: Amelioration of renal toxicity by mannitol diuresis. Cancer 39:1372–1381.

Hreshchyshyn MM, Holland JF (1962): Chemotherapy in patients with gynecologic cancer. Am J Obstet Gynecol 83:468–489.

Hreshchyshyn MM (1963): Vincristine treatment of patients with carcinoma of the uterine cervix. Proc Am Assoc Clin Oncol 4:29.

Jones HW, Plymate S, Gluck FB, Miles PA, Greene SF Jr (1976): Small cell non-keratinizing carcinoma of the cervix associated with ACTH production. Cancer 38:1629–1635.

Kalra J, Cortes E, Chen S, Krumholz B, Rovinsky G, Flores J, Lee J, Molho L, Lee Y (1983): Effective multimodality treatment for advanced epidermoid carcinoma of the female genital tract. Proc Am Soc Clin Oncol 2:152.

Katz ME, Glick JH (1979): Nitrosoureas: A reappraisal of clinical trials. Cancer Clin Trials 2:297–316.

Krakoff IH, Cvitkovic E, Carrie V, Yeh S, LaMonte C (1977): Clinical pharmacologic and therapeutic studies of bleomycin given by continuous infusion. Cancer 40:2027–2037.

Kramer, JK, Bateman JC, Berry GN, Kennelly JM, Klop CT, Platt LI (1952): Use of intraarterial nitrogen mustard therapy in the treatment of cervical and vaginal cancer. Am J Obstet Gynecol 63:538–548.

Krebs HB, Girtanna RE, Nordquist SR, Mineau I, Helmkamp BF, Livingston R (1980): Treatment of advanced cervical cancer by combination of bleomycin and mitomycin C. Cancer 46:2159–2161.

Lefrak EA, Pitha J, Rosenheim S, Gottlieb JA (1973): A clinicopathologic analysis of adriamycin cardiotoxicity. Cancer 32:302–314.

Legha SS, Slavik M, Carter SK (1976): Hexamethylmelamine: An evaluation of its role in therapy of cancer. Cancer 38:27–35.

Leichman LP, Baker LH, Stanhope CR, Samson MR, Fraile RJ, Vaitkevicius UK, Hilgers R (1980): Mitomycin C and bleomycin in the treatment of far-advanced cervical cancer. A Southwest Oncology Group pilot study. Cancer Treat Rep 64:1139–1140.

Malkasian GD Jr, Decker DG, Jorgensen EO (1977): Chemotherapy of carcinoma of the cervix. Gynecol Oncol 5:109–120.

Masuda H, Sumiyoshi Y, Shiojma Y, Suda T, Kikyo T, Iwata M, Fujiyoma N, Machida Y, Nagai K (1981): Local therapy of carcinoma of the uterine cervix. Cancer 48:1899–1906.

Merwe AV, duToit J, Smit B (1983): Combination chemotherapy in stage III B cervical cancer: Comparative five year survival results of cis-diamminedichloroplatinum, methotrexate, bleomycin, and radiotherapy. Proc Am Soc Clin Oncol 2:146.

Miyamoto T, Takabe Y, Watanabe M, Terasima T (1978): Effectiveness of a sequential combination of bleomycin and mitomycin C on an advanced cervical cancer. Cancer 41:403–414.

Morrow CP, DiSaia PJ, Mangan CF, Lagasse LD (1977): Continuous pelvic arterial infusion with bleomycin for squamous cell carcinoma of the cervix recurrent after radiation. Cancer Treat Rep 61:1403–1405.

Myers CE (1982): Anthacyclines in pharmacologic principles of cancer treatment. In Chabner BA (ed): "Pharmacologic Principles of Cancer Treatment." Philadelphia: WB Saunders, pp 416–434.

Omura GA, Velez-Garcia E, Birch R (1981): Phase II randomized study of doxorubicin, vincristine, and 5-FU versus cyclophosphamide in advanced squamous cell carcinoma of the cervix. Cancer Treat Rep 65:901–903.

Orwell ES, Kiessling PJ, Patterson JR (1978): Interstitial pneumonia from mitomycin. Ann Intern Med 89:352–355.

Papavasiliou C, Pappas J, Arauantinos D, Kaskarelis D (1978): Treatment of cervical carcinoma with adriamycin combined with methotrexate. Cancer Treat Rep 62:1387–1388.

Pazdur R, Bonomi P, Slayton R, Gould VE, Miller A, Jao W, Dolan T, Wilbanks G (1981): Neuroendocrine carcinoma of the cervix: Implications for staging and therapy. Gynecol Oncol 12:120–128.

Petrilli ES, Castaldo TW, Ballon SC, Roberts JA, Lagasse LD (1980): Bleomycin-mitomycin C therapy for advanced squamous carcinoma of the cervix. Gynecol Oncol 9:292–297.

Petrilli ES, Castaldo TW, Matutat RJ, Ballon SS, Gutierrez ML (1982): Bleomycin pharmacology in relation to adverse effects and renal function in cervical cancer patients. Gynecol Oncol 14:350–354.

Piver MS, Barlow JJ, Vongtoma N, Blumenson L (1977): Hydroxyurea as a radiation sensitizer in women with carcinoma of the uterine cervix. Am J. Obstet Gynecol 129:379–383.

Piver MS, Barlow JJ, Xynos FP (1978): Adriamycin alone or in combination in 100 patients with carcinoma of the cervix or vagina. Am J Obstet Gynecol 131:311–313.

Piver MS, Barlow JJ, Dunbar J (1980): Doxorubicin, cyclophosphamide, and 5-fluorouracil in patients with carcinoma of the cervix or vagina. Cancer Treat Rep 64:549–551.

Reagan JW, Hamonic MJ, Wentz WB (1957): Analytic study of the cells in cervical squamous cell cancer. Lab Invest 6:241–250.

Rutledge F (1976): Management: Treatment failures in carcinoma of the cervix. In Rutledge F, Boronow RC, Wharton JT (eds): "Gynecologic Oncology" New York: John Wiley, pp 74–760.

Smith JP, Rutledge F, Burns BC Jr, Soffar S (1967): Systemic chemotherapy for carcinoma of the cervix. Am J Obstet Gynecol 97:800–807.

Solidoro AS, Esteves L, Castellano C, Valdivia E, Barrigo O (1966): Chemotherapy of advanced cancer of the cervix: Experience in 55 cases treated with cyclophosphamide. Am J Obstet Gynecol 94:208–213.

Sullivan RD, Wood AM, Clifford P, Duff JK, Trussel R, Nary DK, Burchenal JH (1960): Continuous intra-arterial methotrexate with simultaneous, intermittent, intramuscular citrovorum factor therapy in carcinoma of the cervix. Cancer 12:1248–1261.

Surwit EA, Alberts DS, Aristazabal S, Deatherage K, Heusinkueld R (1983): Treatment of primary and recurrent advanced squamous cell cancer of the cervix with mitomycin C and vincristine and bleomycin plus cisplatin. Proc Am Soc Clin Oncol 2:153.

Swenerton KD, Evers JA, White GW, Boyes DE (1979): Intermittent pelvic infusion with vincristine, bleomycin, and mitomycin C for advanced recurrent carcinoma of the cervix. Cancer Treat Rep 63:1379–1381.

Thigpen T, Shingleton H, Homesley H, LeGasse L, Blessing J (1979): Cis-dichlorodiammine platinum (11) in the treatment of gynecologic malignancies. Phase II trials by the Gynecologic Oncology Group. Cancer Treat Rep 63:1549–1555.

Thigpen T, Vance RB, Balducci L, Blessing J (1981): Chemotherapy in the management of advanced or recurrent cervical cancer. Cancer 48:658–665.

Trope C, Johnson JE, Grundsell H, Mattson W (1980): Adriamycin-methotrexate combination chemotherapy of advanced carcinoma of the cervix. A third look. Obstet Gynecol 55:488–491.

Trope C, Johnson JE, Simonson E, Sigurdsson K, Stendahl U, Mattson W, Gullberg B (1983): Bleomycin-mitomycin in advanced carcinoma of the cervix. A third look. Cancer 51:591–593.

Vogl SE, Moukhtar M, Kaplan BH (1979): Chemotherapy for advanced cervical cancer with methotrexate, bleomycin, and cis-dichlorodiammineplatinum. Cancer Treat Rep 63:1005–1006.

Vogl SE, Moukhtar M, Calanog A, Greemld EH, Kaplan BH (1980): Chemotherapy for advanced cervical cancer with bleomycin, vincristine, mitomycin, cis-diamminedichloroplatinum II (BOMP). Cancer Treat Rep 64:1005–1007.

Vogl SE, Seltzer V, Camacho F, Calanog A (1982): Dianhydragalactitol and cisplatin in combination for advanced cancer of the cervix. Cancer Treat Rep 66:1809–1812.

Wallace HJ, Hreshchyshyn MM, Wilbanks GD, Boronow RC, Fowler WC, Blessing JA (1978): Comparison of the therapeutic effects of adriamycin alone versus adriamycin plus vincristine versus adriamycin plus cyclophosphamide in the treatment of advanced carcinoma of the cervix. Cancer Treat Rep 62:1435–1441.

Wasserman TH, Carter SK (1977): The integration of chemotherapy into combined modality treatment of solid tumors. VIII. Cervical cancer. Cancer Treat Rev 4:25–26.

Yagoda A, Mukherji B, Young C, Etcubanas E, LaMonte C, Smith JA, Tan CT, Krakoff IH (1972): Bleomycin—An antitumor antibiotic. Ann Intern Med 7:861–870.

Zelen M (1973): Keynote address on biostatistics and data retrieval. Cancer Chemother Rep 4:31–42.

Zwelling LA, Kohn KW (1982): Platinum complexes in pharmacologic princples of cancer treatment. In Chabner BA (ed): "Pharmacologic Principles of Cancer Treatment." Philadelphia: WB Saunders, pp 309–339.

Sex Steroid Receptors and Hormonal Treatment of Endometrial Cancer

R. Mortel, R. Zaino, and P.G. Satyaswaroop

Departments of Obstetrics and Gynecology (R.M., P.G.S.) and Pathology (R.Z.), The Milton S. Hershey Medical Center, Pennsylvania State University, Hershey, Pennsylvania 17033

During the past decade or more, a wide variety of experimental evidence has been generated in support of the concept of receptor-mediated mechanism of hormone action. It is now generally accepted that the interaction of the steroid with intracellular receptor protein is the primary event which triggers specific hormonal responses within target tissues. The presence of receptor molecules within the cell ensures the selective sequestration and retention of the steroid hormone. The physicochemical characteristics of the steroid receptors as well as the sequential steps involved in hormone-specific responses within the cell have been elucidated. The findings from these investigations form the basis for using steroid receptor measurements as another valuable laboratory tool in the clinician's understanding of some of the disease processes, especially the endocrine-related tumors, and in his choice of appropriate method of treatment.

Studies in experimental animal models and cell culture systems indicate a positive correlation between the concentration of receptors within the tissue and the magnitude of steroid response. In particular, cells devoid of receptors do not respond to steroids. On the basis of these findings, the measurement of receptors for estradiol and progesterone has been shown to be of clinical value in the management of patients with carcinoma of the breast [McGuire et al., 1975]. Breast cancers which are estradiol and progesterone receptor-positive are more likely to respond to hormonal therapy, either additive or ablative [Allegra et al., 1978], whereas those tumors lacking receptors are less likely to benefit from endocrine manipulation [McGuire, 1978].

Chemotherapy of Gynecologic Cancer, pages 125-138

ENDOMETRIAL CARCINOMA AND RECEPTOR MEASUREMENTS

Studies of Kelley and Baker [1960] demonstrated that metastatic endometrial carcinoma could be effectively treated with progestational agents. Objective response to progestin (17α-hydroxyprogesterone caproate, Delalutin) therapy was observed in about 35% of these patients. Since then, progestins have been generally used in the treatment of recurrent and metastatic adenocarcinoma of the endometrium with essentially similar response rates [Reifenstein, 1974; Kistner et al., 1965; Bonte, 1972; Kohorn, 1976]. A significant number of patients are unresponsive to hormonal therapy and must be provided other forms of treatments—for example, chemotherapy. It would be ideal to have a test with high predictive value for selecting patients for hormonal therapy. Unfortunately, there is no accurate test at the present time for distinguishing progestin-responsive carcinomas from nonresponsive ones; there is therefore an acute need for developing such a test.

Human endometrium is an exquisitely sensitive target tissue for ovarian steroids. And, similar to other steroid responsive tissues, endometrium also contains high-affinity, steroid-specific receptors for estradiol and progesterone [Brush et al., 1967; Evans and Hahnel, 1971; Tseng and Gurpide, 1972; Trams et al., 1973; Weist and Rao, 1971; Bayard et al., 1978; Haukkamaa and Luukkainen, 1974]. From the receptor studies in breast cancer, many investigators have explored the potential usefulness of steroid receptor status of endometrial carcinoma as an index in selecting patients for hormonal therapy. Since presence of receptor is a prerequisite for steroid action, it was inferred that the endometrial carcinomas most likely to respond to progestin treatment are those that contain receptor for progesterone.

Numerous investigators have reported on the estradiol and progesterone receptor concentration in endometrial carcinoma [Young and Cleary, 1976; Pollow et al., 1977; Janne et al., 1979; MacLaughlin and Richardson, 1976; Hunter et al., 1980; Feil et al., 1979; Prodi et al., 1979; Mortel et al., 1981]. There is considerable variation in the receptor concentrations in neoplastic endometrium reported by various investigators. Such a variation is primarily due to methodologic differences and assay conditions such as 1) measurement of total binding sites by exchange assays vs. determination of only available or unoccupied receptor sites; 2) single-point assay vs. Scatchard analysis; 3) cytoplasmic vs. total (nuclear + cytoplasmic) receptors; and 4) inclusion or noninclusion of compounds in the reaction mixture to prevent the binding of radioactive ligand to serum-binding proteins—for example, excess dihydrotestosterone in estradiol receptor assay and excess cortisol in progesterone receptor assay. Surprisingly, in spite of these differences a general pattern of receptor levels in endometrial carcinoma has emerged. The estradiol receptor concentration in the tumors examined is in the same range as in late proliferative phase of normal endometrium [Tseng et al., 1977; Mortel et al., 1981]. And essentially all carcinoma tissues are positive for estradiol receptor. The values for progesterone receptor are relatively low and comparable to those found in the secretory phase of normal menstrual cycle. A systematic study of receptor levels in both cytoplasmic and nuclear compartments of endometrial carcinoma carried out by one of us [Mortel et al., 1981] further indicates that when present, most of the receptors for estradiol and progesterone are found in the cytosol fraction, not a surprising finding since the circulating steroid levels in these postmenopausal women are low.

STABILITY OF PROGESTERONE RECEPTOR UNDER FROZEN CONDITIONS

One of the technical limitations confronting receptor laboratories is the preservation of the progesterone receptor activity of endometrial carcinoma under frozen conditions. Since facilities for PR measurement may not be available at all institutions, there is urgent need to develop a simple procedure for preserving endometrial tumor specimen without loss of PR concentrations. Freezing tumor samples and cytosol preparations has been shown to be adequate for maintaining receptor concentrations in breast cancer specimen. These procedures, although effective in normal endometrium, proved to be unsatisfactory for endometrial carcinoma. A successful method for preserving endometrial carcinoma samples for several days without appreciable loss of receptor sites is to pulverize fresh tumor specimen in liquid nitrogen and freeze the tissue powders in liquid nitrogen. Determination of PR concentrations in fresh tissue, freshly pulverized powder, and tissue powder preserved in liquid nitrogen for 7 days indicate that under these conditions, the number of P-specific binding sites were maintained without appreciable change in K_d, which ranged from 1 to 5 nM (Table I). This method of preservation not only maintains the receptor concentration in endometrial cancer specimen, but also overcomes the problem of heterogeneous distribution of PR within the sample and is being routinely used in our laboratories.

RECEPTOR CONCENTRATION AS A FUNCTION OF TUMOR GRADE

The relationship between steroid receptor concentrations and the grade of tumor differentiation has been widely studied. While there is no definite

TABLE I. Stability of Progesterone Receptor in Pulverized Endometrial Tumor Tissue Powders

	Fresh tissue		Fresh pulverized powder		Frozen tissue powder	
Specimen	fmol/mg protein	K_d (nM)	fmol/mg protein	K_d (nM)	fmol/mg protein	K_d (nM)
1	270	2.0	51	4.0	45	2.6
2	1,210	2.8	470	1.4	720	2.4
3	590	2.5	—	—	480	0.8
4	400	2.2	280	1.2	250	1.6
5	94	2.5	106	4.0	86	4.5

Surgical specimen of carcinoma of endometrium is transported chilled in nutrient medium, cut into tiny fragments, and immediately frozen in stainless steel tissue pulverizer, maintained in liquid nitrogen. The frozen pieces are then pulverized and the tissue powder is kept frozen in freeze tubes in liquid nitrogen containers. The progesterone receptor concentrations were estimated in 1) fresh, unfrozen tissue, 2) the freshly pulverized tumor tissue powder, and 3) after 7 days freezing of powder. The 105,000g supernatant of the tissue homogenates in TED buffer (20 mM Tris buffer, pH 7.8, containing 3 mM EDTA, 1 mM dithiothreitol, and 0.01% sodium azide). The cytosol fractions were incubated at 0°C for 3 h with 1–10 nM concentrations of (1,2,6,7-^{3}H) progesterone (90 Ci/mmol), either alone or in the presence of 100-fold excess unlabeled progesterone. All tubes contained 100-fold excess cortisol. Separation of bound and free ^{3}H-progesterone was effected by DCC treatment. The receptor concentrations and the apparent dissociation constant, K_d, were determined by Scatchard plot analysis of specific binding data.

pattern in the estradiol receptor levels, the progesterone receptor concentrations vary with the degree of differentiation of the tumor. Among the neoplastic endometrial tissues, the well-differentiated carcinomas contain high progesterone receptor concentrations while there is a decrease in this receptor level as the tumor appears anaplastic [Ehrlich et al., 1978; McCarty et al., 1979; Martin et al., 1979; Mortel et al., 1981; Creasman et al., 1980]. Although there is a general agreement regarding the relationship between progesterone receptors and the histologic differentiation of the tumor, the correlation is far from perfect. Several highly differentiated adenocarcinomas with low progesterone receptor concentrations and poorly differentiated tumors with significant levels of this receptor have been regularly reported. The complexity of tissue and tumor heterogeneity may be the underlying reason for such discordant results, and this is discussed in detail in a later section.

We have recently proposed a model of epithelial cell differentiation in human endometrium and its derangement leading to endometrial carcinomas of different histologic grade [Satyaswaroop and Mortel, 1981]. The relationship between the progesterone receptor concentrations and the degree of differentiation referred to above is consistent with the proposed scheme (Fig. 1). The normal endometrial differentiation is shown in the left-hand portion of the figure. According to this concept, with each menstrual cycle, the putative stem cells, presumably located in the lamina basalis, undergo sequential proliferation and differentiation resulting in the formation of progressively specialized cell populations, responsive at different stages to estradiol and progesterone, which are eventually sloughed off during menstruation. The derangement of this process leads to carcinomas of varying degree of differentiation (right-hand portion of the scheme). Neoplastic transformation may originate at any level of the hierarchy of progressively specializing cells. Malignant transformation leads to an enhanced proliferation with simultaneous diminution of differentiative potential. When the stem cell or its immediate descendant is the target cell for neoplastic transformation, the continued proliferation of this primitive cell gives rise to a poorly differentiated tumor. At the other end of the spectrum, a well-differentiated carcinoma suggests that the stem cell differentiation is preserved to a considerable degree. This concept not only provides the basis for the occurrence of endometrial carcinomas of different histologic grades, but also predicts the following pattern of distribution of receptors for estradiol and progesterone and sensitivity to these steroids in varying de-

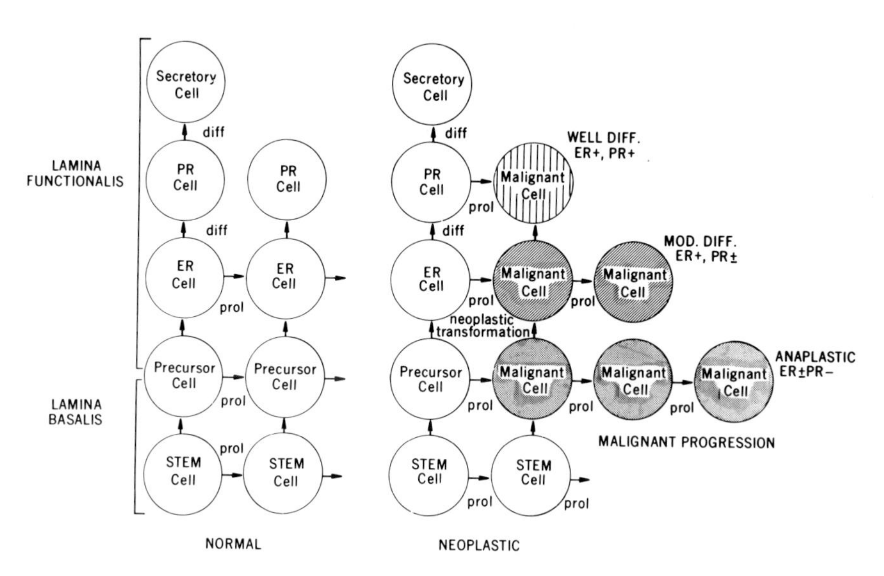

Fig. 1. Scheme of endometrial carcinoma as a defect in stem cell differentiation. Reprinted with permission from Am J Obstet Gynecol 140:620, 1981.

grees of differentiation:

Well differentiated:	ER +, PR +, E_2- and P-responsive
Moderately differentiated:	ER +, PR ±, E_2- and P-responsive (?)
Poorly differentiated:	ER ± PR −, E_2-responsive and P-nonresponsive

These predictions are borne out by the receptor measurements referred to above.

Recently, correlative studies on the progesterone receptor concentration in tumor biopsy specimen of patients and their response to progestin therapy has been carried out with a limited number of patients [McCarty et al., 1979; Martin et al., 1979; Creasman et al., 1980; Benraad et al., 1980; Kaupilla et al., 1982]. These preliminary studies suggest that although a significantly higher response rate is observed in patients with progesterone receptor-positive tumor, there is a variable response in both receptor-positive as well as receptor-negative groups.

FUNCTIONAL RECEPTORS AND DYNAMIC TESTS

The simple existence of progesterone receptor within the tumor, in itself, does not ensure that the tumor will be responsive to administered progestin. There are several steps between the initial binding of progesterone to the cytoplasmic receptor and its final effect(s) in the responsive tissue. These include 1) transformation of the progesterone-receptor complex followed by its translocation to the nucleus, 2) interaction of the progesterone-receptor complex with the chromatin resulting in gene activation, 3) synthesis of mRNAs for progestin-specific products and its transport to the cytoplasm, and 4) synthesis of progestin-specific proteins (enzymes). A defect at any of these steps will result in failure to elicit any response. Therefore, many workers have suggested that dynamic tests, tests which demonstrate the presence of functional receptor by monitoring the end effect of progesterone action, must be performed along with receptor determination.

Several investigators have carried out a variety of in vivo and in vitro dynamic tests. The in vivo approach involves the determination of specific responses of endometrial carcinoma before and after administration of progestin to the patient. In the in vitro methods, the carcinoma explants are cultured in nutrient medium in the presence and absence of progestin for 2–3 days and the progestin-specific biochemical or morphologic effects are examined in the cultured tissue fragments. The biochemical end points of progestin action investigated in these systems are glycogen accumulation [Hughes et al., 1974; Fukuma et al., 1983] and induction of the enzyme, estradiol-17β-hydroxy steroid dehydrogenase [Pollow et al., 1975; Gurpide et al., 1977; Mortel et al., 1981; Satyaswaroop and Mortel, 1982]. The progestin-induced secretory differentiation of the glandular epithelium, microscopically visualized as subnuclear vacuolization in stained sections, has also been examined [Kohorn and Tchao, 1968]. It must be pointed out that all these parameters are essentially extensions of normal endometrial responses to neoplastic tissue. Therefore, it is difficult to establish that the effects observed in biopsy specimen after progestin exposure are indeed the response of neoplastic cells only. In addition to the complexity of heterogeneity, discussed in a later section, the in vitro tests have also to consider whether or not progesterone receptor is stable under culture conditions [Satyaswaroop and Mortel, 1982]. While investigating the reason for the repeated failure of the endometrial carcinoma explants to respond to progestin in vitro, we discovered that the progesterone receptor in this tissue is surprisingly unstable under the culture conditions. About 60–75% of the original binding sites for progesterone receptor are lost within 2 h of culture and by 24 h there are no detectable receptor sites. In contrast, the proges-

TABLE II. Distribution of Cytoplasmic PR in Isolated Glands and Stroma of Human Proliferative Endometrium

	Whole tissue		Glands		Stroma	
Endometrium (proliferative)	Specific ^{3}H-P binding (fmol/mg protein)	K_d (nM)	Specific ^{3}H-P binding (fmol/mg protein)	K_d (nM)	Specific ^{3}H-P binding (fmol/mg protein)	K_d (nM)
1	416	1.4	981	1.3	118	1.1
2	171	2.2	477	2.5	13	4.0
3	1,849	3.0	1,959	3.5	70	1.6
4	910	2.8	3,287	5.0	255	3.9
5	622	1.8	1,995	3.0	50	4.8

Endometrial tissue was digested with 0.25% collagenase solution in the Ham F-10 nutrient medium for 60–90 min at 37°C as previously reported. Aliquots of cytosol fractions (105,000g supernatant) from intact tissue, isolated glands, and stroma were incubated at 0°C for 3 h with 1–10 nM concentrations of (1,2,6,7-^{3}H) progesterone (90 Ci/m mol), either alone or in the presence of 100-fold excess unlabeled P. All tubes contained 100-fold excess cortisol. Separation of bound from free ^{3}H-P was effected by DCC treatment. The receptor concentrations and the apparent dissociation constant, K_d, were determined by Scatchard plot analysis of specific binding data.

Reprinted with permission from Endocrinology 111:743, 1982.

terone receptors in normal proliferative-phase explants are remarkably maintained up to 48 h and the explants consistently respond to added progestin, as determined by a more than twofold increase in the estradiol-17β-hydroxy steroid dehydrogenase activity.

HETEROGENEITY IN ENDOMETRIAL CARCINOMA

One of the major complicating factors in all studies directed toward the development of predictive tests of progestin sensitivity of endometrial carcinoma is the complexity of multiple levels of heterogeneity commonly encountered in endometrial carcinoma. We have identified four levels of heterogeneity, and these are individually discussed below.

Cell Heterogeneity

The endometrium consists of two major cell types—glandular epithelium and stroma. Since endometrial carcinoma is of epithelial cell origin, it is necessary to first establish that receptors for estrogen and progesterone are indeed present in this cell population. We have utilized the gland isolation procedure [Satyaswaroop et al., 1978, 1979] and recently demonstrated a tenfold enrichment of receptors for progesterone within the epithelial cells (Table II) [Satyaswaroop et al., 1982]. Application of the same technique

TABLE III. Distribution of Cytoplasmic PR in Isolated Glands and Stroma of Carcinoma of Endometrium

	Whole tissue		Glands		Stroma	
Tumor grade	Specific ^{3}H-P binding (fmol/mg protein)	K_d (nM)	Specific ^{3}H-P binding (fmol/mg protein)	K_d (nM)	Specific ^{3}H-P binding (fmol/mg protein)	K_d (nM)
I	46	2.4	266	6.0	—[a]	—
I	284	1.8	388	1.2	—	—
II	182	2.9	189	1.0	48	1.6
II	98	1.7	234	1.5	—	—

Endometrial carcinoma tissue was digested with 0.25% collagenase solution in the Ham F-10 nutrient medium for 60–90 min at 37°C as previously reported. Aliquots of cytosol fractions (105,000g supernatant) from intact tissue, isolated glands, and stroma were incubated at 0°C for 3 h with 1–10nM concentrations of (1,2,6,7-^{3}H) progesterone (90 Ci/m mol), either alone or in the presence of 100-fold excess unlabeled P. All tubes contained 100-fold excess cortisol. Separation of bound from free ^{3}H-P was effected by DCC treatment. The receptor concentrations and the apparent dissociation constant, K_d, were determined by Scatchard plot analysis of specific binding data.

[a]Undetectable.

and isolation of intact glands, free of stromal cells in endometrial adenocarcinomas, shows a similar enrichment of progesterone binding sites in the cytosol fraction of the epithelial cells (Table III), in comparison with that present in the undissociated tissue [Mortel et al., 1984]. Such receptor distribution in normal and malignant endometrium suggests that progesterone receptor measurement in carcinoma tissue does indeed reflect the receptor status of cancer tissue and that stromal tumors arising from the endometrium may be devoid of progesterone receptor.

Tissue Heterogeneity

In all studies reported, receptor measurements are performed on endometrial fragments dissected from specimens obtained from patients undergoing endometrial sampling or hysterectomy for carcinoma of the endometrium. The receptor levels in the specimen assayed may not be entirely attributable to tumor, since both neoplastic and nonneoplastic tissue are usually found in the same uterus (Fig. 2) [Sommers, 1973]. Normal and hyperplastic endometria contribute variably to the receptor levels of the sample, and it

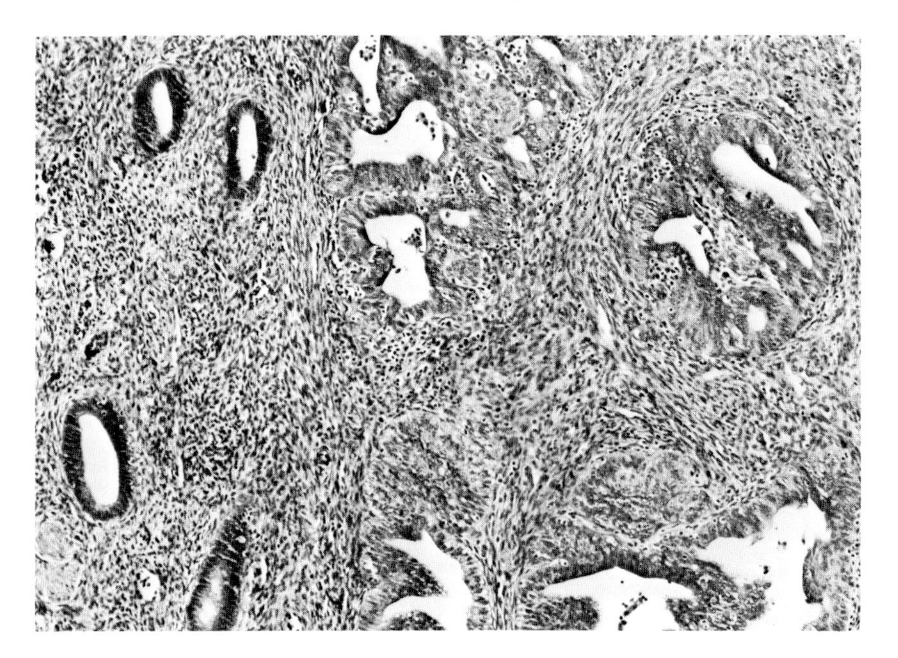

Fig. 2. Endometrium containing proliferative-phase glands adjacent to well-differentiated adenocarcinoma (hematoxylin-eosin, 58×). Reprinted with permission from Cancer 53:113, 1984.

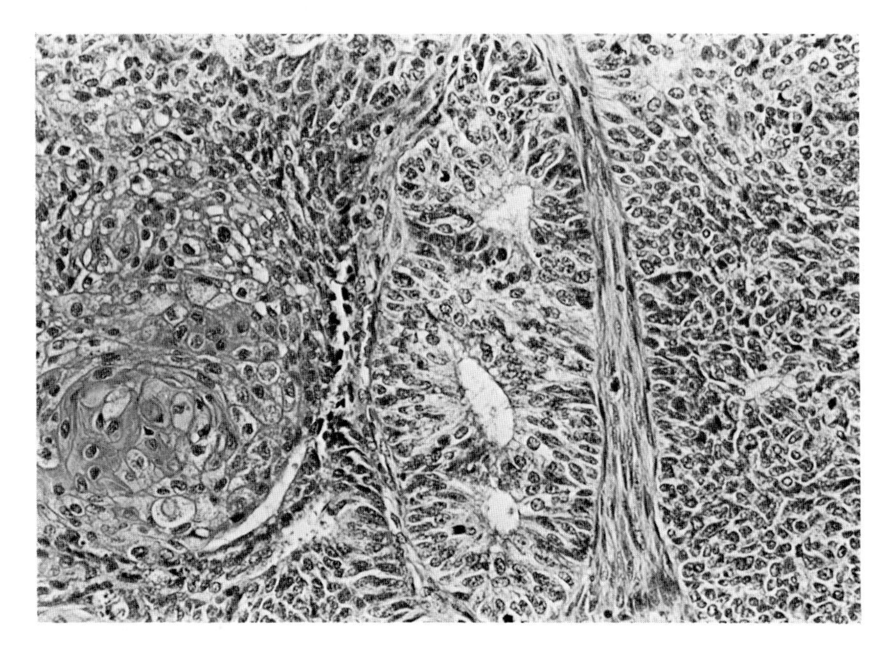

Fig. 3. Endometrium with poorly differentiated adenocarcinoma, well-differentiated adenocarcinoma, and squamous carcinoma in close juxtaposition (hematoxylin-eosin, 147×). Reprinted with permission from Cancer 53:113, 1984.

is unreliable to separate malignant from benign endometrium by gross examination alone. The epithelial cells comprise about 50% of the normal endometrium and, as shown earlier, essentially all progesterone receptor present in the proliferative endometrium is localized to this cell population. Therefore, the presence of even a small fragment of normal endometrium in the tumor specimen can significantly alter the receptor concentrations. This is quite in contrast with the determination of receptor status in breast carcinoma. In the normal breast, the epithelial cells comprise a very small portion of the total volume, and contribution to the receptor concentrations by normal tissue within the breast cancer specimen is usually negligible.

Tumor Heterogeneity

Histologic examination of endometrial carcinoma usually reveals heterogeneity within a single tumor. Using conventional architectural and cytologic criteria of differentiation, it is not uncommon to observe subpopulations of neoplastic cells with varying degrees of differentiation in different portions of the uterine tumor. For example, well-differentiated

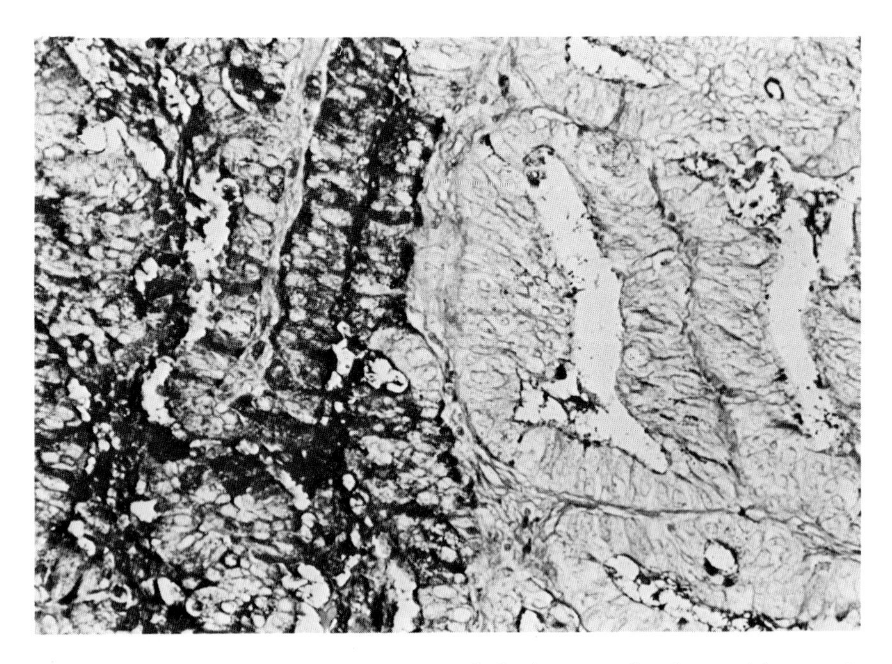

Fig. 4. Well-differentiated adenocarcinoma with focal staining for glycogen/glycoprotein (PAS without diastase, 147×). Reprinted with permission from Cancer 53:113, 1984.

adenocarcinoma is sometimes identified adjacent to foci of moderately and/or poorly differentiated tumors (Fig. 3). Under these circumstances, it is almost impossible to determine if the biologic behavior of these tumors is related to one or the other tumor cell populations present.

Microheterogeneity

Histochemical staining of tumor sections for mucins, glycogen, and glycoproteins generally reveals accumulation of these differentiated products in the cytoplasm of some neoplastic cells, in the lumen of some glands and totally absent in other areas of the tumor (Fig. 4). It is particularly interesting that the presence of these cell products does not necessarily correspond to the regions of greatest histologic differentiation as conventionally defined.

CONCLUSIONS

The various levels of heterogeneity described herein seriously interfere with the receptor determination as well as dynamic tests of progestin sensitivity of endometrial carcinoma. Surprisingly, there is very little recognition of this problem. Unlike studies in breast cancer, where receptor measurements truly reflect the endocrine status of tumor tissue, in endometrial carcinoma the presence of even a small portion of normal tissue can significantly affect the results and lead to erroneous interpretation. The ramifications of the problem of heterogeneity in endometrial carcinoma are far-reaching, and therefore receptor results from various studies must be carefully interpreted with awareness of this problem. Thus, we believe that in endometrial carcinoma it is the absence of progesterone receptor that is more meaningful for arriving at therapeutic decisions.

REFERENCES

Allegra JC, Lippman ME, Thompson EB, Simon R, Bartock A, Green L, Huff KK, Do HMI, Aitken SC, Warren R (1978): Relationship between the progesterone, androgen, and glucocorticord receptor and response rate to endocrine therapy in metastatic breast cancer. Cancer Treat Rep 62:1281–1286.

Bayard F, Damilano S, Robel P, Baulieu EE (1978): Cytoplasmic and nuclear estradiol and progesterone receptors in human endometrium. J Clin Endocrinol Metab 46:635–648.

Benraad TJ, Friberg LG, Koenders AJM, Kullander S (1980): Do estrogen and progesterone receptors in metastasizing endometrial cancers predict the response to gestagen therapy? Acta Obstet Gynecol Scand 59:155–159.

Bonte J (1972): Medroxyprogesterone in the management of primary and recurrent or metastatic uterine adenocarcinoma. Acta Obstet Gynecol Scand (Suppl) 19:21.

Brush MG, Taylor RW, King RJB (1967): The uptake of [6,7-^{3}H]-oestradiol by the normal human female reproductive tract. J Endocrinol 39:599–607.

Creasman WT, McCarty KS Sr, Barton TS, McCarty KS Jr (1980): Clinical correlates of estrogen and progesterone binding proteins in human endometrial adenocarcinoma. Obstet Gynecol 55:363–370.

Ehrlich EC, Cleary RE, Young PCM (1978) The use of progesterone receptors in the management of recurrent endometrial cancer. In Brush MG, King RJB, Taylor RW (eds): "Endometrial Cancer." London: Bailliere-Tindall, 258–264.

Evans LH, Hahnel R (1971): Oestrogen receptors in human uterine tissue. J Endocrinol 50:209–229.

Feil P, Mann W Jr, Mortel R, Bardin CW (1979): Nuclear progestin receptors in normal and malignant human endometrium. J Clin Endocrinol Metab 48:327–334.

Fukuma K, Mimori H, Matsuo I, Nakahara K, Maeyama M (1983): Hormone dependency of carcinoma of the human endometrium: Effect of progestogen on glycogen metabolism in the carcinoma tissue. Cancer 51:288–294.

Gurpide E, Tseng L, Gusberg SB (1977): Estrogen metabolism in normal and neoplastic endometrium. Am J Obstet Gynecol 129:809–816.

Haukkamaa M, Luukkainen T (1974): The cytoplasmic progesterone receptor of human endometrium during the menstrual cycle. J Steroid Biochem 5:447–452.

Hughes EC, Csermely TV, Jacobs RD, O'hern PA (1974): Biochemical parameters of abnormal endometrium. Gynecol Oncol 2:205–220.

Hunter RE, Longcope C, Jordan VC (1980): Steroid hormone receptors in adenocarcinoma of the endometrium. Gynecol Oncol 10:152–161.

Janne O, Kauppila A, Kontula K, Syrjala P, Vihko R (1979): Female sex steroid receptors in normal, hyperplastic and carcinomatous endometrium. Int J Cancer 24:545–554.

Kauppila A, Kujansuu E, Vihko R (1982): Cytosol estrogen and progesterone receptors in endometrial carcinoma of patients treated with surgery, radiotherapy and progestins. Clinical correlates. Cancer 50:2157–2162.

Kelley RM, Baker WH (1960): Progestational agents in the treatment of carcinoma of the endometrium. N Engl J Med 264:216–222.

Kistner RW, Abbott WP, Wall JA (1965): The use of progestational agents in the management of endometrial cancer. Cancer 18:1563.

Kohorn EI, Tchao R (1968): The effect of hormone on endometrial carcinoma in organ culture. J Obstet Gynaecol Br Commonw 75:1262.

Kohorn EI (1976): Gestagens and endometrial cancer. Gynecol Oncol 4:398–411.

MacLaughlin DT, Richardson GS (1976): Progesterone binding by normal and abnormal human endometrium. J Clin Endocrinol Metab 42:667–678.

Martin PM, Rolland PH, Gammerce M, Seyment H, Toga M (1979): Estradiol and progesterone receptors in normal and neoplastic endometrium: Correlations between receptors, histopathological examinations and clinical responses under progestin therapy. Int J Cancer 23:321–329.

McCarty KS Sr, Barton TK, Fetter BF, Creaseman WT, McCarty KS Jr (1979): Correlation of estrogen and progesterone receptors with histology and differentiation in endometrial adenocarcinoma. Am J Pathol 96:171–184.

McGuire WL, Carbone PO, Vollmer EP (1975): "Estrogen Receptors in Human Breast Cancer." New York: Raven Press.

McGuire WL (1978): "Hormones, Receptors and Breast Cancer." New York: Raven Press.

Mortel R, Levy C, Wolff J-P, Nicolas J-C, Robel P, Baulieu EE (1981): Female sex steroid receptors in postmenopausal endometrial carcinoma and biochemical response to antiestrogen. Cancer Res 41:1140–1147.

Mortel R, Zaino R, Satyaswaroop PG (1984): Heterogeneity and progesterone receptor distribution in endometrial adenocarcinoma. Cancer 53:113.

Pollow K, Boquoi E, Lubbert H, Pollow B (1975): Effect of gestagen therapy upon 17β-hydroxysteroid dehydrogenase in human endometrial adenocarcinoma. J Endocrinol 67:131–132.

Pollow K, Schmidt-Gollwitzer M, Nevinny Stickel J (1977): Progesterone receptor in normal human endometrium and endometrial carcinoma. Prog Cancer Res Ther 4:313–325.

Prodi G, DeGiovanni C, Galli MC, Grilli S, Rocchetta R, Orlandi C (1979): 17β-estradiol, 5α-dihydrotestosterone, progesterone and cortison receptors in normal and neoplastic human endometrium. Tumor 65:241–253.

Reifenstein EC (1974): The treatment of advanced endometrial cancer with hydroxyprogesterone caproate. Gynecol Oncol 2:377–414.

Satyaswaroop PG, Fleming H, Bresler RS, Gurpide E (1978): Human endometrial cancer cell cultures for hormonal studies. Cancer Res 38:4367–4375.

Satyaswaroop PG, Bressler RS, DelaPena MM, Gurpide E (1979): Isolation and culture of human endometrial glands. J Clin Endocrinol Metab 48:639–641.

Satyaswaroop PG, Mortel R (1981): Endometrial carcinoma: An aberration of endometrial cell differentiation. Am J Obstet Gynecol 140:620–623.

Satyaswaroop PG, Mortel R (1982): Failure of progestins to induce estradiol dehydrogenase activity in endometrial carcinoma, in vitro. Cancer Res 42:1322–1325.

Satyaswaroop PG, Wartell DJ, Mortel R (1982): Distribution of progesterone receptor, estradiol dehydrogenase and 20-α-dihydroprogesterone dehydrogenase activities in human endometrial glands and stroma: Progestin induction of steroid dehydrogenase activities in vitro is restricted to the glandular epithelium. Endocrinology 111:743–749.

Sommers SC (1973): Carcinoma of endometrium. In Norris HJ, Hertig AT, Abell MR (eds): "The Uterus." Baltimore: Williams and Wilkins, pp 276–297.

Trams G, Engel B, Lehmann F, Maass H (1973): Specific binding of oestradiol in human uterine tissue. Acta Endocrinol (Copenhagen) 72:351–360.

Tseng L, Gurpide E (1972): Nuclear concentration of estradiol in superfused slices of human endometrium. Am J Obstet Gynecol 114:995–1001.

Tseng L, Gusberg SB, Gurpide E (1977): Estradiol receptor and 17β-dehydrogenase in normal and abnormal human endometrium. Ann NY Acad Sci 286:190–198.

Weist WG, Rao BR (1971): Progesterone binding proteins in rabbit uterus and human endometrium. Adv Biosci 7:251–261.

Young PCM, Cleary RE (1974): Characterization and properties of progesterone-binding components in human endometrium. J Clin Endocrinol Metab 39:425–439.

Chemotherapy of Endometrial Carcinoma

Gunter Deppe

Division of Gynecologic Oncology, Department of Obstetrics and Gynecology, Wayne State University School of Medicine, Detroit, Michigan 48201

Endometrial carcinoma is now the most common invasive gynecologic cancer in the United States. It is estimated that in 1982 39,000 new cases were detected and 3,000 deaths occurred. Patients with localized disease are often cured with surgery and radiation therapy. A significant number of patients, however, will develop metastases that require systemic treatment with either hormonal or cytotoxic chemotherapy.

HORMONAL CHEMOTHERAPY

Kelley and Baker [1961] first reported that patients with advanced endometrial carcinoma responded to treatment with a progestational agent. In their original series they gave 17α-hydroxyprogesterone acetate (150–1000 mg weekly) to 21 patients and observed an objective response in six patients lasting from 9 months to 4½ years. They obtained a response among the patients with pulmonary metastases and well-differentiated tumors.

Hormonal treatment of metastatic endometrial adenocarcinoma became popular because of the following: 1) easy administration; 2) minimal toxicity; and 3) subjective benefit.

This frequently led to prophylactic use of progestational agents in the treatment of patients with endometrial carcinoma. Among the most frequently tested progestational agents are hydroxyprogesterone caproate, medroxyprogesterone acetate, and megestrol acetate. Objective response rates are in the range of 30% (Table I). Kohorn [1976] reviewed the literature and surveyed the members of the Society of Gynecologic Oncologists to determine the clinical use and effects of progestational agents in endometrial

Chemotherapy of Gynecologic Cancer, pages 139–150

TABLE I. Progestational Agents in Endometrial Carcinoma

Agent	No. patients	Objective response rate (%)	Reference
Hydroxyprogesterone caproate	381	32	Reifenstein, 1974 Piver et al., 1980a
Medroxyprogesterone acetate	188	31	Anderson, 1965 Kistner et al., 1965 Bonte, 1972 Smith et al., 1966 Peck and Boyes, 1969 Rozier and Underwood, 1974 Piver et al., 1980a
Megestrol acetate	125	33	Geisler, 1973 Rozier and Underwood, 1974 Wait, 1973

TABLE II. Progestational Therapy for Advanced Endometrial Carcinoma: Frequently Used Schedules

Agent	Schedule (maintenance dose)	Reference
Hydroxyprogesterone caproate	1,000 mg IM weekly	Reifenstein, 1974 Piver et al., 1980a
Megestrol acetate	40–160 mg PO daily	Geisler, 1973 Rozier and Underwood, 1974
Medroxyprogesterone acetate (oral)	200–300 mg PO daily	Anderson, 1965 Kohorn, 1980
parenteral	400–1,000 mg IM weekly	Bonte, 1972 Piver et al., 1980a

cancer. His conclusions were the following: 1) Patients with endometrial carcinoma respond to high-dose progestational agents in a third of patients; 2) most of the responders have well-differentiated tumors; 3) 15% of poorly differentiated tumors also showed a response; 4) high loading dose of progestins seems desirable; and 5) progesterone probably acts directly on the carcinomatous epithelial cells.

Various progestational agents in different doses have been tried (Table II). Geisler [1973] suggested that 160 mg of megestrol acetate per day is superior to either 40 or 80 mg per day. Sall et al. [1979] compared serum medroxyprogesterone acetate concentrations by the oral and intramuscular routes in 22 patients with recurrent endometrial carcinoma. The mean serum level in the oral group was noted to be consistently higher; however, this study did not evaluate the clinical effectiveness of the oral versus the parenteral route.

Kohorn [1980] recommends a minimal loading dose for the first 3 weeks of therapy: hydroxyprogesterone caproate (1 g per week), medroxyprogesterone acetate (1 g per week), and megestrol acetate (160 mg daily). After 3 weeks this treatment should be continued with a maintenance dose indefinitely while a response is sustained. The limiting factors may be the cost of medication and such rare side effects as fluid retention, phlebitis, or embolization.

Piver et al. [1980a] embarked on a prospective trial and allocated women with metastatic or recurrent endometrial carcinoma to either medroxyprogesterone acetate (1 g intramuscularly weekly) or 17α-hydroxyprogesterone caproate at a similar dose. Of the 114 patients 15.8% achieved an objective response with 7.0% being complete. There was no significant difference between the two regimens. The effectiveness of both regimens was not influenced by tumor size, number and site of metastases, histologic grade, or prior radiotherapy. The only significant finding was that patients whose tumor recurred 3 or more years after initial treatment responded significantly better than those with tumor recurrence less than 3 years after original therapy. There have been no reports of interference when progestational agents are used concomitantly with radiotherapy or cytotoxic chemotherapy.

The introduction of techniques for measurement of estrogen and progesterone receptors may be helpful in determining which endometrial carcinoma is progestin-responsive. Based on concepts of steroid receptor function in breast carcinoma it has been hypothesized that the antiestrogen tamoxifen could block the proliferative stimulus of estrogen in patients with advanced endometrial carcinoma. Bonte et al. [1981] used secondary tamoxifen treatment and achieved two complete regressions and seven partial regressions with a mean duration of 3 months in 17 patients with recurrent endometrial carcinoma who had previously been treated with progestins. Swenerton [1980] treated 12 patients with tamoxifen in an oral dose of 10 mg twice daily on a continuous basis. Of ten evaluable patients, one demonstrated a complete response and two a partial response with all responding patients having disease-free intervals of more than two years. Age, site of disease, or response to prior cytotoxic chemotherapy had no effect on tamoxifen response. No toxicity attributable to tamoxifen was observed. One patient who had failed progestin therapy achieved a complete response with tamoxifen. This observation suggests that the antiestrogen tamoxifen and progestins may exert their effect through different steroid receptor mechanisms and may have a synergistic inhibiting effect. Based on this theoretical consideration Swenerton treated five patients with a tamoxifen and megestrol acetate combination. Two patients had a partial response. It appears that lack of toxicity of tamoxifen would permit its use in combination with cytotoxic chemotherapy or radiotherapy.

SINGLE-AGENT CHEMOTHERAPY

Cytotoxic chemotherapy of endometrial adenocarcinoma has not been used as frequently as that of other solid tumors because of the following: 1) responsiveness of the tumor to radiation therapy and progestins; 2) limited bone marrow tolerance because of previous radiation therapy; 3) difficulty of drug delivery and evaluation of response due to postsurgical and postradiation scarring and fibrosis; and 4) patients are a poor risk for cytotoxic chemotherapy because of age and, frequently, associated medical problems (obesity, diabetes mellitus, and hypertension).

Several drugs have been tried as single agents in the treatment of patients with advanced or recurrent endometrial carcinoma. In 1974 Donovan reviewed the literature and found 186 patients who had been treated with 16 different chemotherapeutic agents, none of them in controlled studies. Among the most active and most frequently used drugs were cyclophosphamide and 5-fluorouracil (Table III). Complete responses were infrequent and, generally, of short duration.

Dvorak [1971] used cytembena in 30 patients and reported an objective improvement in ten of the patients. However, the author did not define his criteria of improvement and no survival data were reported.

Since Donovan's review the same drugs have been tried more frequently and new agents have also been studied as single agents in the treatment of advanced endometrial cancer. The data in Table IV show that adriamycin, hexamethylmelamine, and cisplatin are the most extensively reported single

TABLE III. Single-Agent Chemotherapy in Endometrial Carcinoma

Drug	Evaluable cases	Response rate (%)
5–Fluorouracil	33	24
Cyclophosphamide	22	28
Chlorambucil	11	9
Cytembena	30	33[a]

[a]Dvorak [1971] reports 33% objective "improvement." "Improvement" is not defined.
Modified from Donovan [1974].

TABLE IV. Single Agents With Activity in Endometrial Carcinoma

Drug	No. patients	Response rate (%)	Reference
Adriamycin	72[a]	32	Donovan, 1974 Thigpen et al., 1979 Horton et al., 1978
Hexamethylmelamine	20[b]	30	Seski et al., 1981c
Cisplatin	80[c]	29	Bruckner et al., 1977 Thigpen et al., 1981 Seski et al., 1981a Deppe et al., 1980 Trope et al., 1980 Loeb et al., 1975

[a]Two patients had prior cytotoxic chemotherapy.
[b]Four patients had prior cytotoxic chemotherapy.
[c]Forty-five patients had prior cytotoxic chemotherapy.

agents with activity against endometrial carcinoma. The response rates are in the range of 30%.

Adriamycin alone was tested in a phase III trial of the Gynecologic Oncology Group (GOG) [Thigpen et al., 1979]. Sixteen of 43 patients (37%) showed an objective response with a median duration of response of 4.4 months for partial responders and 7.4 months for complete responders. Previous therapy, site of metastasis, and differentiation of tumor did not appear to influence the response rate.

The Eastern Cooperative Oncology Group (ECOG) treated 21 patients with adriamycin at a dose of 50 mg/m^2 every 3 weeks with a response rate of 19% [Horton et al., 1978].

Hexamethylmelamine is a synthetic agent structurally related to triethylenemelamine. The M.D. Anderson Hospital and Tumor Institute investigated its use in a prospective single-agent clinical trial for the treatment of disseminated endometrial cancer [Seski et al., 1981c]. Hexamethylmelamine 8 mg/kg/day was given orally to 20 patients. Six patients (30%) had a partial response with a median duration of 3.5 months. No complete responders were reported. Nausea, vomiting, and neurotoxicity were the most common side effects noted. The authors stated that neurotoxicity is the limiting factor to prolonged and continuous administration of hexamethylmelamine in high doses, and if used in the treatment of endometrial cancer hexamethylmelamine should be administered intermittently, at a lower dose, and as part of a combination regimen.

Cisplatin has also been used in the management of advanced or recurrent endometrial carcinoma (Table IV). The activity of the drug has been evaluated in different dosage schedules with varying results. The Gynecologic Oncology Group [Thigpen et al., 1981] studied cisplatin at a dose of 50 mg/m^2 every 3 weeks in 23 patients with advanced endometrial cancer, 20 of whom had received prior chemotherapy. The response rate was only 4%. Seski et al. [1981a] treated 26 patients with cisplatin at a dose of 50, 70, or 100 mg/m^2 every 4 weeks. One patient demonstrated a complete response and ten patients had partial responses with the median duration of remission reported to be 5 months. The study found equivalent antitumor activity when given these different dosage levels. Twenty-one of the 26 patients with advanced or recurrent endometrial cancer had not received previous chemotherapy. Deppe et al. [1980b] administered cisplatin as a second-line agent at a dose of 3 mg/kg by 4-hour intravenous infusion. Four of 13 patients (31%) showed an objective response, with two complete responses noted. The median duration of response was 4 months.

Cisplatin was used as a first-line agent in a study of 11 patients and administered at a dose of 50 mg/m^2. A 36% response rate with one complete and three partial responses was reported [Trope et al., 1980]. Reports in the literature show wide variations in response rates to cisplatin. A realistic estimate of the true response rate may be 30%. The optimal dose and administration schedule are still not known. Although cisplatin is an attractive drug because of its lack of myelosuppressive activity, its potential nephrotoxicity and neurotoxicity may preclude prolonged administration.

COMBINATION CHEMOTHERAPY

Several combination chemotherapy regimens have been evaluated in the treatment of patients with advanced or recurrent endometrial carcinoma. Unfortunately, the majority of these studies included a progestational hormone in addition. Progestational hormones were included in all initial studies because most patients referred for cytotoxic chemotherapy had already received such agents as initial treatment. The results obtained and the dose schedules are summarized in Tables V, VI, and VII.

In a recent controlled clinical trial of 257 patients, studied by the Gynecologic Oncology Group [Cohen et al., 1983], melphalan, 5-fluorouracil, and megestrol acetate were compared to adriamycin, cyclophosphamide, 5-fluorouracil, and megestrol acetate. The dosage and schedules are listed in Table VI. The overall objective response rate was 30.8%. Response rates, duration of response, progression-free interval, and survival were nearly

TABLE V. Combination Chemotherapy and Hormones for Endometrial Carcinoma

Combination	No. patients	Response rate (%)	Reference
Melphalan 5-Fluorouracil Progestin	127	37	Cohen, 1981 Piver et al., 1980b Horton et al., 1982 Cohen et al., 1983
Adriamycin Cyclophosphamide 5-Fluorouracil Progestin	169	34	Bruckner et al., 1977 Deppe et al., 1981 Horton et al., 1982 Cohen et al., 1983
Cyclophosphamide Adriamycin Progestin	55	27	Horton et al., 1982

TABLE VI. Advanced Endometrial Carcinoma: Frequently Used Chemotherapy Schedules

Regimen	Schedule		Reference
Adriamycin	60 mg/m^2 IV	q 3 wks	Thigpen et al., 1979
Cisplatin	50–100 mg^2 IV	q 4 wks	Seski et al., 1981a
Adriamycin Cyclophosphamide	60 mg/m^2 IV 500 mg/m^2 IV	q 3 wks	GOG[a], 1983
Adriamycin Cyclophosphamide 5-Fluorouracil Megace	40 mg/m^2 IV 400 mg/m^2 IV 400 mg/m^2 IV 180 mg daily PO	q 3 wks	Cohen et al., 1983
Adriamycin Cyclophosphamide Cisplatin	50 mg/m^2 IV 600 mg/m^2 IV 60 mg/m^2 IV	q 3–4 wks	Turbow et al., 1982
Melphalan 5-Fluorouracil Medroxyprogesterone acetate	0.2 mg/kg/day PO for 3–4 days 15 mg/kg/day IV for 3–4 days 400 mg IM three times weekly	q 4 wks	Cohen, 1981

[a]Unpublished data from Gynecologic Oncology Group Annual Report 1983.

identical in the two regimens. While the overall objective response rate for these combination regimens was not higher than the objective response rate for adriamycin alone as reported in the GOG's previous study, the trend suggested a better response to combination chemotherapy in patients with poorly differentiated cancers and those with a performance status worse than 1.

TABLE VII. Combination Chemotherapy in Advanced Endometrial Carcinoma

Combination	No. patients	Response rate (%)	Reference
Adriamycin Cyclophosphamide	34	38	Muggia et al., 1977 Seski et al., 1981b
Cisplatin Adriamycin Cyclophosphamide	21	48	Turbow et al., 1982 Deppe et al., 1983
Cisplatin 5-Fluorouracil Cyclophosphamide	11	72	Bayer and Koch, 1982

In a study of the Eastern Cooperative Oncology Group [Horton et al., 1982], patients with advanced endometrial carcinoma were randomized to the following treatment schedules: 1) megestrol 80 mg, three times daily by mouth and cyclophosphamide 400 mg/m^2 IV on day 1 and doxorubicin 40 mg/m^2 IV on day 1 every 4 weeks; 2) megestrol 80 mg, three times daily by mouth, and cyclophosphamide 250 mg/m^2 IV on day 1, doxorubicin 30 mg/m^2 IV on day 1, and 5-fluorouracil 300 mg/m^2 IV on days 1–3 every 4 weeks. There was no significant difference in response rates between the two regimens. The overall response rate was 22% and the overall median survival time was 27 weeks. Patients who were unsuitable for treatment with doxorubicin received megestrol 80 mg three times daily by mouth and melphalan 6 mg/m^2 by mouth on days 1–3 and 5-fluorouracil 350/mg/m^2 IV on days 1–3 every 4 weeks. This combination produced two out of 12 objective responses. The authors concluded that the response rates of these three combinations were too low and that additional studies were needed to find drugs with greater activity.

Only a few investigators have evaluated the efficacy of combination chemotherapy without progestins in patients with advanced endometrial carcinoma. These combinations and their response rates and schedules are summarized in Tables VI and VII. Muggia et al. [1977] gave adriamycin (37.5 mg/m^2) and cyclophosphamide (500 mg/m^2) intravenously every 3 weeks to 11 patients. There were five objective responses in eight patients receiving adequate therapy.

Seski et al. [1981b] used the same drug combination but administered 40–50 mg/m^2 of adriamycin and 400–500 mg/m^2 of cyclophosphamide intravenously every 4 weeks. Eight of 26 patients showed a partial response, and

TABLE VIII. Chemotherapy of Advanced Endometrial Carcinoma

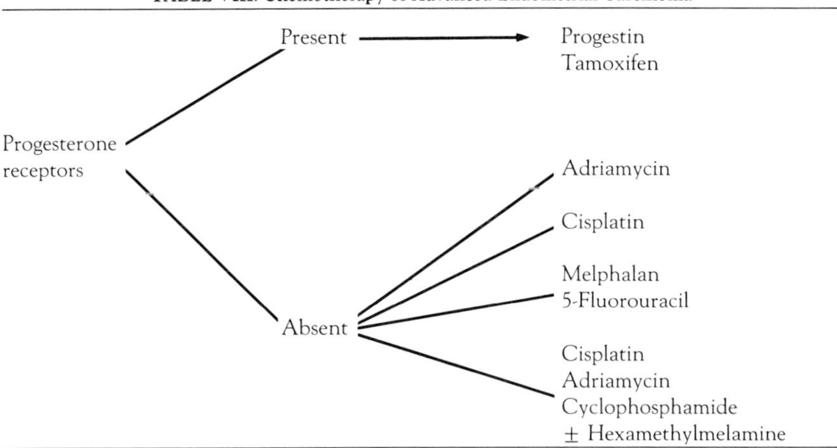

no complete responses were reported. The median duration of response was 4 months.

Turbow et al. [1982] combined adriamycin (50 mg/m^2) with cyclophosphamide (600 mg/m^2) and cisplatin (60 mg/m^2) given every 3–4 weeks intravenously. Of 20 evaluable patients seven had a partial response and two a complete response. The median duration of response was 8 months, with two patients responding longer than 18 months.

Cyclophosphamide, 5-fluorouracil, and cisplatin were given every 4 weeks to 11 patients [Bayer and Koch, 1982]. There were three complete responses and five partial responses with a median duration of 6 months. All of the above reports of combination chemotherapy are subject to obvious criticism because of the small number of patients in the studies and their lack of control; thus no definitive conclusions can be drawn.

The various reports cited in this review established the usefulness of nonhormonal cytotoxic chemotherapy in the treatment of patients with advanced endometrial carcinoma. Future areas of investigation into possible cure of advanced endometrial carcinoma with chemotherapy should include the following: 1) improved dosage schedules of known active agents; 2) evaluation of new cytotoxic drugs; 3) in vitro cell culture drug sensitivity techniques; and 4) the role of cytoplasmic progesterone and/or estradiol receptors for identification of progestin or tamoxifen response.

The Gynecologic Oncology Group has an ongoing phase II program to evaluate new agents in endometrial carcinoma. The GOG is also studying in a therapeutic trial the response to oral progestins in patients with advanced or recurrent endometrial carcinoma. Patients with documented failure to hormonal therapy will be randomized to either a single-agent adriamycin regimen or to combination chemotherapy, consisting of adriamycin and cyclophosphamide.

Several tentative conclusions might be drawn from the limited experience with chemotherapy of advanced endometrial adenocarcinoma:

1) The most active drugs are adriamycin, hexamethylmelamine, and cisplatin.
2) Combination chemotherapy has not shown a statistically significant increase of response rates in controlled trials.
3) Progestins alone have an overall response rate of 30%. However, only 15% of poorly differentiated endometrial carcinomas respond.
4) Progestins have been included in many regimens; although its toxicity is minimal, its contribution to response is uncertain.
5) Tamoxifen, an antiestrogen, merits further study.

These observations would suggest that in the absence of progesterone receptor binding sites and lack of response to tamoxifen, the most active agents should be used alone or in combination. Hexamethylmelamine appears to have limited usefulness as a single agent because of neurotoxicity when administered over a prolonged period. Until randomized prospective multi-institutional trials can give us a definite answer to the question of the best chemotherapeutic protocol for patients with advanced endometrial cancer, the approach recommended is that presented in Table VIII.

REFERENCES

Anderson DG (1965): Management of advanced endometrial adenocarcinoma with medroxyprogesterone acetate. Am J Obstet Gynecol 92:87–99.

Bayer GK, Koch PD (1982): High response rate with combination chemotherapy for advanced endometrial carcinoma. Proc Am Assoc Cancer Res 1:121.

Bonte J (1972): Medroxyprogesterone in the management of primary and recurrent or metastatic uterine adenocarcinoma. Acta Obstet Gynecol Scand (Suppl) 19:21–24.

Bonte J, Ide P, Billiet G, Wynants P (1981): Tamoxifen as a possible chemotherapeutic agent in endometrial adenocarcinoma. Gynecol Oncol 11:140–161.

Bruckner HW, Cohen CJ, Deppe G, Kabakow B, Wallach RC, Greenspan EM, Gusberg SB, Holland JF (1977): Chemotherapy of gynecological tumors with platinum II. J Clin Hematol Oncol 7:619–632.

Bruckner HW, Deppe G (1977): Combination chemotherapy of advanced endometrial adenocarcinoma with adriamycin, cyclophosphamide, 5-fluorouracil and medroxyprogesterone acetate. Obstet Gynecol 50:10s–12s.

Cohen CJ (1981): Advanced (FIGO stages III, IV) and recurrent carcinoma of endometrium. In Coppleson M (ed): "Gynecologic Oncology, Fundamental Principles and Clinical Practice," Vol 2. New York: Churchill Livingstone, pp 578–587.

Cohen CJ, Bruckner HW, Deppe G, Blessing JA, Homesley H, Lee JH, Watring W (1983): A randomized study comparing multi-drug chemotherapeutic regimens in the treatment of advanced and recurrent endometrial carcinoma: A Gynecologic Oncology Group study. Am J Obstet Gynecol (in press).

Deppe G, Jacobs AJ, Cohen CJ (1980a): Second-look operation in endometrial cancer. Diagn Gynecol Obstet 2:193–195.

Deppe G, Cohen CJ, Bruckner HW (1980b): Treatment of advanced endometrial adenocarcinoma with cis-dichlorodiammineoplatinum (II) after intensive prior therapy. Gynecol Oncol 10:51–54.

Deppe G, Jacobs AJ, Bruckner HW, Cohen CJ (1981): Chemotherapy of advanced and recurrent endometrial carcinoma with cyclophosphamide, doxorubicin, 5-fluorouracil and megestrol acetate. Am J Obstet Gynecol 140:313–316.

Deppe G (1982): Chemotherapeutic treatment of endometrial carcinoma. Clin Obstet Gynecol 25:93–99.

Deppe G, Liu TL (1983): Treatment of advanced endometrial carcinoma with cisplatin, cyclophosphamide and doxorubicin. (Submitted.)

DiSaia PJ, Creasman WT (1981): Adenocarcinoma of the uterus. In DiSaia PJ, Creasman WT (eds): "Clinical Gynecologic Oncology." St. Louis: CV Mosby, pp 128–152.

Donovan JF (1974): Nonhormonal chemotherapy of endometrial adenocarcinoma: A review. Cancer 34:1587–1592.

Dvorak O (1971): Cytembena treatment of advanced gynaecological carcinomas. Neoplasma 18:461–464.

Geisler HE (1973): The use of megestrol acetate in the treatment of advanced malignant lesions of the endometrium. Gynecol Oncol 1:340–344.

Horton J, Begg CB, Arseneault J, Bruckner HW, Creech R, Hahn RG (1978): Comparison of adriamycin with cyclophosphamide in patients with endometrial cancer. Cancer Treat Rep 62:159–161.

Horton J, Elson P, Gordon P, Hahn R, Creech R (1982): Combination chemotherapy for advanced endometrial cancer. An evaluation of three regimens. Cancer 49:2441–2445.

Kelley RM, Baker WH (1961): Progestational agents in the treatment of carcinoma of the endometrium. N Engl J Med 264:216–222.

Kistner RW, Griffith CT, Craig JM (1965): The use of progestational agents in the management of endometrial cancer. Cancer 18:1563–1579.

Kohorn EI (1976): Gestagens and endometrial carcinoma. Gynecol Oncol 4:398–411.

Kohorn EI (1980): Hormonal and nonhormonal chemotherapy of endometrial carcinoma. In Sciarra JJ, Buchsbaum HJ (eds): "Gynecology and Obstetrics," Vol 4. Hagerstown, Maryland: Harper and Row, pp 1–19.

Loeb E, Hill JM, MacLellan A (1975): Cis-platinum (II) diammine dichloride treatment of squamous cell carcinoma. Wadley Med Bull 5:281–285.

Muggia FM, Chia G, Reed LJ, Romney SL (1977): Doxorubicin-cyclophosphamide: Effective chemotherapy for advanced endometrial adenocarcinoma. Am J Obstet Gynecol 128:314–319.

Peck JG, Boyes DA (1969): Treatment of advanced endometrial carcinoma with a progestational agent. Am J Obstet Gynecol 103:90–91.

Piver MS, Barlow JJ, Lurain JR, Blumenson LE (1980a): Medroxyprogesterone acetate (Depo-Provera) vs. hydroxyprogesterone caproate (Delalutin) in women with metastatic endometrial adenocarcinoma. Cancer 45:268–272.

Piver MS, Lele S, Barlow JJ (1980b): Melphalan, 5-fluorouracil, and medroxyprogesterone acetate in metastatic or recurrent endometrial carcinoma. Obstet Gynecol 56:370–372.

Reifenstein EC Jr (1974): The treatment of advanced endometrial cancer with hydroxyprogesterone caproate. Gynecol Oncol 2:377–414.

Rozier JC Jr, Underwood PB Jr (1974): The use of progestational agents in endometrial adenocarcinoma. Obstet Gynecol 44:60–64.

Sall S, DiSaia P, Morrow CP, Mortel R, Prem K, Thigpen T, Creasman W (1979): A comparison of medroxyprogesterone serum concentrations by the oral or intramuscular route in patients with persistent or recurrent endometrial carcinoma. Am J Obstet Gynecol 135:647–650.

Seski JC, Edwards CL, Herson J, Rutledge FN (1981a): Cisplatin chemotherapy for disseminated endometrial cancer. Obstet Gynecol 59:225–228.

Seski JC, Edwards CL, Gershenson DM, Copeland LJ (1981b): Doxorubicin and cyclophosphamide chemotherapy for disseminated endometrial cancer. Obstet Gynecol 58:88–91.

Seski JC, Edwards CL, Copeland LJ, Gershenson DM (1981c): Hexamethylmelamine chemotherapy for disseminated endometrial cancer. Obstet Gynecol 58:361–363.

Smith JP, Rutledge F, Soffar SW (1966): Progestins in the treatment of patients with endometrial adenocarcinoma. Am J Obstet Gynecol 94:977–984.

Swenerton KD (1980): Treatment of advanced endometrial adenocarcinoma with tamoxifen. Cancer Treat Rep 64:805–811.

Thigpen T, Buchsbaum HJ, Mangan C, Blessing JA (1979): Phase II trial of adriamycin in the treatment of advanced or recurrent endometrial carcinoma. A Gynecologic Oncology Group study. Cancer Treat Rep 63:21–27.

Thigpen T, Vance RB, Balducci L, Blessing J (1981a): Chemotherapy in the management of advanced or recurrent cervical and endometrial carcinoma. Cancer 48:658–665.

Thigpen T, Blessing J, DiSaia P, Lagasse L (1981b): Phase II trial of cis-diamminedichloroplatinum (CDDP) in the management of advanced or recurrent endometrial carcinoma. Proc Am Soc Clin Oncol 22:469.

Trope C, Grundsell H, Johnsson J-E, Cavallin-Stohl E (1980): A phase II study of cis-platinum for recurrent corpus cancer. Eur J Cancer 16:1025–1026.

Turbow MM, Thornton J, Ballon S, Koretz MM, Torti FM (1982): Chemotherapy of advanced carcinoma with platinum, adriamycin and cyclophosphamide (PAC). Proc Am Assoc Cancer Res 1:108.

Varga A, Henriksen E (1965): Histologic observations on the effect of 17-alpha-hydroxyprogesterone-17-n-caproate on endometrial carcinoma. Obstet Gynecol 26:656–664.

Wait RB (1973): Megestrol acetate in the management of advanced endometrial carcinoma. Obstet Gynecol 41:129–136.

Chemotherapy: The Common Epithelial Ovarian Carcinomas

Howard Warren Bruckner

Departments of Medicine and Neoplastic Diseases, Mount Sinai School of Medicine of the City University of New York, New York, New York 10029

Ovarian cancer claims a life every 15 minutes in the United States. The number of new cases increases each year. Fortunately innovations in diagnosis (staging), surgery, and chemotherapy may, with wide application, shortly counter this trend. Evolving therapeutic investigations have curative potential and therefore make changes in therapy of immediate critical importance. As little as a 10% increase in survival can save more than 1,000 women each year in the United States alone.

PROGNOSIS

Prognostic characteristics identify specific patients who may be cured by specific treatments. An examination of prognostic characteristics and their relationship to the results of therapy suggests that ovarian cancer is in fact a heterogeneous disease. Current treatments can ideally be compared and improved in the group of patients who currently have a good prognosis—e.g., patients with both well-differentiated (grade 1 and 2 and possibly grade 3 tumors) and small (less than 1, 2, or 3 cm) residual tumors. These patients have a 50–90% chance of achieving surgically proven complete remission with 6–12 months of combination chemotherapy. Single agents are less effective in producing surgical complete remission. The combination regimen of choice is unknown because there have been few direct comparisons. In contrast patients with grade 4 or large tumors can be offered innovative investigational therapy because they continue to have only a poor 10–20%

Chemotherapy of Gynecologic Cancer, pages 151-193

prognosis for cure in spite of the 70–90% response rates achieved with many combination chemotherapy cis-platin regimens. Age over 50, incomplete surgery, and severe symptoms due to disease are also poor prognostic characteristics; however, they are relatively unimportant compared to tumor grade and size. Cis-platin combination therapy has produced the best palliative results as measured by response rate and progression-free interval of any combinations for patients with a poor prognosis.

Pathological information is of major prognostic importance—particularly accurate grading and sizing of tumors. Griffiths [1975], Wharton et al. [1980], Dembo et al. [1982], and Deligdisch et al. [1982] found the four common epithelial tumors serous, mucinous, endometrioid, and solid adenocarcinomas to have identical prognosis. Clear cell carcinomas, however, have a markedly worse prognosis than the common tumors.

Undifferentiated or rare morphology tumors require special pathological examinations. Some 5% of all "ovarian" tumors are metastatic from the breast, rectum, cecum, appendix, uterus, or stomach. This is an especially important consideration if patients are young or have an early stage of disease or if there is an atypical distribution of metastases. Nadji et al. [1983] used special histochemical and immunochemical stains and found as many as 10% of all ovarian tumors originally considered to be epithelial in origin to be germ cell or other non-epithelial tumors.

GRADE

Borderline tumors are probably refractory to standard intensive single-agent or combination chemotherapy. Experience is anecdotal. Sixty percent of patients with stage III borderline tumors will survive 5 years. These patients are optimum candidates for complete and elective second or third resections. Serial laparoscopy as recommended by the author is under GOG investigation in order to evaluate these patients for objective evidence of progression. Only half the patients with stage III–IV disease will demonstrate progression and require any therapy after surgery. These patients are in theory optimum candidates for tests of biologic modifiers, redifferentiation agents, or monoclonal antibodies, systemically or as intraperitoneal treatment.

Grade 1 epithelial tumors approach the borderline tumors in prognosis. Wharton et al. [1980] concluded that, unlike borderline tumors, grade 1 tumors almost consistently responded to chemotherapy. Patients with grade 1 tumors in chemotherapy studies for advanced carcinoma should be reported separately, because the exceptional survival of a small number of such patients may produce a misleading result not applicable to the other patients. Tumor grade individually affected survival, P 0.0001. Sixty-one percent of 13 patients with grade 1 tumors were alive at 48 months compared to 19% of 62 patients with grade 2 tumors and only 9% of 102 patients with grade 3 tumors. (Only tumor grade and age retained prognostic significance.) With adjustment for tumor grade and length of follow-up, tumor diameter tended to lose its prognostic significance. Only 25% of patients with tumors 2 cm or smaller were alive at 48 months. This analysis provides a strong note of caution against single-agent chemotherapy for small tumors. The distinction between borderline and grade 1 tumors is unclear in this report. Wharton's analysis also found that melphalan was a superior single agent compared to hexamethylmelamine, adriamycin, and 5FU. It was too early to provide a comparison between melphalan and cis-platinum. Each effected survival P 0.003.

Griffiths [1975] employed multiple regression equation methods in a period of suboptimum single-agent chemotherapy and radiotherapy in order to identify the prognostic characteristics of patients with stage II and III ovarian carcinoma. Clear cell carcinoma ($P < 0.001$) and the histologic grade ($P < 0.001$) had a greater adverse effect then residual tumor size ($P = 0.02$). Tumor grade was the dominant prognostic characteristic.

Ozols et al. [1979, 1980] found combination chemotherapy with HexaCAF to produce only a marginal statistical advantage compared to L-PAM (grade 2, unevaluable; grade 3, $P < 0.1$). It was not possible to make a clear distinction between the prognostic significance of tumor grade and tumor size because 8/8 patients with tumors 2 cm or smaller survived as did 5/6 (1 leukemia death) patients with borderline "grade 1–2" tumors. Unlike others, these investigators implied a possible role for chemotherapy of borderline tumors.

Grade 3 and 4 tumors appear very responsive to platinum regimens as described by Bruckner et al. [1981f, 1983a]. AP was superior to standard drugs TSPA/MTX and CHAP I was superior to AP for patients with poorly differentiated tumors independent of tumor size. Median survival was 28 (CHAP) and 18 (AP, P) months. CHAP was not superior to AP in its ability to produce complete remission proven by second-look surgery. In contrast Bruckner et al. [1983b] found AP equal to CAP in all prognostic subsets defined by grade or size of tumor. Deligdisch et al. [1983] confirmed that cisplatin overcomes the historical poor prognosis for patients with poorly differentiated tumors at least for the first 24 months of follow-up.

Ehrlich et al. [1983] found that patients with well-differentiated grade 1–2 tumors have significantly better median survival (33 vs. 21 months, $P = 0.04$) than patients with grade 3–4. This is similar to the advantage based on tumor size (smaller than 3 cm), 39 vs. 22.5 months for patients with larger tumors. Neijt et al. [1983] also found that optimum survival with CHAP V was demonstrable in patients with well-differentiated tumors. Small tumor size was the dominant and independent confounding prognostic characteristic.

RESIDUAL TUMOR SIZE

Griffiths et al. [1975, 1979] examined survival by diameter of largest residual tumor in 102 patients treated with standard alkylating agents and divided patients into good-risk and bad-risk prognostic groups on the basis of the size of the single largest residual tumor size. The median survival was 18 months if tumors were larger than 1.5 cm. However, 28 patients whose tumors were 0.5 cm or less had a median survival of 29 months, and patients with no visible residual disease had a median survival of 39 months. The effect of grade was not discussed; however, it was identified as the dominant prognostic characteristic in the 1975 analysis.

Griffiths [1980] provided a dramatic demonstration of the impact of tumor size on the chance of achieving surgically proven complete response by combining his experience with that of Wharton et al. [1979], and Parker et al. [1980]. Single agents were inferior to combination therapy only against small tumors. With tumors of 2 cm or less, 18% of 17 patients achieved surgical complete remission with hexamethylmelamine and 18% of 11 patients achieved surgical complete remission with melphalan (L-PAM). With tumors larger than 2 cm 0/37 achieved complete remission with HMM and 15% of 26 achieved complete remission with L-PAM. In contrast, with adriamycin plus cyclophosphamide 90% of 12 patients, and with HexaCAF 100% of 8 patients with small tumors achieved surgical complete remission. With larger tumors 16% of 32 with HexaCAF and 3% of 29 with adriamycin-Cytoxan achieved surgical complete remission.

This demonstrates combining maximum cytoreductive surgery and intensive adjuvant combination chemotherapy as the only current strategy with curative potential. However, these were selected series and the sample sizes are too small to allow comparison of these regimens to other combinations.

Interim collaborative group survival analysis of the GOG trials by Omura et al. [1981] testing CTX-HMM, ADM-CTX, and L-PAM, and ECOG trials by Bruckner et al. [1979, 1983b] testing L-PAM, TSPA/MTX, and CYT-ADM-5FU find only patients with tumors of 0.5 cm or less to have any prognostic advantage defined by tumor size.

Griffiths et al. [1979] debulked 79% of 28 consecutive patients demonstrating the technical feasibility of this strategy. The patients were presumably selected for optimum age and general health because debulking requires extensive surgery and supportive care often including hyperalimination. Parker et al. [1983] failed in an attempt to apply these results prospectively in conjunction with CAP combination therapy. Only some 20% of patients were optimally debulked by performing additional early surgery once patients achieved partial remissions. It appeared that "debulking would be valueless unless all tumor masses larger than 1.5 cm in diameter were removed." Neijt et al. [1983] have similarly failed to demonstrate an advantage for "early" debulking during chemotherapy of patients with good partial remissions. Both trials lacked "no early surgery" controls. At best, 20% of patients may benefit from this additional surgery. However, these may be the same patients who will achieve surgical complete remission or excellent palliation without further surgery.

Cis-platin regimens are also clearly affected adversely by tumor size. Decker et al. [1982] and Bell et al. [1982] examined regimens consisting of cyclophosphamide 1,000 or 750 mg/m^2 respectively in combination with cis-platin 50 mg/m^2. The former treated well-debulked patients and the latter poorly debulked patients. The trials provided evidence that CP is superior to CYC and CLB respectively; however, overall results worsen drastically with increasing tumor size. Although CP produced a significantly better response rate, Bell's median survivals were equal at 16 months. Decker found that only 5/21 patients achieved surgical complete response although 19 were well debulked initially. Median progression-free survival time was only 28 months. These results may be inferior to those achieved with other cis-platin combinations in similar patients. Direct comparative testing is now in progress.

Some platinum combinations appear to improve the patient's prognosis compared to L-PAM or standard combinations, especially when patients have poor prognostic features. Bruckner et al. [1981f, 1983a] in a study of AP vs. CHAP, Mangioni et al. [1980, 1981] in a study of PAC vs. HAC, Vogl et al. [1982] in a study of CHAD vs. L-PAM, and Cohen et al. [1983] in a further analysis of AP and CHAP all found that the platinum regimens improve surgical complete response or survival compared to conventional non-cis-platin regimens if residual tumors are larger that 2 cm, up to 5–6 cm in the case of PAC and CHAP, and possibly up to 10 cm in the case of CHAD. Patients with large tumors have a 10–15% chance of achieving surgically proven complete remission with platinum combination therapy. The chance may improve progressively as the tumor decreases in size from

10 toward 2 cm. It is unclear if this justifies suboptimum debulking because chemotherapy is 80–90% effective in a palliative role. Nevertheless, debulking is the only strategy for improving results with current chemotherapy regimens.

Greco et al. [1981a,b, 1982] describe a single institutional phase II experience for patients with tumors of 3 cm or less, treated with a day-1,8 CHAP regimen, which is more intensive than the conventional CHAP or CHAD regimens: 14/16 (87%) had surgically proven complete remissions. Patients with large tumors had a 3/29 (10%) surgical complete remission. Second-look surgery was performed after only 6 months of treatment. Remissions have been maintained without treatment for some 2 years.

Neijt et al. [1983] found that CHAP V was superior to HexaCAF only in the subgroup with tumors of 1 cm or less. All reports require a confirmatory trial and further direct comparison to regimens such as HexaCAF or ADM/CYC and even L-PAM. The number of patients is too small and the description of prognostic factors is inadequate to allow any conclusive comparison between cis-platin and non-cis-platin combinations. There is no cause for accepting any one of the cis-platin regimens as entirely satisfactory or accepting the regimens as equal. Several platinum combinations are only 20–30% effective in producing surgical complete response even for patients with small tumors (e.g., Ehrlich et al. [1979, 1980, 1983] CAP I and CAP V, Decker et al. [1982], Vogel et al. [1982] CHAD, Cohen et al. [1983] AP and CHAP). The upper limit of optimum tumor size cannot be defined. Additional factors are not described including the relation between size and number and location of nodules and grade of tumor. Various authors report the critical cutoff at 0.5–1, 1.5, 2, or 3 cm. Only the CHAP V regimen and CHAP 1,8 and the most intensive versions of HexaCAF and AC produce attractive surgical complete response rates. Smaller size is always better, and complete removal of visible tumor is the only certain optimum debulking.

AGE

Young age is associated with a good prognosis but is confounded by a higher proportion of patients with low-grade tumors and less advanced stages of disease.

Wharton [1980] found age below 45 to be a favorable prognostic factor, but far less important than tumor grade and treatment. L-PAM, DDP, and HAC (hexamethylmelamine plus adriamycin plus cyclophosphamide) tend to overcome age as a prognostic factor. Griffiths [1975] did not find age to be a significant prognostic characteristic. Edmondson et al. [1979] observed a significant negative prognostic effect associated with perimenopausal status. In postmenopausal patients treated with CYC or AC, survival improved further after adjustment for performance status. This has not been observed by others.

Bruckner et al. [1980a, 1981d] demonstrated that patients older than 60 failing prior chemotherapy had a significantly better rate of response to cis-platinum regimens than younger patients. This was independent of other patient characteristics. Vogl et al. [1982] reported that patients over 50 treated with cis-platin combinations have better response rates and survival without excessive toxicity than patients treated with L-PAM. Age over 60 is definitely not a contraindication to cis-platin therapy, and is possibly an indication for cis-platin therapy because age has less adverse an impact on cis-platin than on conventional regimens.

Bruckner et al. [1979, 1983b] also found that age influences response rates. Young patients have higher rates of response than older patients when treated with L-PAM, TSPA/MTX, or CAF. Age is a stratification variable for prospective trials and for analysis of treatments.

Performance status remains important for stratification and analyses of clinical trials. Completely ambulatory patients do best both in response rate and in survival. Bruckner et al. [1981f and unpublished] found that AP and CHAP tend to diminish the adverse prognostic significance of poor performance status compared to conventional drug combinations. However, the cis-platin regimens do not abolish the prognostic impact of performance status.

In summary, HexaCAF is only marginally superior to L-PAM for grade 2 and 3 tumors, and an adriamycin cis-platium combination is superior to TSPA-MTX for patients with grade 3 and 4 tumors. The case for AP or CHAP cis-platin combinations as palliative treatment compared to standard alkylating agents improves as the prognosis associated with the grade of or size of tumor or the age of the patient worsens. However, only the most alkylating agent–intensive cis-platin regimens CHAP 1,8 and CHAP V are competitive with and possibly superior to the best results reported with HexaCAF and ADM-CYC for patients with small well-differentiated tumors. Direct comparative trials are required in order to clarify the relationship between good prognostic characteristics and choice of treatment.

STAGING—CHEMOTHERAPEUTIC IMPLICATIONS

Optimum surgical and pathological staging requires increasingly extensive exploration. The findings determine the choice of treatment for patients with stage I, II, and III with small residual disease. Past general treatment strategies are largely obsolete and possibly ineffective or even harmful. These have been replaced by treatments based on information derived from optimum staging.

The availability of effective (perhaps 80%) curative therapy for microscopic disease makes full staging efforts which identify microscopic disease imperative, because 80% of understaged patients will not be saved by later treatment. Chemotherapy will only cure 10–20% if treatment is delayed until there is clinical recurrence because recurrence implies large tumors. Efforts at early diagnosis of recurrence are currently unreliable. Serial laparoscopy has not been tested.

Only patients with stage I or II disease (Table I) require complete staging because stage and choice of treatment can change with further tests. Proof of residual disease will clearly indicate the need for combination chemotherapy. Complete staging procedures include 1) preoperative staging with laparoscopy, 2) four-quadrant cytology, 3) examination of the diaphragms, 4) sampling of retroperitoneal lymph nodes, and 5) a complete BSOH and omentectomy.

Extensive staging will identify many of the 20–40% of falsely understaged stage I and (40–60%) of understaged stage II patients. Young et al. [1979] reported that many will be identified by radiologic tests and laparoscopy in

TABLE I. Staging of Ovarian Carcinoma (International Federation of Gynecology and Obstetrics)

Stage I:	Growth limited to ovaries
	A. Growth limited to one ovary; no ascites
	1. No tumor on the external surface; capsule intact
	2. Tumor present on the external surface and/or capsule
	B. Growth limited to both ovaries; no ascites
	1. No tumor on the external surface; capsule intact
	2. Tumor present on the external surface and/or capsule(s)
	3. Tumor stage either Ia or Ib, but with ascites present or positive peritoneal washings
Stage II:	Growth involving one or both ovaries with pelvic extension
	A. Extension and/or metastases to the uterus and/or tubes
	B. Extension to other pelvic tissues
	C. Tumor stage either IIa, IIb, but with ascites present or with positive peritoneal washings
Stage III:	Growth involving one or both ovaries with intraperitoneal metastases outside the pelvis and/or positive retroperitoneal nodes; limited to the true pelvis, histologically proven malignant extension to small bowel or omentum
Stage IV:	Growth involving one or both ovaries with distant metastases. If pleural effusion is present, there must be positive cytology to allot a case to stage IV; parenchymal liver metastases equal stage IV
Special category—V—or explored cases thought to be ovarian carcinoma	

NCI-GOG trials. Some 20% of "stage I or II" patients have lymph node involvement demonstrated either by lymphangiography and selective biopsy or simply by random biopsy. Some 20% of "stage II" patients will have disease usually on the right diaphragm demonstrated by systematic staging laparoscopy with selective cytologic and biopsy techniques. Chen et al. [1983] found that patients with poorly differentiated or lymphocyte-depleted tumors are at especially high risk and that further staging procedures may reveal metastatic lymph node involvement.

For poorly staged patients single-agent chemotherapy with L-PAM as described by Hreshchyshyn et al. [1980] only tends to reduce the risk of recurrence. L-PAM and various sequences of radiotherapy and single-agent chemotherapy are probably not cost-effective, especially after weighing the risk of late leukemia described by Reimer et al. [1977], Einhorn et al. [1982], and Green et al. [1982]. Intraperitoneal ^{32}P and L-PAM are about equally effective in an ongoing trial for early well staged low risk patients. The logical choices, by extrapolation, are short courses of combination chemotherapy or whole abdominal radiotherapy.

Young et al. [1983] found that optimally staged patients with Ia, Ib resected low-grade tumors probably require no further treatment.

Patients must be restaged if they are not adequately staged at primary surgery. Patients with low potential "borderline" malignancies appear to be the only exception. Laparoscopy may be a useful baseline and follow-up test.

Diagnostic Considerations

Diagnostic and staging tests short of surgery have become increasingly superfluous because the need for adequate debulking to allow curative and adjuvant chemotherapy has made surgery both the definitive staging test and the initial therapy. As response rates approach 90%, diagnostic testing is relegated to the difficult role of detecting early failures 6–12 months into treatment, small persistent residual disease which may require a change in therapy, and an as yet largely unsuccessful role in influencing decisions related to second-look surgery.

Routine tests include a urine analysis, complete blood count, and chemistry profile with determinants of renal and liver function. In the presence of anatomically normal kidneys, and a normal BUN and creatinine, there is no indication for creatinine clearance determinations before or during conventional cis-platin therapy. Renal function is also important in deciding the dosage of methotrexate. Liver function is important in deciding the dosage of adriamycin and possibly the dosage of vinblastine or 5-fluorouracil.

Noninvasive cardiac function tests are required during the course of treatment with adriamycin even in young patients. Dysfunction may be discovered at 300 mg/m^2 and may rarely be fatal at 400 mg/m^2. Bruckner et al. [1982] were able to continue ADM therapy (based on serial normal cardiac function tests) to 600–800 mg/m^2 in some patients with responsive tumors.

The *chest x-ray* does not determine operability. A pleural effusion in the absence of clinical symptoms need rarely be removed to optimize pulmonary function. Follow-up films are rarely useful, in the absence of clinical findings, except at treatment decision points, because 95% of effusions respond completely or patients have other evidence of disease. Only bleomycin and possibly methotrexate produce clinically silent pulmonary side effects which may be discovered with serial chest x-rays.

Cytologic studies are required to prove that patients with pleural effusions have stage IV disease. These patients will undergo surgery for removal of the pelvic tumor and optimum debulking regardless of the cytologic findings. The finding has no prognostic or therapeutic implications for primary or second-look surgery or choice of chemotherapy.

Sonography and CAT scans are of marginal value unless one must confirm the presence or location of a mass before primary surgery. Serial tests have not clearly facilitated decisions or cost-effective management regarding operability, results of chemotherapy, or optimum time for second-look surgery, or predicted the findings of second-look surgery. A baseline study is required immediately after surgery to provide operative correlation if these tests are to be used for follow-up or assessing the results of chemotherapy. The tests are particularly ineffective (false-negative) in dealing with tumors in the rectosigmoid and the iliac fossa.

Second-look surgery may be indicated in patients with partial responses and residual disease. This further reduces the usefulness of serial CAT scans and sonography.

The *IVP* has become a two-edged sword because the dehydration and contrast material used for the IVP or CAT scan may damage the cis-platin-compromised kidney. Adequate hydration is important at all points in the diagnostic and therapeutic management of patients with ovarian cancer.

It is important to identify ureteral obstruction, in order to preserve renal function. Nephrotoxic drugs can be used with safety provided the nephrotoxic drug regimen is preceded by optimum hydration. Mild obstruction requires early chemotherapy. Severe obstruction may require a temporary ureteral stent. The IVP, except in the case of the pelvic kidney, which may be diagnosed by sonography or other tests, will not influence the decision to perform surgery.

The *barium enema* continues to be important, especially in early stages of disease. Patients may develop additional primary tumors of the rectum and colon. The patients usually come to surgery for removal of the primary colorectal tumor. The barium enema is recommended before second- or third-look surgery and at 1- to 2-year intervals in order to detect new primary tumors and occult progression with obstruction of the rectosigmoid.

Laparoscopy should be used only if the findings will effect a significant change in therapy which can clearly benefit the patient. It facilitates the staging of patients with stage I or II disease. It is possibly a useful screening test before second-look surgery. It is not a substitute for second-look surgery and has little value if strategy dictates a second debulking. Research has not defined a safe and optimum frequency of laparoscopy in order to identify the optimum time for second-look laparotomy. Other uses include confirmation of 1) no gross disease before second-look surgery, in order to stop all treatment; 2) progressive disease requiring a change in treatment; and 3) objective response, sufficient to attempt debulking (which was not previously possible) or intraperitoneal treatment with isotopes, cytotoxic drugs, or immune modulators.

Lymphangiography is rarely cost-effective. It has a 20% false-negative rate and can probably be replaced by systematic intraoperative biopsies. Such sampling of lymph nodes is relevant to stage I–II patients, especially with tumors of poor histologic grade, only if the physician requires evidence of metastases in order to offer adjuvant investigational treatment. Other patients will require chemotherapy regardless of the lymph node status. It has no general role at the time of second-look surgery because eligible patients are in clinical complete remission and are unlikely to have detectable lymph node involvement. All patients will require intraoperative lymph node biopsy at second-look surgery.

The *liver scan* was once thought to be a superfluous test. Its value remains unproved; however, the author has observed parenchymal liver involvement (even as an only site of failure) among patients relapsing after cisplatinum combination chemotherapy. The liver may represent a sanctuary from current cytotoxic therapy, and deserves systematic reporting as a possible "new" site of failure.

Tumor Markers

The *nonimmunological tumor assays* as a group do not have a useful role as yet. They duplicate more reliable tests of response and do not provide a substitute for either laparoscopy or second-look surgery. These assays have not yet provided a method of early diagnosis of failure for the 20% of patients who have recurrence of disease postsurgically proven complete remission or the 16–25% who "fail" primary cis-platin chemotherapy.

The human chorionic gonadotropin (HCG) and alpha feta protein (AFP) assays may represent useful diagnostic screening tests in order to identify germ cell tumors falsely diagnosed as ovarian cancer, especially in young patients. The author [unpublished] found a high serum CEA to have bad prognostic implications. A markedly elevated CEA is an indication to search for a nonovarian primary site although 70% of mucinous and, less often, 35% of serous tumor may produce an elevation in serum CEA.

Immunological assays continue to have the same shortcomings as described above and continue to have a high frequency (20%) of false-negative tests as described by Bast et al. [1983b,c]. The assays may in theory increase diagnostic accuracy in difficult cases and thereby increase the precision of trials and choice of therapy. Currently, if the differential diagnosis includes ovarian cancer, patients will be treated for ovarian cancer. With the possible exception only if the differential diagnosis includes a germ cell tumor, this strategy offers the best chance of long-term remission.

Primary Surgery—Chemotherapeutic Considerations

Optimum surgery with debulking has increased in importance as a result of the availability of effective intensive combination chemotherapy. Griffiths [1980] reports that the surgical complete response rate in optimally debulked patients approaches 80+% with subsequent combination chemotherapy. Effective adjuvant therapy increases the indications for extensive staging and surgery. However, the best long-term successes for debulking are demonstrated only in patients subsequently treated with dosage-intensive combination chemotherapy regimens with less than conventional dosage modification.

Radical surgery should be performed only if there is a reasonable chance that the tumor can be reduced to less than 3 cm. However, tumor reduction to as small as 0.5 cm or preferably to microscopic size may be necessary to demonstrate dramatic improvement in surgical complete remission and survival, especially with the more conventional chemotherapy regimens. Dembo et al. [1979a,b, 1983] found that complete debulking with BSOH including complete hysterectomy is required in order to consider radiotherapy as the subsequent adjuvant treatment. In this case the type of operation may indirectly reflect the degree of debulking. Wharton et al. [1980] demonstrated the relatively modest benefit of debulking if patients are treated with conventional drugs. Tumor size lost prognostic significance at 4 years.

Radiotherapy

Radiation does not carry the 5–9% risk of late leukemia associated with 12 months of alkylating agent therapy as reported by Reimer et al. [1977], Green et al. [1982], and Einhorn [1982b]. It therefore deserves further trial against stage I, stage II, and possibly stage III tumors provided patients have a complete BSOH, optimum surgery, and absolutely no gross residual disease. Whole abdominal RT may achieve about 80% 5-year survival for these patients. Methodology is critical and requires special equipment, personnel, and supportive care. Combination chemotherapy has not been tested.

Conventional attempts to combine radiotherapy and chemotherapy with standard alkylating agents, simultaneously or in sequence, are obsolete. They uniformly fail to show any advantage compared to the best single modality results. To date the sequential treatment strategy compromises the advantages of both treatments and provides the cumulative toxicities of both treatments.

Intraperitoneal isotopes demand scrupulous attention to documentation of adequate distribution. Buchsbaum et al. [1975] and others reported phase II trials with 73–94% survival. It remains to be determined if this is a true treatment effect or the result of selection of patients with superior staging compared to prior experience. Young et al. [1979, 1983] described an NCI-GOG collaborative trial currently addressing this question. P32 isotopes were equal to L-PAM in early analyses.

In stage I disease pelvic radiotherapy is ineffective. Whole abdominal RT plus pelvic RT by extrapolation may be effective for patients with poorly differentiated tumors. Although chemotherapy and radiotherapy appear equal, a short course of combination chemotherapy has not been tested. Its risk of producing leukemia is unknown.

Fuks [1975] provides a detailed review of the case for conventional radiotherapy in stage II desease. Radiation may contribute 10–15% to 5-year survival. Survival approaches 45%. In theory an untested sequence of systemic combination chemotherapy to eradicate occult microscopic stage III disease with subsequent pelvic irradiation offers the best of both options for bulky residual stage II disease. If radiation precedes chemotherapy it will compromise chemotherapy.

Delclos and Smith [1975] compared 12 cycles of melphalan to whole abdominal pelvic radiation plus a pelvic boost and found no differences in survival with stage I, stage II, and limited stage III disease where the residual tumor mass was 2 cm or less in size. There was no gross tumor in shielded areas. This study marked a turning point identifying chemotherapy as the treatment of choice because it apparently had a superior therapeutic index. It is now recognized that the radiotherapy was in theory suboptimum, and that the late toxicities of chemotherapy may balance the early risks of radiotherapy.

Hreshchyshyn and Norris [1979] and Hreshchyshyn et al. [1980] have described the Gynecologic Oncology Group experience with a controlled trial comparing 18 cycles of melphalan vs. 5,000 rads of pelvic irradiation vs. observation for patients with stage Ia and Ib ovarian carcinoma. Pelvic radiation alone treated an inadequate field. The chemotherapy tended to decrease the risk of recurrence 2/34 vs. 5/29 control and 7/23 radiotherapy, P 0.03. The study is flawed by incomplete descriptions of patient characteristics and many failures to accept the assigned treatment.

Brady et al. [1979] reported no significant advantage for stage III patients treated with 18 cycles of melphalan compared to whole abdomimal radiation plus pelvic radiation followed by melphalan, or to melphalan followed by radiation, or to no treatment (control). However, the control group tended to have inferior survival.

The techniques of radiotherapy employed in early studies were inadequate in terms of current understanding of the total abdominal distribution of disease; understaging of patients; the theoretical limits of radiotherapy against large tumor volume; the inability of a moving strip technique to deal with free-moving tumor cells in the abdomen; failure to include the diaphragm; and excessive shielding of tumor in the process of shielding the liver and the kidneys. Technical criticisms of early studies indirectly support new studies of radiation therapy. Dembo et al. [1979, 1980] address these theoretical considerations.

They described the treatment of 231 patients with stages Ib, II, and "asymptomatic" III. Analysis of this complex multistage, multitreatment trial found whole abdominal RT (combined with pelvic radiotherapy) to be superior to pelvic radiotherapy followed by 2 years of CLB, P = 0.02, with 80% vs. 55% 5-year survival in stage 1b, II, and III asymptomatic patients. This was true only if surgery included a BSOH. Incomplete BSOH presumably was an indirect measure of incomplete removal of large tumors. Results were strengthened by limiting the analysis to patients with no visible residual disease (P = 0.006 with 95% vs. 60% 5-year survivors). The treatment appeared particularly advantageous for the patients with poorly differentiated tumors because patients tended to do equally well regardless of tumor grade. Patients with stage Ia poorly differentiated tumors did worse—70% vs. 100% 5-year survival—than patients with well-differentiated tumors because treatment was inadequate. It consisted of pelvic RT, alone without whole abdominal radiotherapy. Similar survival of stage Ia patients would be expected without any postoperative treatment. The investigators concluded that the benefit of abdominal pelvic radiation was independent of stage or histology and possibly effective even in the presence of small amounts of disease in the upper abdomen.

Dembo's [1983] analyses suggest that radiotherapy will prove substantially less effective for patients with any visible residual disease, especially patients with poorly differentiated tumors. Nevertheless the overall 81% 5-year survival and 55% survival in patients with some small residual disease is a strong argument in favor of testing this method of radiation. It will require scrupulous attention to technical detail, optimum surgical staging and stratification by tumor stage, grade, distribution (pattern), and size. The Gynecologic Oncology Group is currently examining the feasibility of this trial.

CHEMOTHERAPY

Chemotherapy for ovarian cancer has been reviewed by Tobias and Griffiths [1976], Young et al. [1982], and Katz et al. [1982]. Their summary tables report similar (about 50%) response rates for melphalan, chlorambucil, thio TEPA (65%), and cyclophosphamide. Somewhat poorer response rates, about 35%, are reported for mechlorethamine, 5-fluorouracil, hexamethylmelamine, doxorubicin (adriamycin), and cis-platin, and 25% for methotrexate. Rates of response fall to about 15% for BCNU, vinblastine, and progesterone. These latter trials included poor-prognosis extensively treated patients.

In spite of achieving respectable response rate, HMM, adriamycin, 5-FU, and methotrexate still do not have an established role as single agents. Investigations do not demonstrate any favorable impact on survival compared to L-PAM.

Alkylating agents are not as active as these response rates suggest. Controlled collaborative trials of single alkylating agents consistently report only 25–35% rates of response. Only selected patients with good prognostic characteristics—ambulatory asymptomatic clinical status, small tumor size, well-differentiated grade of tumor, and possibly young age—have 50%–60% rates of response. The impact of prognostic characteristics for single agents and combinations was confirmed by Bruckner et al. [1980, 1981d, 1983b]. Only 25% of a general patient population has a "good prognosis." This observation represents a strong argument against delaying chemotherapy until patients become symptomatic or tumors increase in size.

The alkylating agents cannot be assumed to be equal because there is no clear correlation between response and survival and there are too few controlled trials and too few reports describing long-term follow-up.

Standard drugs, particularly L-PAM and CLB, have not been used optimally. Oral drugs are unreliable owing to poor patient compliance and erratic absorption in 25% of dosage tests. Parenteral and intraperitoneal therapy with these drugs await first clinical tests. Wilson and Neal [1981] provided in vitro data favoring high-dose TSPH and DDP for systemic and intraperitoneal therapy compared to other alkylating agents. Vistica et al. [1981] described several types of amino acid interaction which may lead to substantially improved therapy with L-PAM.

Overall results with alkylating agents (usually L-PAM) include a 10- to 14-month median survival and a 5–9% 5-year survival. For responders these end points tend to improve by 50%, and for clinical complete responders they improve by 100%. A best estimate places the overall surgical complete response (negative second look) rate at less than 10%. This comprises some one-third of the clinical complete responders. Surgically proven complete responders may approach an 80% 5-year survival. Patients with microscopic residual may approach 30–80% 5-year survival with continuation of the same chemotherapy depending on the grade of the tumor, as described by Gershenson et al. [1983] and Copeland et al. [1983]. Best results were observed in young, under 40, good histology, grade 1,2 patients with initial optimum surgery and microscopic residual disease.

Single-Agent Trials

Melphalan (L-PAM) is the only well-tested alkylating agent and is therefore the single agent of choice. Chlorambucil (CLB), by comparison across studies, tends to produce inferior survival. Rossof et al. [1976] described CLB as inferior to L-PAM in an early ECOG comparative trial. Cyclophosphamide (CYC), in spite of its better biologic availability as a parenteral drug, also appears to be inferior to L-PAM. Patients have rapid relapse after complete remissions. Buckner et al. [1974] found that very intensive therapy with cyclophosphamide had a poor therapeutic index and no long-term benefit.

Cis-platin (DDP, P, D) is the most active single agent which is largely non-cross-resistant with standard alkylating agents. It has the highest order of in vitro activity of any tested drug as either primary or secondary therapy. Responders, 35–50% of previously untreated patients, survive longer than nonresponders.

Wiltshaw et al. [1976] first described a 35% rate of clinical responses to 30 mg/m^2 dosages in patients previously failing radiotherapy and chlorambucil.

Bruckner et al. [1976] confirmed this, employing a single dose of 50 mg/m^2 every 3 weeks. Patients were at poor risk for further chemotherapy because of poor bone marrow reserve and intensive multidrug prior chemotherapy. Subsequently Bruckner [1978a, 1981a] and Wiltshaw [1979] independently reported 50% response rates with high-dose, 100–120 mg/m^2, cis-platin. The patients were an optimum group treated with only a single prior alkylating agent. Young et al. [1979] reviewed the status of cis-platin as a single agent for primary and secondary treatment.

Any advantage of high-dose DDP is too small to identify in the conventionally sized primary or secondary trials described by Wiltshaw [1979, 1980] or Gershenson et al. [1981]. With conventional doses surgical CR rates are low, 10%, and with high doses clinical response rates are low, about 50%. These results tend to be worse, lower than those achieved with cis-platin in combination chemotherapy.

DDP in all doses produces a median survival comparable to other single agents and combinations. The additive effect of subsequent treatment with a single alkylating agent may be substantial and add to median survival.

Although cis-platin is described as a marrow-sparing drug, the author has sometimes observed marked sensitivity to subsequent chemotherapy and, rarely, very sudden dangerous anemia or thrombocytopenia during primary therapy. DDP produces dose-dependent peripheral and rare CNS toxicity. Very rarely conventional doses produce fatal adrenal insufficiency.

DDP also produces several types of nephrotoxicity largely preventable by saline diuresis. Damage can range from acute renal failure, which is reversible and in some respects similar to acute tubular necrosis, to deteriorating creatinine clearance, which is also usually reversible, to tubular defects with electrolyte abnormalities such as hypomagnesemia, hypokalemia, and hypocalcemia. Although saline diuresis alone is adequate to virtually prevent serious damage, supplementary treatment with diuretics is helpful if it is difficult to monitor the diuresis due to cardiac disease or overcommitted nursing resources. Mannitol may possibly provide extra protection if the kidneys are mechanically or physiologically compromised.

Doxorubicin (adriamycin) (ADM, A) as a primary treatment may achieve a response rate equal to that of L-PAM. In vitro studies confirm that ADM has a high order of activity as primary therapy, but demonstrate that tumors frequently develop rapid cross resistance during chemotherapy. This suggests that its role if any will be as part of early courses of primary therapy. Its possible synergism with other drugs has not been tested in vitro. De Palo et al. [1975, 1977] described responses comparable to L-PAM in a small number of patients in a single institution study employing high doses of 75 mg/m^2 adriamycin. These doses do not lend themselves to secondary treatment or to primary combination treatment; because of the risk of severe toxicity one must compromise the dosages of ADM. ADM as an optimally used single drug has an inferior therapeutic index compared to L-PAM. There were some fatalities due to myelosuppression.

Hexamethylmelamine (HMM, H) is a broadly active drug of unknown mechanism of action. Reports by Wampler et al. [1972] and Wharton et al. [1979] indicated a 32–45% rate of response. It is never a single agent of choice. Little is known concerning the quality of the responses, especially their impact on survival. However, trials do not suggest any advantages compared to standard L-PAM alkylating agents.

HMM produces a wide variety of gastrointestinal and neurologic side effects which are largely dose-dependent and reversible. Myelosuppression is relatively mild compared to other cytotoxic drugs. Its cumulative myelosuppressive or neurological side effects may sometimes be severe when the drug is employed as a secondary treatment. Parathesias may persist. The use of vitamin B_6 to lessen the incidence of neurotoxicity, tested by Smith et al. [1975b] and employed by several investigators including the author, needs further evaluation in order to establish its efficacy.

Methotrexate (MTX, amethopterin) is a highly schedule-dependent drug. Response rates are poor and of short duration, with schedules ranging from daily low-dose oral treatment by Greenspan and Bruckner [1976] to high-dose methotrexate with leucovorin rescue by Parker et al. [1979]. The high-dose regimen produced only a 13% rate of response.

The safety of methotrexate is dependent on adequate renal clearance. Methotrexate is an infrequent (5–10%) but sometimes serious nephrotoxin at any dose, but particularly in high-dose regimens. In the author's [unpublished] experience, secondary treatment with moderate 160 mg/m^2 methotrexate and high-dose methotrexate, 1–5 g/m^2, was entirely ineffective even in the presence of treatment limiting toxicity. "Responses" were of poor quality and short duration. Methotrexate has a low order of in vitro activity, a poor therapeutic index, and may be very dangerous to combine with other nephrotoxic drugs such as cis-platin.

Vinblastine (VLB, V) has been only minimally tested as a single agent. Vaitkevicius et al. [1961] first reported 2–10 responses. Activity was confirmed in a review by Tobias and Griffiths [1976]: Vinblastine has achieved an increasingly important role in investigational combination therapy because of its marked synergism with cis-platin and bleomycin, the demonstrated cure of germ cell tumors, and a high order of activity in vitro.

Single-agent treatment with vinblastine does not appear to offer the patient any substantial benefit except as a secondary therapy based on in vitro tests predicting activity against the specific tumor. Although vinblastine is schedule-dependent, in the author's unpublished experience, escalating dosages of vinblastine infusions produced only one response in ten patients. The response occurred at a dosage which produced unacceptable bone marrow toxicity. Other alkaloids are inactive: VP 16-213, 2 out of 38 responded; VM 26, 0 of 16; and vincristine, 0 out of 22. Vincristine is generally considered to be an unsatisfactory drug in spite of its relative sparing of the bone marrow because it can produce ileus.

Fluorouracil trials have largely been limited to treatment of patients failing conventional therapy. Fluorouracil produces a 20% response rate. These responses were generally of short duration.

Combination Chemotherapy

The apparent ability to achieve complete response in some 80% of patients with small residual stage III tumors has led to recommending combination chemotherapy as a general treatment of choice. The high surgical complete response rates have yet to be confirmed and further information is required in order to define other prognostic characteristics and long-term survival. Although several combinations consistently improve clinical response rates and progression-free intervals, especially cis-platin regimens, surgical complete response and survival advantages represent only trends demonstrated in subgroup rather than overall analyses. There is no proof that some drugs contribute to combination therapy. These include methotrexate, high-dose methotrexate, hexamethylmelamine, adriamycin, and perhaps even "standard" cyclophosphamide at 500–750 mg/m^2 dosage schedules.

Single agents in combination chemotherapy. *Cytoxan* is commonly used because it spares the bone marrow compared to other alkylating agents. It need not be cross-resistant with other drugs including conventional alkylating agents. It does not appear to be the alkylating agent of choice. If Cytoxan is inferior to L-PAM, there may be reason for concern about the practice of equating CTX and L-PAM in order to compare an active drug combination with Cytoxan to L-PAM alone and then concluding that the drug used in combination with Cytoxan is valueless. Aroneyi et al. [1981], in a direct comparison of L-PAM and CTX as MAF vs. CAF (adriamycin A, fluorouracil F), illustrate the reason for this concern in that the duration of responses to CAF was inferior. Other trials except by Bruckner et al. [1983b] have not made CTX the phase III variable. There is no evidence that CTX 750 mg/m^2 or less contributes to any combination: AP $\pm$ C, HAP $\pm$ C, A $\pm$ C. It is questionable if Cytoxan at the dosage tested has adequate phase II activity or produces adequate quality of response against large tumors in order for its contribution, if any, to be detected in phase III combination chemotherapy trials. Perhaps even the trial of Decker et al. [1983] employing 1,000 mg/m^2 dosages is inconclusive because there was no DDP control for the good-risk patients.

Cis-platin combination chemotherapy has been reported systemically by Bruckner et al. [1977a,b, 1981f, 1983a,b] and reviewed by Holland et al. [1980a,b] and Cohen et al. [1983]. Trials included the initial controlled prospective tests of cis-platinum as primary therapy alone and in combination chemotherapy: cis-platin (P); adriamycin/cis-platin (A/P vs. P); followed by trials of thiotepa/cis-platin (TP vs. AP), Cytoxan/hexamethylmelamine/adriamycin/cis-platin (CHAP vs. AP); and cyclophosphamide/adriamycin/cis-platin (CAP vs. AP). Platinum alone at 50 mg/m^2 produced a 20% response rate. Subsequent treatment with thiotepa produced additional responses and probably contributed to an overall median survival of some 18 months for the DDP regimen. The platinum-adriamycin combination produced a 76% response rate, and 22% of these patients are surgically proven complete responders. AP, CHAP, and CAP produce similar response rates, surgical complete response, and overall survival identical to all similar two-, three-, and four-drug regimens regardless of dosage variations. For poor-prognosis patients, especially patients with poorly differentiated tumors, analysis by Bruckner et al. [1981f, 1983a] identify these regimens as superior to a thiotepa, methotrexate regimen which is equivalent to L-PAM in separate controlled trials reported by Bruckner et al. [1979, 1983c]. As described, the CHAP regimen produced further advantage in median survival for patients with poorly differentiated tumors compared to AP. This was demonstrable even after adjustment for residual tumor size.

Only cis-platin combinations have clearly succeeded in demonstrating superiority to other regimens in some controlled trials—e.g., CHAP V vs. HexaCAF, CP vs. CTX, and AP and CHAP I in subsets. The addition of either adriamycin 50 mg/m^2 as described by Bruckner et al. [1981f] or cyclophosphamide 1,000 mg/m^2 or DDP 50 mg/m^2 as described by Decker et al. [1982] more than doubles response rates as compared to single agents. CP may exert its best effect in good-prognosis patients and AP in poor-prognosis patients. Neither regimen is proven to be superior to P alone in sequence with an alkylating agent. Barker and Wiltshaw [1981] described trials of low-dose cis-platin and chlorambucil plus or minus adriamycin. Wiltshaw's low-dose cis-platin regimens (20–30 mg/m^2) appear to produce a somewhat lower response (50%) and complete response (28%) rate and a shorter median length of remission, 13–16 months than the more cis-platin-intensive AP regimens. The preliminary surgical complete remission rates for these regimens was half that of the AP (24%) series described by Bruckner [1978a, 1981f] and Cohen [1983]. These data suggest an advantage, albeit inconclusive, for either adriamycin and/or the larger dosage of cis-platin. These trials have been replaced by trials of high-dose cis-platin which cannot be compared directly to others because there is little discussion of the patient's prognostic characteristics. However, many patients have large residual tumors. Response rates are about 50% for high-dose cisplatin. The surgical complete response rates are low but not clearly inferior to other regimens.

The CHAP V and CAP regimens tested in controlled trials by Neijt et al. [1983] and Sturgeon et al. [1982] were superior to HexaCAF in survival at 5 years and therapeutic index respectively. The advantage in survival was most apparent in good-prognosis patients with tumors less than 1 cm in size. Surgical complete response rates are consistently about 20%. As discussed, CHAP 1,8 may produce the best surgical complete response rate in patients with intermediate-size tumors, 1–3 cm. Bruckner et al. [1981f, 1983a] and Vogl et al. [1982] also described CHAP regimens as tending to have advantages for the elderly, poor-histology, and suboptimum (large) tumor size subsets.

Vogl et al. [1982] and Omura et al. [1982] provide a note of caution against equating cis-platin combinations or concluding that their superiority to single agents is proved for all patients. In comparison to L-PAM, CHAD and CAP significantly increase response rate and progression-free interval but overall survival and surgical complete response were not different. Follow-up was incomplete. The best conclusion appears to be that cis-platin regimens give better early results. Although they may be "saved" for use as salvage treatment after L-PAM and still contribute to overall survival, this strategy compromises the chance of surgical complete response—a rarity with second-line cis-platin regimens, and therefore cure.

Adriamycin's contribution to overall survival and its relative merit compared to other drugs (platinum or any combination chemotherapy) remain controversial. Wiltshaw et al. [1980] found a cis-platinum/chlorambucil combination equal to a cis-platinum/chlorambucil/adriamycin 20/50 mg/ m^2 combination.

Four lines of investigation support consideration of adriamycin. Bruckner et al. [1979] found that adriamycin/platinum regimens produce twice as many responses as cis-platin alone. As primary therapy the adriamycin/ platinum regimen and the AC regimens described by Schwartz et al. [1982] tend to improve survival compared to cis-platinum or HC respectively for patients who have poor-histology tumors. Edmonson et al. [1979] found that the combination of adriamycin plus cyclophosphamide tended to produce superior survival compared to cyclophosphamide alone when patients have small residual tumors. Trope et al. [1983, personal communication] found adriamycin plus melphalan to produce superior 5-year survival compared to melphalan alone.

Doxorubicin's relative merit compared to other drugs remains unproved. It is recommended only for controlled investigations. (Pfleiderer et al. [1982] observed that the cytotoxic effect of adriamycin in vitro predicts a response to standard alkylating agents in clinical practice. This suggests that adriamycin and cyclophosphamide may in large part be effective only in the same patients and that adriamycin may not substantially broaden the spectrum of responding patients.)

Hexamethylmelanine (HMM) is part of several combinations all of which produce about 50% secondary rates of response: HP, HAD, CHAD, CHAP I, CHAP II, HP Velban, bleomycin. Only HD reported by Davis et al. [1980] directly tests the contributions of HMM to DDP. (It appeared to improve response rates compared to historical experience with DDP alone.) However, the test group consisted of optimum patients likely to have a high response rate.

Wiltshaw [1980] tested HMM as a part of primary therapy with disappointing (response [50%] and median duration of complete response [11 months]) results compared to cis-platin plus CLB. HMM is entirely ineffective as primary therapy in non-cis-platin regimens with the possible exception of HexaCAF, discussed elsewhere.

Fluorouracil in conventional bolus schedules does not have a satisfactory therapeutic index and therefore cannot serve as a building block for combination therapy because of suppression of the bone marrow. All combinations that include bolus FU have failed except HexaCAF. However, the "success" of HexaCAF cannot be attributed to 5FU. Unsuccessful combinations include CMF, CAF, CHEX UP, and CHFP.

Villasanta [1980] tested an infusion of FUDR 2 mg/kg/day ×5 in combination with cyclophosphamide 7–8 mg/kg day ×5. He reported a surprising 34% CR rate, 18% PR rate, and 60% 5-year survival in patients with stage III disease. However, some two-thirds of the "responders" had residual tumors of less than 2 cm, suggesting the treatment's benefit may be limited to good-risk patients. Izbicki et al. [1977] reported that 5FU infusion plus Cytoxan significantly improved survival compared to Cytoxan alone.

The author in unpublished work has examined a 5-fluorouracil 30 mg/kg/day infusion both alone and in combination with mitomycin C. The infusion is bone marrow–sparing except sometimes after months of DDP. Some one-third respond, and response improves survival by some 6 months. It is especially useful if compromised bone marrow prevents treatment with more cytotoxic drugs.

Methotrexate's contribution to combination therapy including HexaCAF is unproved. Barlow and Piver's [1979] test of a second-line "MeCY" regimen provided the only and as yet unconfirmed positive report.

Conclusions

Combination chemotherapy is a potentially curative treatment. It represents the chemotherapy of choice which will be selected by many properly informed patients. Several types of patients comprising a large percentage of the overall patient population achieve greater palliation and a greater chance of cure with combination chemotherapy regimens. The ability to achieve surgically proven complete remission for some 80% of patients with small residual advanced disease has led to recommending combination chemotherapy as treatment for high-risk patients with early stages of occult microscopic residual disease. These extrapolations have not been tested.

Only a few combination regimens appear to compete as a treatment of choice for specific good-prognosis patients with small tumors: AC; HexaCAF; CHAP 1,8; and CHAP V for patients with small tumors. For the general population the treatment of choice may be AP, CP, CHAP I, CHAP V, or possibly ADM/L-PAM. None of these trials have been confirmed.

The following studies illustrate important general principles and specific applications for combination chemotherapy. Response rates prove to be unimportant. Only superior survival and possibly superior surgical complete response rates may identify a superior treatment.

Young et al. [1978] tested HexaCAF adding 14 days of oral hexamethylmelamine to 14 days of oral cyclophosphamide while methotrexate (amethoptherin) and fluorouracil were given IV on days 1 and 8. This small trial differed from preceding trials in that the patients were younger and chemotherapy was given in a very aggressive fashion for 6 months with little dosage modification. Response was assessed by laparoscopy rather than by second-look surgery. HexaCAF produced a 75% overall response rate, 33% complete by laparoscopy, and L PAM produced a 54% response rate, 16% complete. The HexaCAF regimen produced an overall survival advantage of P 0.02 compared to melphalan. The advantage with further analysis was only marginal and limited to patients with grade 2 or 3 small tumors as discussed under prognostic factors. In subsequent controlled trials of CHAP

V by Neijt et al. [1979, 1980, 1983] and Sturgeon et al. [1980], the HexaCAF regimen was inferior to both in response rate, to CAP in therapeutic index, and to CHAP V in 5-year survival. It was particularly inferior to CHAP V in patients with small, 0- to 1-cm tumors.

Carmo-Pereira et al. [1981] found HexaCAF with CTX reduced from 150 to 100 mg/m^2 daily equal to high-dose parenteral Cytoxan 40 mg/kg D1 q 3 W. However, HexaCAF was largely ineffective for patients with a poor prognosis as defined by large tumor, high (poor) grade, or poor performance status. Median survival was only 10 months. Delgado et al. [1979] examined a less toxic version of HexaCAF, deleting methotrexate and reducing CTX to 100 mg/m^2. This HexaCF regimen has produced a preliminary response rate similar to that of the original HexaCAF. Dosages of methotrexate may probably be sacrificed in preference to doses of the other drugs in the HexaCAF regimen.

Hexamethylmelamine plus cyclophosphamide as tested by Smith et al. [1979] produced response rates superior to melphalan, fluorouracil, adriamycin, or hexamethylmelamine. Subsequent analysis of these trials by Wharton et al. [1980] found that the combination had no survival advantage compared to melphalan. Omura et al. [1981] tested hexamethylmelamine plus melphalan vs. melphalan alone and also found the now familiar pattern of an early response rate advantage for the combination, but no subsequent evidence of improved survival. The Medical Research Council [1981] also failed to find any advantage for cyclophosphamide/hexamethylmelamine compared to only 100 mg of CTX daily. Median survival was poor compared to other regimens. It was only 12 and 18 months for the overall group and the clinically nonmeasurable patients respectively. These studies did not attempt to determine if the combination was particularly effective for good-prognosis patients.

Adriamycin plus Cytoxan regimens continue to be candidate treatments only for selected good-prognosis patients with tumors less than 1.5 cm in size, as described by Griffiths [1979, 1980]. With the exception of a marginally confirmatory controlled trial reported by Edmonson et al. [1979] for patients with stage II–III residual tumors of less than 3 cm, a half dozen trials of ADM/CTX in a variety of dosage schedules, with or without 5-fluorouracil, fail to find any hint of a survival advantage compared to single alkylating agents. The combinations consistently produce better response rates than single alkylating agents, however.

Attempts to combine adriamycin with other alkylating agents have been few and disappointing with the exception of a ADM + L-PAM vs. L-PAM first reported by Trope [1981]. In a 1983 personal communication he described advantages in response rate and 35% survival at 5 years. DePalo et al. [1977] found no advantage for the combination in response rate or survival and a disadvantageous therapeutic index. However, the control treatment was ADM, not L-PAM.

Immunotherapy employing BCG in combination with AC and in confirmatory trial with AC and with CAP has been compared to AC and CAP respectively by Alberts et al. [1979b]. This large study found both a response P 0.05 and survival P 0.004 advantage for immunotherapy with 12% CR, 40% PR, and 23.5 month median survival. These results are similar or slightly inferior to those achieved with cis-platin regimens except that the surgical complete response rate is dismal.

Vinblastine-bleomycin–cis-platinum combinations tested as PVB remain the subject of anecdotal reports. They are not clearly better than P alone. Surwit et al. [1983] described PHVB. The rate and quality of responses tend to be better than achieved with PH by others or PHFC by the same investigators.

Best results with any combination have yet to be confirmed. Only HexaCAF vs. L-PAM and cis-platinum/cyclophosphamide vs. cyclophosphamide produced significant overall survival advantages. Both were small controlled trials, and benefit may be limited to good-prognosis patients with small tumors and good histology. Cohen et al. [1983] reported that platinum combination regimens tend to be superior to other combinations in that they produce a 20% rate of complete surgically proven remission in patients with large, 2- to 6-cm, possibly even 6- to 10-cm, residual tumors. The cis-platin regimens in their most alkylating agent–intensive forms, CHAP V, and the day 1,8 CHAD regimen appear to produce more improvement in surgically proven complete remissions than is achieved with other cis-platin combinations.

Intensification of therapy has been examined in phase II and only indirectly in phase III trials. Although it remains attractive in theory and preclinical models, it has failed several tests. Escalating cyclophosphamide to 40 mg/kg described by Buckner et al. [1974] increased response rates but failed to produce unmaintained remissions and had an exceptionally poor therapeutic index. Phase II attempts to use intensive cis-platin (100–120 mg/m^2 q 3 weeks by Bruckner et al. [1981a] or 50 mg/m^2 weekly by Piver et al. [1980]) possibly increase secondary rates of response from 30% to 50%. These trials involve selected good-prognosis patients; therefore the improved response rates may reflect patient characteristics. O'Connell et al. [1983] failed to improve overall results by intensifying both adriamycin/cis-platin in a 20 mg/m^2 weekly schedule. CHAP II, an attempt to escalate all drugs except cis-platin, provides an unclear test because it also examines a schedule and a route of administration change. Preliminary results suggest that CHAP II as both primary and secondary therapy increases response rates and clinical CR rates.

The CHAD day 1,8 regimen described by Greco et al. [1981a,b] is an intensive regimen which may produce frequent (about 87%) complete responses for patients with tumors of less than 3 cm. The results appear better than those achieved with other cis-platin regimens only for patients with small tumors, but this requires confirmatory trials.

SECONDARY THERAPY

Secondary trials can at best identify an active regimen and may produce false-negative results or underestimate a regimen's value as primary therapy. The patients are usually too few and too heterogeneous, all failing prior alkylating agent or multidrug treatments, to allow any direct comparison of phase II trials. Complications associated with progression diminish even further the prognosis for response and survival. Bruckner et al. [1981d, 1983f] described these characteristics which include diminished ambulatory status, age, extensive prior chemotherapy, and large size of tumors. Partial bowel obstruction and poor bone marrow tolerance also prevent testing of optimum doses of new drug regimens. Prognostic characteristics continue to determine response more than the choice of treatment. All the cis-platin regimens (P, AP, CAP, CHAP) produce similar results as secondary therapy. Analyses of HAP by Vogl et al. [1980] and PH by Davis et al. [1980] suggest that these treatments overcome some of these prognostic factors, but this is unlikely.

Only cis-platin regimens improve survival as secondary treatment. Crossover to cis-platin combination treatment after L-PAM fails is credited with obscuring survival advantages for CAP or CHAD versus L-PAM.

New studies must be examined closely because results may improve owing to early change of treatment. "Failure" is possibly identified earlier because of wide use of new tumor-imaging methods and second-look surgery. Patients with small residual tumors at second-look surgery who never progressed during prior drug therapy may now be perhaps incorrectly treated as failures.

Stanhope et al. [1977] described an overall response rate of only 8% for secondary treatments at the M.D. Anderson Hospital. Tobias and Griffiths [1976], Griffiths et al. [1979], and Katz et al. [1981] reviewed similar poor results. This pre-cis-platin experience demonstrates the importance of testing and utilizing drugs as primary therapy and finding alternate means of testing drugs to replace secondary therapy trials. Secondary therapy will often underestimate the efficacy of a drug or combination.

Hexamethylmelamine alone produces 15–20% rates of response. Some alkylating agents and antimetabolites approach this rate of response, but the trials are small or otherwise unconvincing. Adriamycin has been disappointing perhaps because it is too toxic to test in adequate dosages. HexaCAF generally produces response rates of only 5–20%.

The results with non-cis-platin secondary adriamycin or hexamethylmelamine combination regimens are largely the same; only 15–20% respond, survival impact is short, and median survival is unchanged at 4–6 months. Only some unconfirmed 5FU regimens and the unconfirmed MeCy ± VCR described by Barlow and Piver [1979] claim response rates of about 35%. In contrast the cis-platin regimens consistently produce response rates of about 35%, and the combinations produce a similar rate; only a few reports describe a 45–60% rate of response: HD, CHAP, PAC, CAP, CHVP. The quality of the cis-platin responses, as measured by their duration and effect on survival, appears better than that achieved with other drugs. However, only a few regimens (CHVP, CHAP II) may improve median survival.

Bruckner et al. [1981d, 1980a] found that secondary cis-platin regimens were essentially identical whether they involved AP, CAP or CHAP. They produced 75% response rates in good performance patients and 35% response rates overall. Adriamycin appears to add to the complete response rates compared to DDP alone. Davis et al. [1980] suggested that hexamethylmelamine in the PH combinations may improve response rates 15–25% compared to those with platinum alone. These poor results should encourage attempts to substitute other drugs for adriamycin, Cytoxan, and perhaps HMM. Surwit et al.'s [1983] tests of the combination of Cytoxan/hexamethylmelamine/Velban/bleomycin represent one such attempt. Of 35 patients with clinical evaluable disease eight achieved complete clinical remission and nine achieved partial remission, for an overall response rate of 49%. Responses were associated with excellent 12+-month survival.

CHAP II tests intensification of the alkylating agent and adriamycin hexamethylmelamine elements of therapy. Escalating treatment is designed to produce nadir white blood counts of 1,000–1,500. It also tests schedule modification based on a series of laboratory observations by the author in which low concentrations of cis-platin produced progressive morphologic changes in cells 24–48 h after treatment. Treatment with adriamycin/cyclophosphamide was delayed 48 h so that these drugs would be present at the time of maximum membrane effect. The CHAP II regimen described by Bruckner et al. [1982] is the first secondary treatment to produce an overall 70% response rate and a median projected survival of 18 months. For the first time responders include 5/7 patients failing chemotherapy with CAP and CHAP. Four additional patients achieved surgically proven complete remissions. Response and surgical complete remissions were not previously observed with other cis-platinum combinations after cis-platinum failed. Decker et al. [1982] and the author have observed complete surgical remission at third-look surgery suggesting that secondary treatment can be curative. This demonstrates the need for close follow-up, early modifications (intensification) in treatment, and perhaps new sequential treatment strategies.

NEW DRUGS

New drug research has been reviewed by several authors including Muggia [1980], Long and Young [1980], Katz et al. [1981], and Young et al. [1982]. Muggia [1980] emphasized the importance of considering tumor characteristics such as histologic grade, residual tumor burden after surgery, performance status, and the method of assessing a response prior to and after chemotherapy. Based on these reviews the drugs are classified in four groups as shown in Table II: 1) active new analogues related in structure or mechanism of action to established active (class of) drugs; 2) new agents,

TABLE II. New Medical Treatments for Ovarian Cancer

Analogues	
	Carboxy platinum (CBCDA), chlorambucil,[a] FUDR infusion, FU infusion, melphalan,[b] penberol, phenesterin, prednimustine, thiotepa,[a] triazinate
New Drugs	
	BCG,[a] bleomycin,[a] cytosine arabinoside (ARA C),[a,b] 13-cis-retinoic acid,[a] interferon,[a] Mullerian regression factor,[a] peptichemio, treosulfan,[a] vinblastine[a]
Unsuccessful trials	
	Actinomycin D,[a] m-AMSA,[c] BCNU, CCNU, C Parvum,[b] cytembena, galactitol, ICRF-159, maytansine, MeCCNU, methyl-GAG,[a] medroxy progesterone,[a] mitomycin,[c] piperazinidine, purazofurin, spirogermanium, vincristine, VM 26, VP 16
To be tested	
	Acridines, anthraquinones, busulfan, chlorazotocin, dichloromethotrexate, hydroxyurea, 6-mercaptopurine,[c] methylprednisolone acetate,[a] mithramycin, norethisterone acetate,[a] PALA,[c] porfiromycin, procarbazine,[a] streptozotocin, vindesine

[a]Active in vitro.
[b]Active as intraperitoneal therapy.
[c]No activity in vitro.

entirely unrelated to past successful agents; 3) unsuccessful drugs; and 4) drugs that are incompletely tested. It includes in vitro evidence of activity and examples of marginally active drugs or drugs with conflicting reports which meet some criteria for further study (preferably supplemented by a new improved study design such as a new route, schedule, or predicted drug interaction).

Some represent problem drugs. Reports on VP 16 and Cytembena conflict. In the case of Phenesterin and Prednimustine it is unknown if the alkylating agents' steroidal carrier conveys specific activity and an improved therapeutic index compared to standard alkylating agents.

Muggia [1980] considered chlorambucil and thiotepa as agents requiring reevaluation against drug-resistant disease because of anecdotal favorable experience. These agents may not be cross-resistant with other alkylating agents.

Treosulfan has had extensive favorable trials outside the United States. Descriptions of patients and reponses in these trials are difficult to compare with other reports. There is no experience with its analogue busulfan.

Peptichemio is also active after standard therapy fails. Favorable results include surgical complete remissions in patients with minimum residual disease at second-look surgery.

Dichloro methotrexate's metabolism is determined by hepatobiliary clearance and binding to serum protein. It is potentially a safer analogue for testing in combination with cis-platin. No such trials for ovarian cancer have been reported. An experimental antifol of the *triazinate* family tested by Corbett et al. [1982] is among the most active drugs against murine ovarian cancer.

Cis-platinum analogues are of great interest because they include nonnephrotoxic analogues such as dicarboxylate 1,2-diaminoi-cycloxenane (CBCDA). CBCDA may be used to maintain responses in patients with compromised renal function and appears to allow treatment at higher molar concentrations of platinum. Only infrequent responses can be expected in patients resistant to conventional cis-platinum. However, Burchenal et al. [1977] reported that some of these analogues are not cross-resistant. Because the drugs can be used in higher molar concentrations than cis-platin CBCDA is particularly attractive for trials of intraperitoneal therapy. CBCDA is more myelosuppressive than cis-platin. Its suppression of the bone marrow may prevent successful application in combination chemotherapy. Wiltshaw et al. [1983] report single-agent activity comparable to cis-platin and a superior therapeutic index.

Hormonal therapy has received new attention because of its relative lack of cytotoxicity, the availability of new antiestrogen agents, demonstrations of hormone receptors, and a demonstration of a variety of risk factors for ovarian cancer related to ovulation and birth control. Progestational agents have been described as producing about 20% response rates. However, the criteria of response fail to meet current standards. Geisler [1983] reported that doses of megestrol acetate of 800 mg/day for 30 days and 400 mg/day thereafter produced a 5/23 rate of long-lasting remission. One responder had a pelvic mesothelioma. Best responses were reported in low-grade tumors. Estrogen and progesterone receptors have been described in epithelial ovarian malignancies by Schwartz et al. [1980a] and others in as many as 50% of tumor specimens. Progesterone receptors are relatively weak compared to those in breast cancer. The receptors appear independent of the tumor's histologic appearance and degree of differentiation, age, and clinical stages. Tamoxifen's role is uncertain. Schwartz et al. [1980b] noted apparent disease stabilization for periods of only 10–30 weeks in patients treated with tamoxifen. This occurred in the absence of objective tumor regression. Schwartz et al. [1982] provided indirect supporting information that tamoxifen may slow tumors; in the absence of therapy with tamoxifen survival was not prolonged in receptor-positive compared to receptor-negative patients. When multiple sites are biopsied receptor assays can be positive in some sites and negative in other sites (usually metastatic) in the same patient.

The tamoxifen, receptor, and epidemiologic studies all imply a need for caution in the use of estrogen, especially as replacement therapy. In theory steroids such as decadron which are used as antiemetic adjuvants to cisplatin therapy are also relatively contraindicated because of the in vitro, preclinical, and clinical BCG trials supporting immunotherapy for ovarian cancer.

CURRENT TREATMENT STRATEGIES

Stage I Disease

Adjuvant therapy is unproved and not indicated except possibly for patients with a poor prognosis. Poorly differentiated tumor, positive cytology, and inadequate staging in theory represent indications for treatment. Extrapolation from the advanced disease experience with combination and single-agent chemotherapy for patients with small residual tumor suggests that only intensive chemotherapy — not single agents — promises the best chance of long-term remission (cure) for the patients with microscopic occult residual disease. Possibly short courses of combination chemotherapy emphasizing antimetabolites (HexaCAF) may reduce the risk of leukemia.

Whole abdominal radiation remains an investigational alternative and does not carry the risk of late leukemia. Second-look surgery is not recommended after adjuvant therapy because the chance of demonstrating residual disease is very small; providing further treatment would be both investigational and without successful precedent.

Stage II Disease

Stage II patients may be considered identical to stage I patients if they have undergone optimum staging exploration and complete surgery including a bilateral salpingo oophorectomy, complete hysterectomy, and omentectomy, provided there is no visible residual disease. Patients with visible residual disease may be considered analagous to patients with stage III residual disease of the same size.

HexaCAF appears most attractive for the patients with well or moderately differentiated, particularly 0.5 cm or smaller tumors. However CHAP V was the superior regimen in a controlled trial for stage III disease. By extrapolation alkylating agent–intensive platinum combinations such as the D 1,8 CHAP appear most attractive for patients with residual tumors 0.5–3 cm in size and patients with poorly differentiated tumors.

Radiotherapy is an alternative for patients especially if they are in the good histologic grade prognostic category. Pelvic radiotherapy is an untested consolidation treatment for stage II patients, with microscopic residual pelvic disease after systemic combination chemotherapy eradicates all extra-pelvic microscopic diseases.

Stage III Disease

In stage III patients with large, 3 cm, residual tumors, the treatment of choice appears to be an alkylating agent–intensive cis-platinum regimen in a sequence of surgery → CT → surgery → regional therapy. A two-drug cis-platin regimen is possibly as effective as a 3- or 4-drug regimen. Nevertheless the best results in phase II and phase III trials involve four drug combinations: CHAP 1 vs. AP, CHAP V vs. HexaCAF, and CHAP 1,8 vs. other trials.

Patient characteristics appear to identify different treatments of choice. The four drug-intensive cis-platin regimens are the only ones that overcome to any degree large residual tumor size, poor tumor differentiation, and age. They are clearly the most palliative regimens as defined by response and progression-free interval, and cure about 10% of these patients. For intermediate tumors 1–3 cm in size only the DDP regimen approaches 50–80% surgical complete response results. It remains to be determined if HexaCAF or AC may have a better therapeutic index for patients with well-differentiated tumors 0.5 cm or smaller. Griffiths' [1980] review of non-cis-platin data must be viewed with extreme caution because of the small numbers of patients and the superiority of CHAP V over HexaCAF for good-prognosis patients as described by Neijt et al. [1983].

Second-look surgery may be considered a routine procedure with high yield because it allows an end to therapy or assists in selecting further therapy. It is recommended after 6–12 cycles of combination chemotherapy provided the patient is in complete remission by clinical and radiologic tests. Patients with small residual tumors given the D 1,8 version of CHAP may require only 6 months of treatment. Smith et al. [1980] preferred 12 months of chemotherapy with a single alkylating agent regimen in order to reduce the risk of recurrence following the end of therapy. There is a 40% chance that a patient in clinical complete remission will have no residual disease at second-look surgery. If patients originally had small residual disease or well-differentiated tumors the chance that second-look surgery will find no tumor may be as high as 70–90%.

Second-look surgery may also be beneficial for patients with only partial remissions. Smith et al. [1980] reported that these patients may have a 30% chance of 5-year survival. The findings at second-look surgery determine the strategy of further chemotherapy. Continuing the same chemotherapy was superior to switching to whole abdominal radiotherapy. Copeland et al. [1983] have confirmed and extended these observations. The advantages of chemotherapy are best in patients with low grade 1–2 and microscopic residual tumors. Patients with only microscopic residual disease and those with gross resectable residual disease have an 80% and 30% chance of 5-year remission respectively. Wiltshaw [1980] also suggested that second-look surgery can be therapeutic for patients with residual disease. Debulking of patients in continued high-quality partial response may allow additional chemotherapy to control or eradicate microscopic foci of residual disease. Both Bruckner et al. [1982] and Decker et al. [1982] have patients with surgically identified residual disease who achieved complete surgical and pathological proven remission at third- and fourth-look surgery. Only some of these patients had complete removal of the visible tumor. Some subsequently underwent more intensive chemotherapy adding intensive alkylating agent(s) to the original chemotherapy. Similar results have been achieved by the postoperative use of intraperitoneal chemotherapy with 5FU, ADM, or DDP.

Second-look surgery also provides an opportunity to obtain tissue for in vitro clonogenic sensitivity testing; however, primary surgery is the optimum time for such prospective drug testing. The tumor specimen available at the time of second-look surgery is often of inadequate size or will not grow, and is already resistent to drugs that would have been effective earlier.

As a group the cis-platinum regimens produce higher response rates than HexaCAF or single-agent regimens. The cis-platin combinations clearly improve palliation by producing very frequent high-quality responses and the longest progression-free and symptom-free intervals compared to other combinations or any single agent. Reserving the cis-platin combination for second-line therapy may produce remissions and survival of substantially worse quality. All trends favor the most intensive cis-platin combinations. Less intensive regimens may be distinctly inferior in achieving surgical complete response for patients with small residual tumors. Surgical complete response currently implies a 75% chance of cure. This is observed in 20% of patients treated with intensive cis-platin regimens and in perhaps 80% of good-prognosis patients. This is fourfold the rate achieved in similar patients with single alkylating agents. This single advantage will have modest impact on interim analyses of median survival, but will have a substantial impact on long-term survival.

REFERENCES

Alberts DS, Hilgers RD, Moon TE, Martimbeau PW, Rivkin, S (1979a): Combination chemotherapy for alkylator-resistant ovarian carcinoma: A preliminary report of a Southwest Oncology Group trial. Cancer Treat Rep 63:301–305.

Alberts DS, Moon TE, Stephens RA, Wilson H, Oishi N, Hilgers RD, O'Toole R, Thigpen JT (1979b): Randomized study of chemoimmunotherapy for advanced ovarian carcinoma: A preliminary report of a Southwest Oncology Group study. Cancer Treat Rep 63:325–331.

Alberts DS, Chen HSG, Soehnlen B, Salmon SE, Surwit EA, Young L (1980): In-vitro cologenic assay for predicting response of ovarian cancer to chemotherapy. Lancet 2:340–342.

Alberts DS, Chen HSG, Salmon SE, Surwit EA, Young L, Moon TE, Meyskens FL (1981): Chemotherapy of ovarian cancer directed by the human tumor stem cell assay. Cancer Chemother Pharmacol 6:279–285.

Aroneyi RS, Levi JA, Dalley DN (1981): Triple drug chemotherapy for advanced ovarian carcinoma. Comparative study of two regimens. Med J Aust 1:633–635.

Barker GH, Wiltshaw E (1981): Randomized trial comparing low-dose cisplatin and doxorubicin in advanced ovarian carcinoma. Lancet 1:747–750.

Barlow JJ, Piver MS (1977): Single agent vs combination chemotherapy in the treatment of ovarian cancer. Obstet Gynecol 49:609–611.

Barlow JJ, Piver MS (1979): Second-line efficacy of intermediate high-dose methotrexate with citrovorum factor rescue + cyclophosphamide in ovarian cancer. Gynecol Oncol 7:233–238.

Barlow JJ, Piver MS, Lele SB (1982): Weekly cis-platinum remission "induction" and combination drug consolidation and maintenance in ovarian cancer. Proc Am Soc Clin Oncol 1:119

Bast RC Jr, Berek JS, Obreist R, Griffiths CT, Berkowitz RS, Hacker NF, Parker L, Lagasse LD, Knapp RC (1983a): Intraperitoneal immunotherapy of human ovarian carcinoma with *Corynebacterium parvum*. Cancer Res 443:1395–1401.

Bast, RC Jr, Klug T, St John E, Jenison J, Niloff, J, Lazarus H, Berkowitz R, Leavitt T, Griffiths CT, Parker L, Zurawski V, Knapp RC (1983b): A radioimmunoassay for monitoring patients with epithelial ovarian carcinoma: Comparison of CA125 and CEA. Proc Am Soc Clin Oncol 2:11.

Bast RC Jr, Klug T, Jenison E, Niloff J, Lazarus H, Berkowitz R, Leavitt T, Griffiths CT, Parker L, Zurawski V, Knapp RC (1983c): Monitoring growth of human ovarian carcinoma with a radioimmunoassay for antigen B1 defined by a murine monoclonal antibody (DC125). Soc Gynecol Oncol 14:12.

Bell DR, Woods RL, Levi JA, Fox RM, Tattersall MHN (1982): Advanced ovarian cancer: A prospective randomised trial of chlorambucil versus combined cyclophosphamide and cis-daimminedichloroplatinum. Aust NZ J Med 12:245–249.

Bolis G, Bortolozzi G, Carinelli G, D'Incalci M, Gramellini F, Morasca L, Mangioni C (1980): Low-dose cyclophosphamide versus adriamycin plus cyclophosphamide in advanced ovarian cancer. A randomized clinical study. Cancer Chemother Pharmacol 4:129–132.

Brady LW, Blessing JA, Slayton RE, Homesley HD, Lewis GC (1979): Radiotherapy, chemotherapy, and combined modality therapy in stage III epithelial ovarian cancer. Cancer Clin Trials 2:111–120.

Bruckner HW, Cohen CJ, Gusberg SB, Wallach RC, Kabakow B, Greenspan EM, Holland JF (1976): Chemotherapy of ovarian cancer with adriamycin (ADM) and cis-platinum (DDP). Proc Am Soc Clin Oncol 17:287.

Bruckner HW, Cohen CJ, Kabakow B, Wallach RC, Greenspan EM, Gusberg SB, Holland JF (1977a): Combination chemotherapy of ovarian carcinoma with platinum: Improved therapeutic index. Proc Am Assoc Cancer Res 18:339.

Bruckner HW, Cohen CJ, Deppe G, Kabakow B, Wallach RC, Greenspan EM, Gusberg SB, Holland JF (1977b): Chemotherapy of gynecological tumors with platinum II. J Clin Hematol Oncol 7:619–632.

Bruckner HW, Wallach RC, Kabakow B, Greenspan EM, Gusberg SB, Holland JF (1978a): Cis-platinum (DDP) for combination chemotherapy of ovarian carcinoma: Improved response rates and survival. Proc Am Soc Clin Oncol 19:373.

Bruckner HW, Cohen CJ, Wallach RC, Kabakow B, Deppe G, Grenspan EM, Gusberg SB, Holland J (1978b): Treatment of advanced ovarian cancer with cis-dichlorodiammineplatinum (II): Poor-risk patients with intensive prior therapy. Cancer Treat Rep 62: 555–558.

Bruckner H, Pagano M, Falkson C, Creech R, Arsenault JC, Horton J, Brodowsky H, Davis TE, Slayton RW, Greenspan EM (1979): Controlled prospective trial of combination chemotherapy with cyclophosphamide, adriamycin, and 5-fluorouracil for the treatment of advanced ovarian cancer: A preliminary report. Cancer Treat Rep 63:297–299.

Bruckner HW, Cohen CJ, Kabakow B, Wallach R, Deppe G, Ratner L, Greenspan EM, Jaffrey I, Goldberg J, Reisman A, Holland JF (1980a): Improving analysis and results: Secondary chemotherapy of ovarian cancer. Am Fed Clin Res 28:412A.

Bruckner HW, Cohen CJ, Goldberg J, Deppe G, Wallach R, Kabakow B, Gusberg SB, Holland JF (1980b): Differentiation of ovarian cancer as a survival determinant for adriamycin and cis-platin (AP) ± cyclophosphamide and hexamethylmelamine (CHAP). Proc Am Assoc Cancer Res 21:428.

Bruckner HW, Wallach R, Cohen CJ, Deppe G, Kabakow B, Ratner L, Holland JF (1981a): High-dose platinum for the treatment of refractory ovarian cancer. Gynecol Oncol 12:64–67.

Bruckner HW, Cohen CJ, Deppe G, Gusberg SB, Holland JF (1981b): Effect of cis-diamminedichloroplatinum chemotherapy on the survival of patients with advanced ovarian cancer. Mt Sinai J Med 48:121–123.

Bruckner HW, Cohen CJ, Deppe G, Kabakow B, Wallach R, Ratner L, Holland JF (1981c): Treatment of chemotherapy-resistant advanced ovarian cancer with a combination of cyclophosphamide, hexamethylmelamine, adriamycin, and cis-diamminedichloroplatinum (CHAP). Gynecol Oncol 12:150–153.

Bruckner HW, Cohen CJ, Kabakow B, Wallach R, Deppe G, Ratner L, Bhardwaj S, Goldberg JD, Resiman A, Holland JF (1981d): Ovarian cancer: Secondary cisplatin regimens and prognostic factors. Proc Am Soc Clin Oncol 22:469.

Bruckner HW (1981e): Therapeutic strategies for ovarian cancer. Ann Intern Med 95:653.

Bruckner HW, Cohen CJ, Goldberg JD, Kabakow B, Wallach RC, Deppe G, Greenspan EM, Gusberg SB, Holland JF (1981f): Improved chemotherapy for ovarian cancer with cis-diamminedichloroplatinum and adriamycin. Cancer 47:2288–2294.

Bruckner HW, Cohen CJ, Deppe G, Bhardwaj S, Zaken D, Storch JA, Goldberg J, Holland JF (1982): Schedule modification and dosage intensification of cyclophosphamide, hexamethylmelamine, adriamycin, cisplatin regimen (CHAP II). Proc Am Soc Clin Oncol 1:107.

Bruckner HW, Cohen CJ, Goldberg JD, Kabakow B, Wallach RC, Deppe G, Reisman AZ, Gusberg SB, Holland JF (1983a): Cisplatin regimens and improved prognosis of patients with poorly differentiated ovarian cancer. Am J Obstet Gynecol 145:653–658.

Bruckner HW, Cohen CJ, Goldberg J, Kabakow B, Wallach R, Holland JF (1983b): Ovarian cancer: Comparison of adriamycin and cisplatin ± cyclophosphamide. Proc Am Assoc Cancer Res 2:35.

Bruckner HW, Dinse G, Falkson G, Creech R, Arseneau JC, Davis TE, Vogel S, Greenspan E (1983c): A randomized comparison of cyclophosphamide, adriamycin and 5-fluorouracil with triethylenethiophosphamide and methotrexate both as sequential and as fixed rotational treatment in patients with advanced ovarian cancer. Cancer (submitted).

Buchsbaum HJ, Keetel WC, Latourette HB (1975): The use of radioisotopes as adjunct therapy of localized ovarian cancer. Semin Oncol 2:247–251.

Buckner CD, Briggs R, Clift RA, Fefer A, Funk DD, Glucksberg H, Neiman PE, Storb R, Thomas ED (1974): Intermittent high dose cyclophosphamide (NSC 26271) treatment of stage III ovarian carcinoma. Cancer Chemother Rep 58:697–704.

Burchenal JH, Kalaher K, O'Toole T, Chrisholm J (1977): Lack of cross-resistance between certain platinum coordination compounds in mouse leukemia. Cancer Res 37:2455–2547.

Carmo-Pereira J, Costa F, Henriques E, Ricardo JA (1981): Advanced ovarian carcinoma: A prospective and randomized clinical trial of cyclophosphamide versus combination cytotoxic chemotherapy (Hexa-CAF). Cancer 48:1947–1951.

Chen S, Lee L (1983): Prognostic significance of morphology of tumor and retroperitoneal lymph node in epithelial carcinoma of the ovary. Soc Gynecol Oncol 14:29.

Clark DG, Hilaris B, Roussis C, Brunschwig A (1973): The role of radiation therapy (including isotopes) in the treatment of cancer of the ovary: Results of 614 patients treated at Memorial Hospital, NY, NY. Prog Clin Cancer 5:227–235

Cohen CJ (1983): Improved therapy with cisplatin regimens for patients with ovarian carcinoma (FIGO stages III and IV) as measured by surgical end-staging (second-look operation). Am J Obstet Gynecol 145:955–967.

Cohen JM (1979): Peritoneoscopy for staging of ovarian cancer (Correspondence). N Engl J Med 300:987–988.

Copeland LJ, Gershenson DM, Wharton JT, Edwards CL, Rutledge FU (1983): Microscopc disease at second look laparotomy in advanced ovarian cancer. Soc Gynecol Oncol 14:18.

Corbett TH, Leopold WR, Dykes DJ, Roberts BJ, Griswold DP Jr, Schabel FM Jr (1982): Toxicity and anticancer activity of a new triazine antifolate (NSC 127755). Cancer Res 42:1707–1715.

Creasman WJ, Gall SA, Blessing JA, Schmidt HJ, Abu-Ghazaleh S, Whisnant JK: (1979): Chemoimmunotherapy in the management of primary stage III ovarian cancer: A Gynecologic Oncology Group study. Cancer Treat Rep 63:319–324.

Davis T, Vogl SE, Kaplan BH, Tunca J, Arseneau J (1980): Diamminedichloroplatinum (D) and hexamethylmelamine (H) in combination for ovarian cancer (OvCA) after failure of alkylating agent (AA) therapy — a phase I–II pilot trial. Proc Am Assoc Cancer Res 21:428.

Decker DG, Fleming TR, Malkasian GD, Webb MJ, Jefferies JA, Edmonson JH (1982): Cyclophosphamide plus cisplatinum in combination: Treatment program for stage III or IV ovarian carcinoma. Obstet Gynecol 60:481–487.

Dedrick RL, Myers CE, Bungay PM, DeVita VT Jr (1978): Pharmacokinetic rationale for peritoneal drug administration in the treatment of ovarian cancer. Cancer Treat Rep 62:1–11.

Delclos L, Smith JP (1975): Ovarian cancer with special regard to types of radiotherapy. Natl Cancer Inst Monogr 42:129–135.

Delgado G, Schein P, McDonald J (1979): L-PAM vs cyclophosphamide, hexamethylmelamine and 5-fluorouracil (CHF) for advanced ovarian cancer. Proc Am Assoc Cancer Res 20:434.

Deligdisch L, Jacobs A, Cohen, CJ (1982): Histologic correlates of virulence in ovarian adenocarcinoma. Am J Obstet Gynecol 144:885–889.

Dembo AJ, Bush RS, Beal FA, Bean HA, Pringle JF, Sturgeon J, Reid JG (1979a): Ovarian carcinoma: Improved survival following abdominopelvic irradiation in patients with completed pelvic operation. Am J Obstet Gynecol 134:793-800.

Dembo AJ, Bush RS, Beale FA, Beale HA (1979b): The Princess Margaret Hospital study of ovarian cancer: Stages I, II, and asymptomatic III presentations. Cancer Treat Rep 63:249–254.

Dembo AJ, Brown TC, Bush RS, Sturgeon JFG (1982): Prognostic significance of pathology subtype and differentiation in epithelial carcinoma of ovary (ECO). Proc Am Soc Clin Oncol 1:105.

Dembo AV (1983): Radiation therapy in the management of ovarian cancer. Clin Obstet Gynecol 10:261–278.

De Palo GM, De Lena M, Di Re F, Luciani L, Valagussa P, Bonadonna G (1975): Melphalan versus adriamycin in the treatment of advanced carcinoma of the ovary. Surg Gynecol Obstet 141:899–902.

De Palo GM, De Lena M, Bonadonna G (1977): Adriamycin versus adriamycin plus melphalan in advanced ovarian carcinoma. Cancer Treat Rep 61:355–357.

De Palo G, Demicheli R, Valagussa P (1981): Prospective study with HEXA-CAF combination in ovarian carcinoma. Cancer Chemother Pharmacol 5:157–161.

Donahoe PK, Swann DA, Hayashi A, Sullivan MD (1979): C.E. Mullerian duct regression in the embryo correlated with cytotoxic activity against human ovarian cancer. Science 205:913–915.

Edmonson JH, Fleming TR, Decker DG, Malkasian GD, Jorgensen EO, Jefferies JA, Webb MJ, Krols LK (1979): Different chemotherapeutic sensitivities and host factors affecting prognosis in advanced ovarian carcinoma versus minimal residual disease. Cancer Treat Rep 63:241–247.

Ehrlich CE, Einhorn L, Williams SD, Morgan J (1979): Chemotherapy for stage III–IV epithelial ovarian cancer with cis-dichlorodiammineplatinum (II), adriamycin, and cyclophosphamide: A preliminary report. Cancer Treat Rep 63:281–288.

Ehrlich CE, Einhorn LH, Stehman FB, Roth L (1980): Response, "second look" status and survival in stage III–IV epithelial ovarian cancer treated with cis-dichlorodiammineplatinum (II) (cis-platinum), adriamycin (ADR), and cyclophosphamide (CTX). Proc Am Assoc Cancer Res 21:423.

Ehrlich, C, Einhorn L, Stehman FB, Blessing J (1983): Treatment of advanced epithelial ovarian cancer using cis platin, adriamycin and cytoxan. The Indiana University experience. Clin Obstet Gynecol 10:325–335.

Einhorn N, Cantell K, Einhorn S, Strander H (1982a): Human leukocyte interferon therapy for advanced ovarian carcinoma. Am J Clin Oncol 5:167–172.

Einhorn N, Eklund G, Franzen S, Lambert BO, Lindsten J, Soderhall, LS (1982b): Late side effects of chemotherapy in ovarian carcinoma. Cancer 49:2234–2241.

Epstein LB, Shen JT, Abele JS, Reese CC (1980): Sensitivity of human ovarian carcinoma cells to interferon and other antitumor agents as assessed by an in vitro semi-solid agar technique. Ann NY Acad Sci 350:228–244.

Fuks Z (1975): External radiotherapy of ovarian cancer: Standard approaches and new frontiers. Semin Oncol 2:253–266.

Fuks Z, Bagshaw MA (1975): The rationale for curative radiotherapy for ovarian cancer. Int J Radiat Oncol Biol Phys 1:21–32.

Fuller AF, Guy S, Budzik GP, Donahoe PK (1982): Mullerian inhibiting substance inhibits colony growth of a human ovarian carcinoma cell line. J Clin Endocrinol Metab 54:1051–1055.

Geisler HE (1983): Megesterol acetate for the palliation of advanced ovarian cancer. Obstet Gynecol 61:95–98.

Gershenson DM, Wharton JT, Herson J, Edwards CL, Rutledge RN (1981): Single-agent cis-platinum therapy for advanced ovarian cancer. Obstet Gynecol 58:487–496.

Gershenson DM, Copeland LV, Wharton JT, Edwards CL, Rutledge FN (1983): Surgically-determined complete responders in advanced ovarian cancer. Soc Gynecol Oncol 14:18.

Greco FA, Oldham RK, Richardson RL, Hande KR, Burnett LS, Julian C (1981a): Limited stage III ovarian cancer — a potentially curable neoplasm. Proc Am Cancer Res 21:422.

Greco FA, Julian CG, Richardson RL, Burnett L, Hande KR, Oldham RK (1981b): Advanced ovarian cancer: Brief intensive combination chemotherapy and second look operation. Obstet Gynecol 58:199–205.

Greco FA, Burnett LS, Wolff SN, Hande KR, Richardson RL, Oldham RK, Jones HW (1982): Limited residual advanced ovarian cancer—a curable neoplasm? Proc Am Soc Clin Oncol 1:106.

Greene MH, Boke VD, Greer BE, Blessing DA, Dembo AJ (1982): Acute non-lymphocytic leukemia (ANL) after alkylating agent (AA) therapy for ovarian cancer. Am Soc Clin Oncol 1:118.

Griffiths CT (1975): Surgical resection of tumor bulk in the primary treatment of ovarian carcinoma. Seminar on ovarian cancer. Natl Cancer Inst Monogr 42:101–104, 113–115.
Griffiths CT, Fuller AF (1978): Intensive surgical and chemotherapeutic management of advanced ovarian cancer. Surg Clin North Am 58:131–141.
Griffiths CT, Parker LM, Fuller AF (1979): Role of cytoreductive surgical treatment in the management of advanced ovarian cancer. Cancer Treat Rep 63:235–239.
Griffiths CT (1980): Cytoreductive surgical treatment in the management of advanced ovarian cancer. In Van Oosterom AT, Muggia FM, Cleton FJ (eds): "Therapeutic Progress in Ovarian Cancer, Testicular Cancer and the Sarcomas." The Hague: Martinus Nijhoff, pp 3–12.
Holland JF, Bruckner HW, Cohen CJ, Wallach RC, Gusberg SB, Greenspan EM, Goldberg J (1980a): Cis-platinum therapy of ovarian cancer. In Prestayko AW, Crooke ST (eds): "Cisplatin: Current Status and New Developments." New York: Academic, pp 383–391.
Holland JF, Bruckner HW, Cohen CJ, Wallach RC, Gusberg SB, Greenspan EM, Goldberg J (1980b): Cisplatin therapy of ovarian cancer. In Van Oosterom AT, Muggia FM, Cleton FJ (eds): "Therapeutic Progress in Ovarian Cancer, Testicular Cancer and the Sarcomas." The Hague: Martinus Nijhoff, pp 41–52.
Hreshchshyn MM, Norris HJ (1979): Postoperative treatment of resectable malignant and possibly malignant epithelial ovarian tumors with radiotherapy, melphalan or no further treatment. Proc XII Int Cancer Congr, Buenos Aires. New York: Pergamon, p 157.
Hreshchyshyn MM, Park RC, Blessing JA, Norris HJ, Levy D, Lagasse LD, Creasman WT (1980): The role of adjuvant therapy in stage I ovarian cancer. Am J Obstet Gynecol 138:139–145.
Izbicki RM, Baker LH, Samson MK, McDonald B, Vaitkevicius VK (1977): 5FU infusion and cyclophosphamide in the treatment of advanced ovarian cancer. Cancer Treat Rep 61:1573–1575.
Julian CG, Woodruff JD (1972): The biologic behavior of low-grade papillary serous carcinoma of the ovary. Obstet Gynecol 40:860–867.
Katz ME, Schwarz PE, Kapp DS, Luikart S (1981): Epithelial carcinoma of the ovary: Current strategies. Ann Intern Med 95:98–111.
Limburg H, Brachetti AKJ (1981): 16 jahrige klinische ergebnisse in der behandlung des ovarialkarzinoms nach dem chemotherapie-resistenztest. Geburtsh. Faeuenheilk 41: 126–135.
Longo DL, Yong RC (1980): Current treatment and new prospects. In Van Oosterom AT, Muggia FM, Cleton FJ (eds): "Therapeutic Progress in Ovarian Cancer, Testicular Cancer and the Sarcomas." The Hague: Martinus Nijhoff, pp 61–75.
Mangioni C, Bolis G, Bortolozzi G, Sessa C, Garrattini S (1980): Cis dichlorodiamine platinum, adriamycin cyclophosphamide (PAC) versus hexamethylmelamine, adriamycin, cyclophosphamide (HAC) in advanced ovarian cancer. Proc Am Assoc Cancer Res 21:149.
Mangioni C, Bolis G, Valente I, Molina P, Sessa CI (1981): Cis-diammine chloroplatinum, adriamycin, cyclophosphamide (PAC) versus hexamethylmelamine, adriamycin and cyclophosphamide (HAC). Proc Am Assoc Cancer Res 22:166.
Mayer RJ, Berkowitz RS, Griffiths CT (1978): Central nervous system involvement by ovarian carcinoma. Cancer 41:776–783.
Medical Research Council's Working Party on Ovarian Cancer (1981): Medical Research Council study on chemotherapy in advanced ovarian cancer. Br J Obstet Gynaecol 88:1174–1185.

Miller AB, Klaassen DJ, Boyes DA, Dodds DJ, Gerulath A, Kirk ME, Levitt M, Pearson JG, Wall C (1980): Combination vs sequential therapy with melphalan, 5-fluorouracil and methotrexate for advanced ovarian cancer. CMA J 123:365–371.

Muggia FM, McGuire WP, Pozencweig M (1979): Rationale, design and methodology of phase II clinical trials. In Busch H, DeVita VT (eds): "Methods in Cancer Research." New York: Academic, Vol XVII, pp 199–214.

Muggia FM (1980): New drugs in the treatment of ovarian cancer. In Van Oosterom AT, Muggia FM, Cleton FJ (eds): "Therapeutic Progress in Ovarian Cancer, Testicular Cancer and the Sarcomas." The Hague: Martinus Nijhoff, pp 129–138.

Nadji M, Ganjei P, Morales A, Averette H (1983): The value of immunoperoxidase technique in histogenetic classification of ovarian tumors. Soc Gynecol Oncol 14:26.

Neijt JP, Van Lindert ACM, Vendrik CP, Roozendaal KJ, Strugvenberg A, Pinedo HM (1979): Hexa-CAF combination chemotherapy and other multiple drug regimens in advanced ovarian carcinoma: Present and future. Neth J Med 22:38–44.

Neijt JP, Van Lindert ACM, Vendrik CPJ, Roozendaal KJ, Struyvenberg A, Pinedo HM (1980): Treatment of advanced ovarian carcinoma with a combination of hexamethylmelamine, cyclophosphamide, methotrexate and 5-fluorouracil (Hexa-CAF) in patients with and without previous treatment. Cancer Treat Rep 64:323–326.

Neijt JP, Ten Bokke J, Huinink WW, Hamersma E, Van de Burg MEL, Van Oosterom AT, Koojman CD, Van Houwelingen J, Pinedo HM (1982): Combination chemotherapy including cis-platinum in previously treated patients with advanced ovarian carcinoma. Proc Am Soc Clin Oncol 18:108.

Neijt JP, Ten Bokke J, Huinink WW, Van de Burg MEL (1983): Chemotherapy with Hexa-CAF and CHAP V in advanced ovarian carcinoma. A randomized study of the Netherlands Joint Study Group for Ovarian Cancer. Proc Am Soc Clin Oncol 2:148.

Neijt JP (1983): Combination chemotherapy in the treatment of advanced ovarian carcinoma. Utrecht, The Netherlands: ICG Printing, Dordtrecht (monograph).

Nevin JE (1983): The use of intravenous phenylalanine mustard followed by supervoltage irradiation in the treatment of carcinoma of the ovary. Cancer 51:1273–1283.

O'Connell GJ, DePetrillo AD, Taylor MH, Scruton J, Turner AR (1983): Pilot study — accelerated weekly combination chemotherapy in advanced epithelial ovarian carcinoma under cotrimoxazole coverage and pretreatment cryo-preservation of host marrow. Mtg Soc Gynecol Oncol 14:17.

Omura GA, Blessing JA, Morrow CP, Buchbaum HJ, Homesley HD (1981): Follow-up of a randomized trail of melphalan vs melphalan plus hexamethylmelamine vs adriamycin plus cyclophosphamide in advanced ovarian adenocarcinoma. Proc Am Soc Clin Oncol 22:470.

Omura GA, Ehrlich CE, Blessing JA (1982): A randomized trial of cyclophosphamide (C) plus adriamycin (A) with or without cis platinum (P) in ovarian carcinoma. Proc Am Soc Clin Oncol 1:104.

Order SE, Rosenshein NB, Klein J, et al (1979): New methods applied to the analysis and treatment of ovarian cancer. Int J Radiat Oncol Biol Phys 5:861–873.

Ozols RF, Garvin AJ, Costa J, Simon RM, Young RC (1979): Histologic grade in advanced ovarian cancer. Cancer Treat Rep 63:255–263.

Ozols RF, Garvin AJ, Costa J, Simon RM, Young RC (1980): Advanced ovarian cancer. Correlation of histologic grade with response to therapy and survival. Cancer 45:572–581.

Parker LM, Griffiths CT, Yankee RA, Knapp RC, Canellos GP (1979): High-dose methotrexate with leucovorin rescue in ovarian cancer: A phase II study. Cancer Treat Rep 63:275–279.

Parker LM, Griffiths CT, Yankee RA, Canellos GP, Gellan R, Knapp RC, Richmann CM, Tobias JS, Weiner RS, Frei E III (1980): Combination chemotherapy with adriamycin-cyclophosphamide for advanced ovarian carcinoma. Cancer 46:669–674.

Parker LM, Griffiths CT, Janis D, Welch WR, Gelman RS, Bast RC, Canellos GP (1983): Advanced ovarian carcinoma: Integration of surgical treatment and chemotherapy with cyclophosphamide (C), adriamycin (A), and cis diamminedichloroplatinum (P). Proc Am Soc Clin Oncol 2:153.

Pesando JM, Come SE, Stark J, Parker LM, Griffiths CT, Canellos GP (1980): Cis-diamminedichloroplatinum (II) therapy for advanced ovarian cancer. Cancer Treat Rep 64:10–11,1147–1148.

Pfleiderer A (1982): Chemotherapy of ovarian carcinoma. Strahlentherapie 158:708–716.

Piver MS, Lele S, Barlow J (1980): Weekly cis-diamminedichloroplatinum (II): Active third-line chemotherapy in ovarian carcinoma—a preliminary report. Cancer Treat Rep 64:1379–1382.

Pretorius GR, Hacker NF, Berek JS, Ford LC, Chamorro T, Lagasse LD (1982): Intraperitoneal cis platinum in patients with ovarian carcinoma. Proc Soc Clin Oncol 1:113.

Reymer RR, Hoover R, Fraumeniu F, Young RC (1972): Acute leukemia following alkylating agent therapy of ovarian cancer. N Engl J Med 297:177–181.

Rosenoff SH, DeVita VT, Hubbard S, Young RC (1975): Peritoneoscopy in the staging and follow-up of ovarian cancer. Semin Oncol 2:223–228.

Rossof AH, Drukker BH, Talley RW, Torres J,, Bonnett, Brownlee RW (1976): Randomized evaluation of chlorambucil and melphalan in advanced ovarian cancer. Proc Am Soc Clin Oncol 17:300.

Salmon SE, Meyskens FL, Alberts DS, Soehnlen B, Young L (1981): New drugs in ovarian cancer and malignant melanoma: In vitro phase II screening with the human tumor stem cell assay. Cancer Treat Rep 65:1–12.

Salmon SE, Meyskens FL, Alberts DS, Soehnlen B, Young L (1981): Update on in vitro testing of new drugs in ovarian cancer and melanoma. Cancer Treat Rep 65:532–533.

Schwartz PE, LaVolsi W, MacLuskey N, Eisenfeld A (1980a): Steroid receptor protein in ovarian malignancies. Gynecol Oncol 10:371.

Schwartz PE, Keating G, MacLusky N, Eisenfeld A (1980b): Tamoxifen therapy for advanced ovarian cancer. Proc Am Assoc Cancer Res 21:430.

Schwartz PE, Smith JP (1980c): Second look surgery in ovarian cancer management. Am J Obstet Gynecol 138:1124–1130.

Schwartz PE, Lawrence R, Katz ME (1981): Combination chemotherapy for advanced ovarian cancer: A prospective randomized trial comparing hexamethylmelamine-cyclophosphamide to adriamycin-cyclophosphamide. Cancer Treat Rep 65:137–171.

Schwartz PE, LaVolsi VA, Hildreth N, MacLusky NJ, Naftolin FN, Eisenfeld AJ (1982): Estrogen receptors in ovarian epithelial carcinoma. Obstet Gynecol 59:229–238.

Sessa C, D'Incalci M, Valente I, Bolis G, Colombo N, Mangioni C (1982): Hexamethylmelamine-CAF (cyclophosphamide, methotrexate, and 5-FU) and cisplatin-CAF in refractory ovarian cancer. Cancer Treat Rep 66:1233–1234.

Smith JP, Rutledge F (1970): Chemotherapy in the treatment of cancer of the ovary. Am J Obstet Gynecol 107:691–703.

Smith JP, Rutledge F, Wharton JT (1972): Chemotherapy of ovarian cancer: New approaches to treatment. Cancer 30:1565–1571.

Smith JP, Rutledge FN, Delclos L (1975a): Postoperative treatment of early ovarian cancer: A random trial between postoperative irradiation and chemotherapy. Natl Cancer Inst Monogr 42:149–153.

Smith JP, Rutledge FN (1975b): Randomized study of hexamethylmelamine, 5-fluorouracil and melphalan in the treatment of advanced carcinoma of the ovary. Natl Cancer Inst Monogr 42:169–172.

Smith JP, Rutledge FN, Delclos L (1975c): Results of chemotherapy as an adjunct to surgery in patients with localized ovarian cancer. Semin Oncol 2:277–281.

Smith JP, Day TG (1979): Review of ovarian cancer at the University of Texas Systems Cancer Center, M.D. Anderson Hospital & Tumor Institute. Am J Obstet Gynecol 135:984–990.

Smith JP, Schwartz PE (1980): Second look laparotomy and prognosis related to extent of residual disease. In Van Oosterom AT, Muggia FM, Cleton FJ (eds): "Therapeutic Progress in Ovarian Cancer, Testicular Cancer and the Sarcomas." The Hague: Martinus Nijhoff, pp 77–93.

Stanhope RC, Smith JP, Rutledge FN (1977): Second trial drugs in ovarian cancer. Gynecol Oncol 5:52–58.

Sturgeon JFG, Fine S, Bean HA, Bush RS, Pringle JF, Beule FA (1980): A randomized trial of melphalan alone versus combination chemotherapy in advanced ovarian cancer. Proc Am Assoc Cancer Res 21:422.

Sturgeon JFG, Fine S, Gospodarowicz MK, Dembo AJ, Bean HA, Bush RS, Beale FA, Pringle JF, Thomas GM, Herman JG (1982): A randomized trial of melphalan alone versus combination chemotherapy in advanced ovarian cancer. Proc Am Soc Clin Oncol 1:108.

Surwit EA, Alberts DS, Jackson R, Leigh, S (1983): Multiagent chemotherapy in relapsing ovarian cancer. Mtg Soc Gynecol Oncol 14:15.

Tobias JS, Griffiths CT (1976): Management of ovarian carcinoma: Current concepts and future prospects. N Engl J Med 294:818–823, 882–887.

Trope C, Mattsson W, Astedt B (1977): A phase II study of combined adriamycin, L-PAM and methotrexate with citrovorum factor rescue in advanced ovarian carcinomas. Tumori 63:469–477.

Trope C (1981): A prospective and randomized trial comparison of melphalan vs adriamycin-melphalan in advanced ovarian carcinoma. Proc Am Soc Clin Oncol 22:469.

Trope C, Sigurdsson K (1981): Use of tissue culture in cancer. Correlation between in vitro results and the response in vivo. Neoplasma 29:309–314.

Turbow MM, Jones H, Yu VK, Greenberg B, Hannigan J, Torti FM (1980): Chemotherapy of ovarian carcinoma: A comparison of melphalan vs adriamycin-cyclophosphamide. Proc Am Assoc Cancer Res 21:196.

Vaitkevicius VK, Talley RW, Brennan MJ, Kelly JE (1961): Chemotherapy of advanced ovarian cancer. J Mich State Med Soc 60:492–496.

Villasanta U (1980): Cyclophosphamide and floxuridine adjuvant chemotherapy for stage III and IV carcinoma of the ovary. Gynecol Oncol 10:44–50.

Vistica DT, Von Hoff DD, Torain B (1981): Uptake of melphalan by human ovarian carcinoma cells and its relationship to the amino acid content of ascitic fluid. Cancer Treat Rep 65:157–161.

Vogl SE, Berenzweig M, Kaplan BH, Moukhtar M, Mulkin W (1979): The CHAD and HAD regimens in advanced ovarian cancer: Combination chemotherapy including cyclophosphamide, hexamethylmelamine, adriamycin, and cis-dichlorodiammineplatinum II). Cancer Treat Rep 63:311–317.

Vogl SE, Kaplan BH, Greenwald E (1980): Prognostic factors for platinum-based combination chemotherapy of advanced ovarian cancer (AdOvCa). Proc Am Assoc Cancer Res 21:429.

Vogl SE, Pagano M, Kaplan B (1981): Cyclophosphamide, hexamethylmelamine, adriamycin and diamminedichloroplatinum "CHAD" vs melphalan for advanced ovarian cancer: A randomized prospective trial of the Eastern Cooperative Oncology Group. Proc Am Soc Clin Oncol 22:473.

Vogl SE, Kaplan B, Pagano M (1982): Diamminedichloroplatinum (D)-based combination chemotherapy (CT) is superior to melphalan for advanced ovarian cancer (OvCa) when age is over 50 and tumor diameter over 2 cm. Proc Am Soc Clin Oncol 1:119.

Wampler GL, Mellette SJ, Kuperminc M, Regelson W (1972): Hexamethylmelamine (MSC-13875) in the treatment of advanced cancer. Cancer Chemother Rep 56:505–514.

Webb MJ, Malkasian GD Jr, Jorgensen EO (1974): Factors influencing ovarian cancer survival after chemotherapy. Obstet Gynecol 44:564–570.

Wernz JC, Speyer JL, Noumoff J, Faig D, Clayton M, Muggia F (1982): Cisplatin (DDP)/cytoxan: A high dose DDP regimen for advanced ovarian carcinoma. Proc Am Soc Clin Oncol 1:112.

Wharton JT, Rutledge F, Smith JP, Herson V, Hodge MP (1979): Hexamethylmelamine: An evaluation of its role in the treatment of ovarian cancer. Am J Obstet Gynecol 133:833–844.

Wharton JT, Herson J, Edwards CL, Seski V, Hodge MD (1980): Longterm survival following chemotherapy for advanced epithelial ovarian carcinoma. In Van Oosterom AT, Muggia FM, Cleton FJ (eds): "Therapeutic Progress in Ovarian Cancer, Testicular Cancer and the Sarcomas." The Hague: Martinus Nijhoff, pp 96–112.

Wharton JT, Herson J, Edwards CLL, Griffith AB (1982): Single agent adriamycin followed by combination hexamethylmelamine-cyclophosphamide for advanced ovarian carcinoma. Gynecol Oncol 14:262–270.

Williams CJ, Whitehouse JMA (1980): Combination chemotherapy of advanced ovarian carcinoma with cis diamminedichloroplatinum (DDP), adriamycin and cyclophosphamide (PACe). Proc Am Assoc Cancer Res 21:36.

Wilson AP, Neal FE (1981): In vitro sensitivity of human ovarian tumours to chemotherapeutic agents. Br J Cancer 44:189–200.

Wiltshaw E, Kroner T (1976): Phase II study of cis-dichlorodiammineplatinum (II) (NSC-119875) in advanced adenocarcinoma of the ovary. Cancer Treat Rep 60:55–60.

Wiltshaw E (1978): A review of clinical experience with cis-platinum diammine dichloride: 1972–1978. Biochemie 60:925–929.

Wiltshaw E, Subramarian S, Alexopoulos C, Barker GH (1979): Cancer of the ovary: A summary of experience with cis-platinum diamminedichloride (II) in the Royal Marsden Hospital. Cancer Treat Rep 63:1545–1548.

Wiltshaw E (1980): Hexamethylmelamine and cisplatinum combinations in the treatment of ovarian cancer. In Van Oosterom AT, Muggia FM, Cleton FJ (eds): "Therapeutic Progress in Ovarian Cancer, Testicular Cancer and the Sarcomas." The Hague: Martinus Nijhoff, pp 53–60.

Wiltshaw E, Evans BD, Jones AC, Baker JW, Calvert AH (1983): JM8, successor to cisplatin in advanced ovarian carcinoma. Lancet 1:587.

Young RC, Chabner BA, Hubbard SP, Fisher RI, Bender RA, Anderson T, Simon RM, Canellos GP, DeVita VT (1978): Advanced ovarian adenocarcinoma: A prospective clinical trial of melphalan (L-PAM) versus combination chemotherapy. N Engl J Med 299:1261–1266.

Young RC (1979): A strategy for effective management for early ovarian carcinoma. In Jones SE, Salmon SE (eds): "Adjuvant Therapy of Cancer II." New York: Grune and Stratton, pp 467–474.

Young RC, Von Hoff DD, Gormley P, et al (1979): Cis-dichlorodiammineplatinum (II) for the treatment of advanced ovarian cancer. Cancer Treat Rep 63:1539–1544.

Young RC, Howser DM, Myers CE, Ozols RF, Fisher RI, Wesley M, Chabner BA (1981): Combination chemotherapy (Chex-UP) with intraperitoneal maintenance in advanced ovarian adenocarcinoma. Proc Am Soc Clin Oncol 22:465.

Young JA, Kroener JF, Lucas WE, Mendelsohn J, Yon JL, Campbell TN, Weiss R, Saltzstein SL, Johnson A, Green MR (1982): Cisplatin (P), adriamycin (Adr), and cyclophosphamide (Ctx) alternating with hexamethylmelamine (Hmm), CTX, methotrexate (Mtx), and 5-fluorouracil (5-FU) for advanced ovary cancer (AdOC). Proc Am Soc Clin Oncol 1:115.

Young, RC, Walton L, Decker D, Major F, Homesley H, Ellenberg S (1983): Early stage ovarian cancer: Preliminary results of randomized trials after comprehensive initial staging. Proc Am Soc Clin Oncol 2:148.

Chemotherapy of Malignant Ovarian Germ Cell Tumors

Robert E. Slayton

Section of Medical Oncology, Department of Internal Medicine, Rush-Presbyterian-St. Luke's Medical Center, Chicago, Illinois 60612

The malignant germ cell tumors of the ovary are uncommon but important tumors since treatment, properly designed and directed, may lead to cure. These tumors range in virulence from the dysgerminoma, usually localized and radiosensitive, to the endodermal sinus tumor, an aggressive tumor frequently incompletely resected and relatively insensitive to radiation therapy. Even though totally resected, most endodermal sinus tumors recur promptly, the majority of patients dying with widespread peritoneal metastases within a year [2]. Progression and survival with immature teratoma are related to the grade of the primary tumor [4]. In mixed germ cell tumors the presence of endodermal sinus elements is the most important factor in determining prognosis [2].

In a 1974 review Malkasian et al. [3] cited eight reports evaluating chemotherapy in 20 patients with ovarian germ tumors, including four with choriocarcinoma. Malkasian added ten patients, eight failing within an average of 5.1 months after pelvic and abdominal radiation. Two treated with vincristine, cyclophosphamide, and dactinomycin (VAC) showed an objective response. A year later Smith and Rutledge [6] reported responses with this drug combination in patients with advanced endodermal sinus tumor of the ovary and urged its use in an adjuvant setting in early disease. In 1979 Gallion et al. [1] reported 17 of 25 (68%) stage I patients alive 2 or more years following treatment with VAC.

At about the same time the Gynecologic Oncology Group (GOG) reported preliminary experience with VAC therapy in germ cell tumors of the ovary [5]. Including 13 patients with pure endodermal sinus tumors, 11 of 19 (58%) were alive and free of disease at 2 years. Since then the GOG has

Chemotherapy of Gynecologic Cancer, pages 195–197

treated 67 patients with endodermal sinus tumors with VAC following resection of all visible tumor. The majority were stage IA. Twenty-three (34%) have failed, including 16 of 44 (36%) with pure endodermal sinus tumors and seven of 23 (30%) with mixed tumors containing endodermal sinus elements. The smallest mixed germ cell tumor was 9.5 cm in diameter. The risk of failure for patients with mixed tumors smaller than 10 cm in diameter [2] may be lower but this could not be confirmed in the GOG study. For immature teratoma grade 2 and 3 VAC appears to be even more effective with only two failures among 37 GOG patients (6%) with grade 2–3 disease who received adjuvant therapy (unpublished data).

Nine patients who failed adjuvant VAC therapy received salvage vinblastine, cisplatin, and bleomycin (VPB) therapy. Six are evaluable, and four have failed; two are clinically free of disease at 11 and 34 months [7].

VAC appears to be less effective against germ cell tumors that cannot be completely resected. Four of eight GOG patients with incompletely resected immature teratoma failed while receiving chemotherapy; the other four were found to have mature teratoma at "second-look" surgery and remain progression-free. Only three of 14 (21%) patients with incompletely resected endodermal sinus tumor are progression-free (unpublished data), and the GOG has abandoned VAC therapy in favor of VPB in this group of patients. Preliminary data [7] show complete responses in 13 and partial responses in four patients with measurable disease treated with this combination. However, VPB is not without serious and life-threatening side effects, and its role as adjuvant therapy for patients with immature teratoma is limited in view of the demonstrated effectiveness of VAC. Should one accept the toxicity of adjuvant VPB therapy as the price of increasing the survival rate for patients with totally resected endodermal sinus tumors? A trial of adjuvant VPB therapy modified to avoid life-threatening toxicity is planned by the GOG.

REFERENCES

1. Gallion H, VanNagell, JR Jr, Powell DF, Donaldson ES, Hanson M: Therapy of endodermal sinus tumor of the ovary. Am J Obstet Gynecol 135:447–451, 1979.
2. Kurman RJ, Norris HJ: Malignant germ cell tumors of the ovary. Hum Pathol 8:551–564, 1977.
3. Malkasian GD, Webb MJ, Jorgensen EO: Observations on chemotherapy of granulosa cell carcinomas and malignant ovarian teratomas. Obstet Gynecol 44:885–888, 1974.
4. Norris HJ, Zirken HJ, Benson WL: Immature (malignant) teratoma of the ovary: A clinical and pathologic study of 58 cases. Cancer 37:2359–2372, 1976.

5. Slayton RE, Hreshchyshyn MM, Silverberg SG, Shingleton HM, Park RC, DiSaia PJ, Blessing JA: Treatment of malignant ovarian germ cell tumors: Response to vincristine, dactinomycin and cyclophosphamide (preliminary report). Cancer 42:390–398, 1978.
6. Smith J, Rutledge F: Advances in chemotherapy for gynecologic malignancies. Cancer 36:669–674, 1975.
7. Williams S: Personal communication.

Chemotherapy of Stromal Tumors of the Ovary

Robert E. Slayton

Section of Medical Oncology, Department of Internal Medicine, Rush-Presbyterian-St. Luke's Medical Center, Chicago, Illinois 60612

Roughly 1–3% of all ovarian tumors are derived from collagen-producing stromal cells including theca cells, granulosa cells, and Sertoli-Leydig cells in various stages of differentiation. Frequently these tumors are hormonally active, producing estrogens, progestogens, and androgens. The embryonic gonad is hormonally bisexual. The gynandroblastoma contains both male and female elements.

The majority of stromal tumors produce estrogens. In younger patients estrogens produced by granulosa cells may produce feminization or precocious puberty; in older women they may produce amenorrhea, bleeding, endometrial hyperplasia, and, occasionally, endometrial carcinoma. Sertoli-Leydig tumors, in contrast, contain structures resembling fetal testis, produce androgens, and cause defeminization or masculinization. Serial measurement of steroid hormone levels may be helpful in detecting recurrence. Fifteen percent of stromal tumors are hormonally inactive.

The majority of stromal tumors are limited to one ovary. The capsule is generally smooth and intact. Factors such as tumor size, stage, degree of differentiation, and histologic pattern are of prognostic importance [3]. Theca cell tumors are rarely malignant. Granulosa cell tumors, although malignant, are indolent tumors with a long natural history. Not uncommonly, patients will have tumors that contain both elements. In adults, recurrence is late and long-term survival the rule. According to Fox et al. [4] patients over 40 have a worse prognosis than younger patients. Sertoli-Leydig cell tumors are generally seen in younger women. Seventy-three of 111 (66%) patients reviewed by Novak and Long [9] were below the age of 30. Like other stromal tumors they are low-grade malignancies. In the

Chemotherapy of Gynecologic Cancer, pages 199–202

Ovarian Tumor Registry, 26 of 90 (28.9%) patients died within 5 years, most of them within 3 years of surgery [9]. On the other hand O'Hern and Neubecker [10] observed only one recurrence among 33 patients with arrhenoblastoma, and suggest that adenocarcinomas were occasionally mistakenly identified as arrhenoblastomas in earlier reports. In GOG trials only one of 11 patients with a Sertoli-Leydig cell tumor has developed recurrence, this patient failing within 3 months following surgery [14].

Because malignant stromal tumors of the ovary are uncommon and indolent, a role of adjuvant therapy has not been defined. Recurrence is generally localized to the pelvis or abdomen. Hematogeneous dissemination is rare [3]. Postoperative irradiation has been given without clear evidence of benefit [5]. Indeed, until risk factors (stage, histologic grade, tumor size, menopausal status) are more clearly defined it is unlikely that drugs currently used for treatment of advanced disease will be used effectively in an adjuvant setting. Estrogens may be indicated for replacement in premenopausal women, but may also be helpful in postmenopausal women on the basis of experiments showing prevention of tumor grafts in mice pretreated with estrogens or androgens [5].

Drugs currently used in advanced disease include cyclophosphamide, vincristine, dactinomycin, 5-fluorouracil, doxorubicin, and bleomycin, alone or in combination. In the early 1970s Malkasian et al. [8] recommended pelvic and abdominal irradiation for patients with advanced disease, reserving cyclophosphamide for radiation failures. Using cyclophosphamide, Malkasian observed partial response in three of 12 patients with recurrent granulosa cell tumors [8]. Lusch [7] reported a complete response to melphalan. Smith and Rutledge [16] reported partial response in six of 15 patients with recurrent granulosa cell tumor; the majority received alkylating agents. DiSaia et al. [2] reported a temporary but dramatic response to doxorubicin alone.

Combination chemotherapy may be more effective. Barlow et al. [1] observed a complete response in stage III disease using doxorubicin plus bleomycin. Jacobs et al. [6] reported complete clinical remission in two patients with cisplatin and doxorubicin. Schulman et al. [11] observed a partial response with cyclophosphamide, doxorubicin, and cisplatin. In a recent GOG trial [13] 13 patients with advanced disease received combined dactinomycin, 5-fluorouracil, and cyclophosphamide (AcFuCy) therapy. Seven had measurable disease; complete clinical response was seen in three. One failed at 21 months; the others remain clinically free of disease at 27 and 45 months. Partial responses were not observed. There were three with stable disease; of these, two are progression-free at 4 and 34 months; one died of other causes at 4 months. One patient progressed at 2 months. Of six patients with advanced but nonmeasurable disease treated with AcFuCy, one progressed at 26 months. In the same GOG trial one patient with metastatic, bulky Sertoli-Leydig cell tumor received three cycles of vincristine, dactinomycin, and cyclophosphamide (VAC) with a partial response continuing at 2½ months. A second patient with recurrent Sertoli-Leydig cell tumor received five cycles of VAC and is clinically free of disease at 6 months.

Finding alkylating agents generally ineffective when used alone, Schwartz and Smith [12] have used the AcFuCy combination for metastatic and recurrent granulosa cell tumors, and the VAC combination for Sertoli-Leydig cell tumors. Finding no advantage in using different regimens, the GOG, encouraged by Smith [15] now uses VAC for both histologic types. It is clear that optimal chemotherapy for these uncommon tumors cannot be established without further evaluation in cooperative group trials.

REFERENCES

1. Barlow JJ, Piver MS, Chuang JT, Cortes CP, Onuma T, Holland JF: Adriamycin and bleomycin alone, and in combination, in gynecological cancer. Cancer 32:735–743, 1973.
2. DiSaia P, Saltz A, Kagan AR, Rich WA: A temporary response of recurrent granulosa cell tumor to adriamycin. Obstet Gynecol 52(3):355–358, 1978.
3. Evans AT III, Gaffey TA, Malkasian GD Jr, Annegers JJ: Clinicopathologic review of 118 granulosa and 82 theca cell tumors. Obstet Gynecol 55:231–238, 1980.
4. Fox N, Agarical K, Langley FA: A clinicopathologic study of 92 cases of granulosa cell tumors of the ovary with special reference to the factors influencing prognosis. Cancer 35:231–241, 1975.
5. Goldston WR, Johnston WW, Fetter BF, Parker RT, Wilbanks GD: Clinocopathologic studies in feminizing tumors of the ovary. I. Some aspects of the pathology and therapy of granulosa cell tumors. Am J Obstet Gynecol 112:244–249, 1972.
6. Jacobs AJ, Deppe G, Cohen CJ: Combination chemotherapy of ovarian germ cell tumors with cis-platinum and doxorubicin. Gynecol Oncol 14:294–297, 1982.
7. Lusch CJ: Delayed recurrence and chemotherapy of a granulosa cell tumor. Obstet Gynecol 51(4):505–507, 1978.
8. Malkasian GD, Webb MJ, Jorgensen EO: Observation on the chemotherapy of granulosa cell and malignant ovarian teratoma. Obstet Gynecol 44:885–888, 1974.
9. Novak ER, Long JH: Arrhenoblastoma of the ovary. A review of the Ovarian Tumor Registry. Am J Obstet Gynecol 92:1082–1093, 1965.
10. O'Hern TM, Neubecker RD: Arrhenoblastoma. Obstet Gynecol 19:758–770, 1962.
11. Schulman P, Cheng E, Cvitkovic E, Golbey R: Spontaneous pneumothorax as a result of intensive cytotoxic chemotherapy. Chest 75:194–196, 1979.
12. Schwartz PE, Smith JP: Treatment of ovarian stromal tumors. Am J Obstet Gynecol 125:402–409, 1976.

13. Slayton R, Brady L, Johnson G, Blessing JA: Role of radiotherapy or combined dactinomycin, 5-fluorouracil, and cyclophosphamide in malignant stromal tumors of the ovary. Proc ASCO/AACR 21:430, 1980.
14. Slayton RE: Unpublished data.
15. Smith JP: Personal communication.
16. Smith JP, Rutledge F: Chemotherapy in the treatment of carcinoma of the ovary. Am J Obstet Gynecol 107:691–700, 1970.

Chemotherapy of Fallopian Tube Neoplasms

Gunter Deppe

Division of Gynecologic Oncology, Department of Obstetrics and Gynecology, Wayne State University School of Medicine, Detroit, Michigan 48201

Primary carcinoma of the Fallopian tube is one of the rarest of all gynecologic malignancies. It accounts for only 0.1–0.5% of all female genital tract neoplasms. To date, approximately 1,300 cases of Fallopian tube carcinoma have been reported. The experience of any one institution is limited [Sedlis, 1978; DiSaia and Creasman, 1981; Park and Parmley, 1978; Merrill, 1982].

The average age of patients with tubal carcinoma is about 55 years. The majority occurs between ages 45 and 60. Two-thirds of the patients with tubal malignancy may present with symptoms such as pain, vaginal discharge or bleeding, adnexal mass, and abdominal distention. Carcinoma of the Fallopian tube is almost never diagnosed preoperatively. Suspected tumor of the ovary or endometrium is the usual indication for surgery. The differentiation between a primary tubal or primary ovarian malignancy may be extremely difficult. Diagnostic criteria suggested by Finn and Javert [1949] may be helpful in determining the tubal origin: 1) The tubal carcinoma should arise from the endosalpinx; 2) the histologic pattern should resemble the epithelium of the tubal mucosa; 3) transition from benign to malignant epithelium should be present; 4) the endometrium and ovaries should be normal, or contain a malignant neoplasm that by its histologic appearance, small size, and distribution appears to be metastatic from a tubal primary.

The natural course of Fallopian tube carcinoma is similar to that of carcinoma of the ovary in that after contiguous growth through the tube to the serosa the dominant spread is by intraperitoneal dissemination. Tamimi and Figge [1981] found a 33% frequency of aortic lymph node metastasis in

Chemotherapy of Gynecologic Cancer, pages 203-212

a small number of patients. They concluded that lymphatic spread, especially to the aortic nodes, is a major pattern of dissemination for adenocarcinoma of the Fallopian tube.

The stage of disease and the modality of treatment are important in determining the survival of patients with Fallopian tube malignancies. There is no official International Federation of Gynecology and Obstetrics (FIGO) staging classification for tubal carcinoma. Several have been suggested but none has been accepted. Because the spread pattern of ovarian and tubal carcinoma is similar, tubal carcinoma can be adequately staged according to the FIGO staging system for ovarian cancer.

Stage IA: Growth limited to one tube; no ascites.
  1) No tumor on the external surface, serosa intact.
  2) Tumor present on the external surface, or serosa ruptured, or both.
Stage IB: Growth limited to both tubes; no ascites.
  1) No tumor on the external surface; serosa intact.
  2) Tumor present on the external surface, or serosa ruptured, or both.
Stage IC: One or both tubes involved with ascites or positive peritoneal fluid cytology.
Stage IIA: Extension and/or metastases to the uterus and/or ovaries.
Stage IIB: Extension to other pelvic tissues.
Stage IIC: Tumor either stage IIA or stage IIB, but with ascites present with positive peritoneal washings.
Stage III: Growth involving one or both tubes with intraperitoneal nodes, or both. Tumor limited to the true pelvis with histologically proven malignant extension to small bowel or omentum.
Stage IV: Growth involving one or both tubes with distant metastases. If pleural effusion is present, there must be positive cytology to allot a case to stage IV. Parenchymal liver metastases indicate stage IV.

Using the above staging classification the overall 5-year survival figures range from 5% to 30%.

Surgery and radiotherapy have been the mainstay of treatment. The use of cytotoxic chemotherapy in the treatment of patients with Fallopian tube cancer is relatively recent. Chemotherapy was employed most often after surgery and irradiation failed to control the tumor [Smith and Rutledge, 1975; Maier, 1978; Phelps and Chapman, 1974; Roberts and Lifshitz, 1982].

In 1973 Boronow reviewed the English-language literature and identified fewer than 50 patients who had been treated with chemotherapeutic agents, none of them in controlled studies (Table I). The majority of these patients received systemic alkylating agents. One patient received intraperitoneal nitrogen mustard without response. The largest experience was accumulated

TABLE I. Single Agents Used in Carcinoma of Fallopian Tube

Agent	No. patients
Nitrogen mustard (systemic)	3
Nitrogen mustard (intraperitoneal)	1
5-Fluorouracil	3
Thiotepa	8
Chlorambucil	1
Melphalan	11
Melphalan and progestin	8

Modified from Boronow [1973].

at the M.D. Anderson Hospital and Tumor Institute. Because of their successful use of alkylating agents in patients with advanced ovarian adenocarcinoma and the histologic similarity of the tubal epithelium to the epithelium of the ovarian serous tumors, they applied these drugs to patients with adenocarcinoma of the Fallopian tube. Progestins were added because of some cyclic response by the tubal epithelium to the normal ovarian cycle. Three of eight patients who were treated with a progestin and melphalan had prolonged responses. One of the three patients survived with residual disease for more than 5 years.

Since 1973 several other drugs have been tried as single agents in the treatment of Fallopian tube carcinoma. The active agents are summarized in Table II. Many of these reports were single case descriptions and failed to define response or duration of response or survival. Staging of the disease was inconsistent.

The alkylating agents are the most extensively reported single agents with efficacy against adenocarcinoma of the Fallopian tube. Raju et al. [1981] evaluated cisplatin alone in two patients with carcinoma of the Fallopian tube. One patient had a partial response but relapsed while on cisplatin. The other patient had a complete response after six courses and had no evidence of disease at second-look operation, but disease recurred 14 months later. There are only a few case reports citing the use of progestins without chemotherapy. The results are equivocal.

For most malignancies effective chemotherapeutic agents used in combination produce higher response rates than single-agent therapy. Cell populations resistant to one drug may be sensitive to another drug in combination. Combinations tested in carcinoma of the Fallopian tube have been, for the most part, alkylating agent–based regimens. Adriamycin and cisplatin were added to the treatment because these drugs had the broadest

TABLE II. Single Agents Active in Carcinoma of Fallopian Tube

Drug	Reference
Cyclophosphamide	Schinfeld and Winston [1980] Turunen [1969]
Chlorambucil	Blaikley [1973], Griffiths [1973] Phelps and Chapman [1974]
Alkeran	Boronow [1973], Smith [1978] Tamimi and Figge [1981] Dodson et al. [1970] Phelps and Chapman [1974]
Thiotepa	Smith [1978]
Progestins	Chalmers and Marshall [1976]
Cisplatin	Raju et al. [1981]
5-Fluorouracil	Erez et al. [1967] Hanton et al. [1966]
Adriamycin	Yoonessi [1979]

range of activity against gynecological tumors. A summary of the experience with combination chemotherapy in the treatment of Fallopian tube carcinoma may be inspected in Table III.

Second-look surgery in Fallopian tube carcinoma has been used for the same reasons as in the management of ovarian cancer. Surgical exploration can prevent excessive chemotherapy with its chronic toxicities and risks if the patient is in complete remission. It also allows objective decisions for modification of treatment or additional resection of tumor. Table IV presents the experience with second-look laparotomy in Fallopian tube carcinoma. The majority of these patients were stage III, although staging of the disease was not always indicated in the particular report. Most of the reported regimens contained alkylating agents, cisplatin, and adriamycin. The majority of patients had a relatively short follow-up period after the second-look operation. As shown in ovarian cancer it seems logical to conclude that modern chemotherapy will improve the response rates and duration of response in patients with Fallopian tube carcinoma.

Several tentative conclusions might be drawn from this limited experience with chemotherapy of adenocarcinoma of the Fallopian tube: 1) The most active drugs appear to be alkylating agents, cisplatin and adriamycin; 2)

TABLE III. Experience With Combination Chemotherapy for Adenocarcinoma of Fallopian Tube

Drug combination	No. patients	Objective regressions	Reference
Cyclophosphamide[a], actinomycin D, 5-fluorouracil	2	1	Henderson et al. [1977]
Adriamycin, cyclophosphamide	1		Guthrie and Cohen [1981]
Cisplatin[a], adriamycin, progestin	1	1	Deppe et al. [1980]
Cisplatin, adriamycin, cyclophosphamide, progestin	1	1	Deppe et al. [1980]
Cisplatin, adriamycin	1	0	Diamond et al. [1982]
Chlorambucil[a], 5-fluorouracil	3	3	Phelps and Chapman [1974], Yoonessi [1979]
Cyclophosphamide[a], vincristine, 5-fluorouracil	1	0	Raju et al. [1981]
Methotrexate[a], chlorambucil	1	0	Raju et al. [1981]
Cisplatin[a], chlorambucil	2	0	Raju et al., [1981]

[a]These patients received radiotherapy prior to chemotherapy.

progestin therapy needs to be further investigated relating responses to the presence or absence of progesterone receptor binding sites on the Fallopian tube cancer cells; 3) the superiority of combination chemotherapy to single agents has not been shown; and 4) the superiority of combination chemotherapy or single-agent therapy to hormonal therapy has not been established.

In summation, management of patients with carcinoma of the Fallopian tube will consist of total abdominal hysterectomy, bilateral salpingo-oophorectomy, peritoneal cytology, and selective pelvic and aortic lymphadenectomy. Debulking of tumor and assaying tumor for progesterone receptors is recommended. The optimal therapy including the role of radiotherapy will be found only by prospective randomized multi-institutional trials. At present, in the absence of proven optimal therapy for Fallopian tube carcinoma, the following recommendations for the use of chemotherapy are suggested (Table V). If the progesterone receptor assay predicts response to progestins,

TABLE IV. "Second-Look" Experience in Adenocarcinoma of Fallopian Tube

Patients	Initial treatment	Chemotherapy	Findings at second look	Subsequent treatment and follow-up	Reference
1	BSO Pelvic RT	Cisplatin Chlorambucil ↓ Cisplatin	NED	Hexamethylmelamine ×4 recurred at 14 months	Raju et al. [1981]
2	TAH, BSO	Melphalan	NED	NED at 52 months	Tamimi and Figge [1981]
3	TAH, BSO omentectomy	Chlorambucil ↓ Cyclophosphamide	Left pelvic sidewall tumor (3×2×1 cm)	Cyclophosphamide Pelvic RT Melphalan ×18 Third-look at 19 months—NED	Schinfeld and Winston [1980]
4	Subtotal hysterectomy BSO pelvic RT	Cisplatin Adriamycin Progestin	NED	NED at 9 months	Deppe et al. [1980]
5	TAH, BSO omentectomy	Cisplatin Adriamycin Cyclophosphamide Progestin	NED	NED at 6 months	Deppe et al. [1980]
6	Right SO	Adriamycin Cyclophosphamide ↓ Cyclophosphamide Progestin	NED	Cyclophosphamide ×5 Progestin Chlorambucil ×7 NED at 12 months	Guthrie and Cohen [1980]
7	TAH, BSO Selective aortic lymphadenectomy	Adriamycin Cisplatin	Microscopic tumor	5-Fluorouracil Mitomycin ×7 Alive at 7 months	Diamond et al. [1982]

Abbreviations: RT: radiotherapy, TAH: total abdominal hysterectomy, BSO: bilateral salpingo-oophorectomy, NED: no evidence of disease.

TABLE V. Chemotherapy for Carcinoma of Fallopian Tube

Stage IA_2, IB, IC	+ PR	Progestins
	− PR	Alkylating agent
Stage II, III, IV	+ PR	Progestins
	− PR	Cyclophosphamide Adriamycin Cisplatin

Abbreviations: PR = progesterone receptor.

a trial with hormonal therapy prior to cytotoxic chemotherapy may be indicated even in the advanced stages.

SARCOMA OF THE FALLOPIAN TUBE

Sarcomas of the Fallopian tube are exceedingly uncommon tumors, fewer than 50 cases having been reported in the literature [Abrams et al., 1958; Blaikley, 1973; Manes and Taylor, 1976; Ullmann and Kallett, 1968; Viniker et al., 1980; Wu et al., 1973]. The ratio of sarcoma to adenocarcinoma of the Fallopian tube is in the order of 1:25. They are found predominantly in postmenopausal women. They may be pure or mixed with carcinomatous elements. Included in this group are leiomyosarcomas, carcinosarcomas, and malignant mixed Müllerian tumors. The prognosis in all sarcomas of the Fallopian tube is extremely poor. Most patients present at a late stage, when metastases are present. The patients usually die within 12 months from the time of diagnosis. The treatment is primarily surgical. Adjunctive radiation therapy has been shown to be of little value. Four patients were identified in the literature who responded to different chemotherapeutic combinations (Table VI). These anecdotal reports do not allow conclusions on optimal therapy. It would seem that in this lethal disease aggressive surgery should be followed by postoperative chemotherapy. With the introduction of better radiotherapeutic techniques the role of postoperative radiotherapy needs to be reevaluated.

CHORIOCARCINOMA OF FALLOPIAN TUBE

Choriocarcinoma of the Fallopian tube is an extremely rare entity. It may arise as a consequence of gestational trophoblastic neoplasia within an ectopic pregnancy located in the Fallopian tube or it may be a nongestational primary germ cell tumor. Ober and Maier [1981] reviewed the world literature and identified 93 reported cases of gestational choriocarcinoma primary in the tube. They only accepted 58 cases and added 18 cases from

TABLE VI. Chemotherapy Used in Patients With Tubal Sarcoma

Regimen	Histology	Response	Reference
Vincristine, actinomycin D, cyclophospamide	Mixed Müllerian	+	Hanjani et al. [1980]
Adriamycin, DTIC	Mixed Müllerian	?	Acosta et al. [1974]
Cyclophosphamide, 5-fluorouracil	Carcinosarcoma	+	Jain [1977]
Adriamycin, cyclophosphamide, vincristine sulfate, DTIC	Rhabdomyosarcoma	+	Piver et al. [1982]
Cyclophosphamide, cisplatin	Mixed Müllerian	+	Deppe et al. [1983]

Abbreviations: DTIC = dimethyl-triazeno imidazole carboxamide.

the Armed Forces Institute of Pathology. Of 47 patients who were treated prior to chemotherapy, 41 died. Of 16 patients who received chemotherapy, 15 survived. Patients with gestational tubal choriocarcinoma can be treated with actinoycin D or methotrexate with high certainty of cure. If risk factors such as liver or brain metastases or HCG titer > 40,00 mIU/ml are present, combination chemotherapy with methotrexate, actinomycin D, and either chlorambucil or cyclophosphamide should be used. To determine the etiology of a tubal choriocarcinoma is important for treatment and prognosis. Unfortunately this is often difficult.

All choriocarcinomas secrete human chorionic gonadotropin (HCG), which can be used as a tumor marker to follow the response to chemotherapy. However, HCG cannot be used to distinguish between gestational and nongestational tubal choriocarcinoma. Histologically it is only possible to diagnose a nongestational primary germ cell tumor of the Fallopian tube if germ cell elements other than choriocarcinoma are present. Patients with nongestational primary choriocarcinoma have a poorer prognosis and should be treated with aggressive combination chemotherapy known to be effective against ovarian germ cell tumors. Combinations consisting of vincristine, actinomycin D, and cyclophosphamide or cisplatin, bleomycin, and vinblastine have been employed successfully.

REFERENCES

Abrams J, Kazal HL, Hobbs RE (1958): Primary sarcoma of the Fallopian tube, review of the literature and report of one case. Am J Obstet Gynecol 75:180–182.

Acosta AA, Kaplan AL, Kaufman RH (1974): Mixed Müllerian tumors of the oviduct. Obstet Gynecol 44:84–90.

Blaikley JB (1973): Advanced adenocarcinoma of the Fallopian tube. J Obstet Gynaecol Br Commonw 80:757–758.

Blaikley JB (1973): Sarcoma of the Fallopian tube. J Obstet Gynaecol Br Commonw 80:759–760.

Boronow RC (1973): Chemotherapy for disseminated tubal cancer. Obstet Gynecol 42:62–66.

Chalmers JA, Marshall AT (1976): Carcinoma of the Fallopian tube. Br J Obstet Gynaecol 83:580–583.

Deppe G, Bruckner HW, Cohen CJ (1980): Combination chemotherapy for advanced carcinoma of the Fallopian tube. Obstet Gynecol 56:530–532.

Deppe G, Friberg I, Friberg J, Thomas W (1983): Combination chemotherapy for malignant mixed Müllerian tumor of the Fallopian tube. Cancer (Accepted for publication).

Diamond SB, Rudolph SH, Lubicz SS, Deppe G, Cohen CJ (1982): Cerebral blindness in association with cis-platinum chemotherapy for advanced carcinoma of the Fallopian tube. Obstet Gynecol 59:84s–86s.

DiSaia PJ, Creasman WT (1981): "Clinical Gynecologic Oncology." St. Louis: CV Mosby, pp 351–356.

Dodson MG, Ford JH, Averette HE (1970): Clinical aspects of Fallopian tube carcinoma. Obstet Gynecol 36:935–939.

Erez S, Kaplan AL, Wall JA (1967): Clinical staging of carcinoma of the uterine tube. Obstet Gynecol 30:547–550.

Finn WF, Javert CT (1949): Primary and metastatic carcinoma of the Fallopian tube. Cancer 2:803–814.

Griffiths CT (1973): Ovary and Fallopian tube. In Holland JF, Frei E III (eds): "Cancer Medicine." Philadelphia: Lea and Febiger, pp 1718–1720.

Guthrie D, Cohen S (1981): Carcinoma of the Fallopian tube treated with a combination of surgery and cytotoxic chemotherapy. Br J Obstet Gynaecol 88:1051–1053.

Hanjani P, Petersen RO, Bonnell SA (1980): Malignant mixed Müllerian tumor of the Fallopian tube. Gynecol Oncol 9:381–393.

Hanton EM, Malkasian GD, Dahlin DC (1966): Primary carcinoma of the Fallopian tube. Am J Obstet Gynecol 94:832–839.

Henderson SR, Harper RC, Salazar OM, Rudolph JH (1977): Primary carcinoma of the Fallopian tube: Difficulties of diagnosis and treatment. Gynecol Oncol 5:168–179.

Jain U (1977): Mixed mesodermal tumor of the Fallopian tube. Report of a case and review of literature. Md State Med J 26:43–46.

Maier JG (1978): Radiotherapy in carcinoma of the Fallopian tube. In McGowan L (ed): "Gynecologic Oncology." New York: Appleton-Century-Crofts, pp 281–282.

Manes JL, Taylor HB (1976): Carcinosarcoma and mixed Müllerian tumors of the Fallopian tube. Cancer 38:1687–1693.

Merrill JA (1982): Lesions of the Fallopian tube. In Danforth DN (ed): "Obstetrics and Gynecology." Philadelphia: Harper and Row, pp 1108–1113.

Ober WB, Maier RC (1981): Gestational choriocarcinoma of the Fallopian tube. Diagn Gynecol Obstet 3:213–231.

Park RC, Parmley TH (1978): Fallopian tube cancer. In McGowan L (ed): "Gynecologic Oncology." New York: Appleton-Century-Crofts, pp 274–280.
Phelps HM, Chapman KE (1974): Role of radiation therapy in treatment of primary carcinoma of the uterine tube. Obstet Gynecol 43:669–673.
Piver MS, DeEulis TG, Lele SB, Barlow JJ (1982): Cyclophosphamide, vincristine, adriamycin and dimethyl-triazeno imidazole carboxamide (CYVADIC) for sarcomas of the female genital tract. Gynecol Oncol 14:319–323.
Raju SK, Barker GH, Wiltshaw E (1981): Primary carcinoma of the Fallopian tube. Report of 22 cases. Br J Obstet Gynaecol 88:1124–1129.
Roberts JA, Lifshitz S (1982): Primary adenocarcinoma of the Fallopian tube. Gynecol Oncol 13:301–308.
Schinfeld JS, Winston HG (1980): Primary tubal carcinoma in pregnancy. Am J Obstet Gynecol 137:512–514.
Sedlis A (1978): Carcinoma of the Fallopian tube. Surg Clin North Am 58:121–129.
Smith JP (1978): Chemotherapy in gynecologic cancer. Surg Clin North Am 58:201–215.
Smith JP, Rutledge F (1975): Advances in chemotherapy for gynecologic cancer. Cancer 36:669–674.
Tamimi HK, Figge DC (1981): Adenocarcinoma of the uterine tube: Potential for lymph node metastases. Am J Obstet Gynecol 141:132–137.
Turunen A (1969): Diagnosis and treatment of primary tubal carcinoma. Br J Gynaecol 7:294–300.
Ullmann SA, Kallet MB (1968): Primary mixed myosarcoma of the uterine tube: A case report and review of the literature. Can Med Assoc J 98:258–261.
Viniker DA, Mantell BS, Greenstein RJ (1980): Carcinosarcoma of the Fallopian tube: A case report and review of the literature. Br J Obstet Gynaecol 87:530–534.
Wu J, Tanner W, Fardal P (1973): Malignant mixed Müllerian tumor of the uterine tube. Obstet Gynecol 41:707–712.
Yoonessi M (1979): Carcinoma of the Fallopian tube. Obstet Gynecol Surv 34:257–270.

Chemotherapy of Gyn Sarcomas and Lymphomas

George A. Omura

Department of Medicine, University of Alabama, Birmingham, Alabama 35294

A multimodal therapeutic approach to gyn sarcomas and lymphomas seems logical, especially in those where survival has been poor after surgery alone, but their rarity precludes definitive statements about adjuvant chemotherapy. A brief review of drug treatment will be presented, recognizing that some extrapolations from the management of those lesions in other sites may be required. In certain gyn lymphomas, cure with drugs may be a realistic goal. There is more information available about sarcomas, which would indicate that chemotherapy is largely investigational, yet with the hope of benefit to individual patients.

GYN SARCOMAS

Uterine Sarcomas

Most of the available information about the chemotherapy of gyn sarcomas relates to lesions of the uterus. The four major cell types are leiomyosarcoma, heterologous mixed mesodermal sarcoma, homologous mixed mesodermal sarcoma (carcinosarcoma), and endometrial stromal sarcoma, the last being the rarest. Before discussing treatment of these specific lesions, a brief survey of chemotherapy of the general group of soft-tissue sarcomas will be made.

Single-agent activity. A number of drugs have been tried in adult soft-tissue sarcomas but few have had a definitive evaluation. Adriamycin has been reported to produce a 27% response (CR + PR) rate [Pinedo and Kenis, 1977; Schoenfeld et al., 1982]. Pinedo and Kenis [1977] tabulated no re-

Chemotherapy of Gynecologic Cancer, pages 213–229

sponse to vincristine in ten cases, 3/6 patients showing some sort of "improvement" with actinomycin, and 2/14 responses to cyclophosphamide.

Methyl CCNU was not active, with one of 11 cases responding [Creagan et al., 1976]. The role of cisplatin in treatment of sarcomas is unclear; Karakousis et al. [1979] reported two complete remissions and one partial remission among 13 metastatic sarcomas, but Samson et al. [1979] observed only one partial remission among 16 leiomyosarcomas. Bramwell et al. [1979] reported no responses in 17 sarcoma patients including three leiomyosarcomas. Brenner et al. [1982] observed two PR of 36 (6%) patients treated with high-dose cisplatin. All of these patients had had extensive prior treatment.

High-dose methotrexate gave only one response among 18 patients with soft-tissue sarcomas as secondary treatment [Karakousis et al., 1980]. Fluorouracil has not been systemically evaluated in recent years, although Malkasian et al. [1967] reported five temporary responses in ten gyn sarcomas. One of seven leiomyosarcomas had a partial response to hexamethylmelamine [Borden et al., 1977].

Dacarbazine had a 16% response rate in the general category of soft-tissue sarcoma, and 25% (6/24) in leiomyosarcoma [Pinedo and Kenis, 1977]. Vindesine was not highly active in previously treated patients but produced two PR in 13 previously untreated patients [Sordillo et al., 1981a]. Chlorozotocin was not active in two trials in previously treated patients [Mouridsen et al., 1981; Sordillo et al., 1981b].

Combinations. With such limited activity of single agents and with few randomized trials in a heterogeneous group of tumors, it is not surprising that variable results have been reported with combination chemotherapy. Uncontrolled studies have reported response rates in the range of 45–71% for adriamycin combinations [Yap et al., 1980; Rivkin et al., 1980; Blum et al., 1980; Bodey et al., 1981]. However, Schoenfeld et al. [1982] found in a randomized study that adriamycin alone at 70 mg/M^2 was more effective than adriamycin 50 mg/M^2 plus cyclophosphamide plus vincristine, and more effective than vincristine, actinomycin, and cyclophosphamide (VAC) in causing temporary regression; the advantage for adriamycin alone (27%) over VAC (115) was significant (P = 0.03).

Creagan et al. [1976] had no responses among 17 patients treated with adriamycin or actinomycin combinations. Yap et al. [1981] had no response among 28 patients treated with actinomycin plus methyl CCNU. Bryant and Wiltshaw [1980] observed only a 13.5% response rate using the five-drug combination of vincristine, actinomycin, cyclophosphamide, adriamycin, and methotrexate. Adriamycin and actinomycin were combined in one study but gave no better result (28% CR+PR) than adriamycin alone [Brenner et al., 1981]. A complex multiagent regimen (CYOMAD) based on adriamycin, decarbazine, and vincristine was disappointing, with a response rate of 32% in previously untreated patients [Lynch et al., 1982].

Different cell types. The assumption has frequently been made that the adult soft-tissue sarcomas could be lumped together with respect to drug testing. That has been based more on the reality of small numbers of different cell types in most trials than on science. However, leiomyosarcoma arising from various sites appears to be at least as responsive (32%) as the entire group of soft-tissue sarcomas (27%) to adriamycin [Pinedo and Kenis, 1977]. The GOG experience (see below) suggests a difference by cell type. As noted above, the results with dacarbazine seem to favor leiomyosarcoma [Pinedo and Kenis, 1977]. It should be mentioned that a rare variant of malignant fibrous histiocytoma, inflammatory fibrous histiocytoma, seems exceptionally responsive to chemotherapy in a small series [Poon et al., 1982].

Advanced uterine sarcoma. Piver et al. [1979] reported one response (6%) of 17 patients treated with adriamycin 90 mg/M^2 every 3–4 weeks, but the cell types were not stated. The same group reported one patient with a stromal sarcoma who had a partial response with adriamycin and then prolonged survival after debulking and pelvic radiotherapy [Yazigi et al., 1979]. Piver et al. [1982] also reported one complete response in a leiomyosarcoma and a partial response in one of three stromal tumors but no response in five previously untreated patients with mixed mesodermal sarcomas who received CYVADIC. Azizi et al. [1979] reported complete reponse in three of six uterine leiomyosarcomas treated with vincristine, adriamycin, and dacarbazine. Omura et al. [1978] observed one CR (leiomyosarcoma) of 12 patients with uterine sarcomas treated with nitrosoureas. Thigpen et al. [1982] treated 28 patients with mixed mesodermal sarcomas with cisplatin and had five (18%) responses.

The GOG has done two randomized trials in advanced or recurrent uterine sarcomas using adriamycin combinations. The first [Omura et al., 1983a] prospectively compared adriamycin 60 mg/M^2 every 3 weeks versus adriamycin plus dacarbazine 250 mg/M^2 $\times$ 5 every 3 weeks. Of 85 patients with measurable disease treated with adriamycin alone, five (5.9%) had a complete respone and ten (11.8%) had a partial response. Of 70 patients randomized to adriamycin plus dacarbazine, seven (19%) had a CR and ten

(14.3%) had a PR. These results were not significantly different; when the individual cell types were examined the response rate for leiomyosarcoma was 27% for one drug and 29% for both drugs. In homologous mixed mesodermal tumors, both regimens gave only a 9% response rate. In heterologous tumors, adriamycin alone produced a response in two of 22 patients (9%) compared with six out of 22 (29%) with the combination. These differences were not significant but the combination regimen produced significantly more gastrointestinal and hematologic toxicity. Lung metastases responded more frequently to combination therapy (8 responses of 21 cases compared with 2 responses of 20 cases for adriamycin alone; P = 0.04), but there was no survival advantage for this group. The seeming advantage of the combination in treating lung metastases must also be tempered by the observation that equally toxic dose regimens were not evaluated. Leiomyosarcomas had a significantly longer survival than other cell types (12.4 months versus 6 months) regardless of the regimen. The response rate in leiomyosarcoma is similar to what has previously been described for adriamycin alone. The very poor result in mixed mesodermal tumors was notable; overall, there were only 11/77 (14%) responses in mixed mesodermal sarcoma patients, none of whom had had prior chemotherapy.

The combination of vincristine plus actinomycin plus cyclophosphamide (VAC), previously popular for the treatment of soft-tissue sarcomas, was evaluated in 41 patients with uterine sarcomas after failing adriamycin with or without decarbazine; there were no responses in that group [Omura et al., 1983a].

A second GOG trial (H. Muss et al., unpublished observations) randomized adriamycin 60 mg/M^2 versus adriamycin plus cyclophosphamide 500 mg/M^2 every 3 weeks. The study was closed prematurely after 52 patients with measurable disease had been evaluated, because the results (19% response rate in each arm) were no more promising than in the previous study. Currently, the GOG is evaluating cisplatin in patients with no prior chemotherapy, based on hints noted above that it may have activity in soft-tissue sarcomas.

Adjuvant therapy in early-stage high-risk patients. It has long been recognized that early-stage uterine sarcomas have a substantial risk of hematogenous spread as well as pelvic and intra-abdominal recurrence. As success was achieved in the adjuvant treatment of certain other types of cancer, "prophylactic" therapy of uterine sarcomas was applied on a small scale using regimens such as VAC [Buchsbaum et al., 1979] or adriamycin [Piver et al.,

1979] with inconclusive results. More recently Hannigan et al. [1983] reported negative results.

The GOG has conducted a prospective trial [Omura et al., 1983b] in stage I and II uterine sarcomas following definitive surgery. Patients were randomized to adriamycin 60 mg/M^2 every 3 weeks × 8 doses or to no further treatment. At the time this study was started (1973), adriamycin was thought to be highly active in advanced sarcomas of various types, and was expected to be even better in micrometastatic disease. A second randomization to radiotherapy was not feasible because of the limited number of cases available, so radiotherapy was allowed as an option prior to the chemotherapy randomization. The drug was started 1–4 weeks after operation or after radiotherapy. Of 159 evaluable patients, 77 received adriamycin, with 29 recurrences to date (38%), compared with 40/82 (49%) recurrences in those receiving no drug. In the leiomyosarcoma category, 8/25 (32%) have recurred after adriamycin compared with 11/23 (48%) on no adjuvant. With homologous tumors (carcinosarcoma), 11/25 (44%) have recurred after adriamycin compared with 12/24 (50%) without this treatment; 26% (5/19) of heterologous tumors have failed after adriamycin compared with 13/27 (48%) recurrences after no adjuvant drug. Unfortunately, although the numbers suggest benefit, they are not significantly different. Moreover, when progression-free interval and survival are examined, there was no statistically significant difference in any category, even after adjusting for any maldistribution of cases. Twenty-eight of 62 cases (45%) treated with optional radiotherapy recurred while 41 of 97 (42%) without radiotherapy recurred. While pelvic radiotherapy did not appear to have an impact on leiomyosarcoma, there was a suggestion that it benefited mixed mesodermal tumors (with regard to local control).

One of the findings in this study was that the risk of recurrence without chemotherapy, while approximately 50% in all three major cell types, is not as high as previously thought [Buchsbaum et al., 1979]. This may be related in part to increased emphasis on careful surgical staging, which tends to improve the prognosis of early-stage cases. Still, a definite need remains for effective adjuvant chemotherapy., New drugs or combinations need to be identified that are highly active in advanced disease and which can then be tested in the adjuvant setting. Regarding adriamycin, although a benefit could not be shown for 60 mg/M^2 every 3 weeks, it should be said that soft-tissue sarcomas appear to have a steep dose-response curve for this drug [Bodey et al., 1981; Schoenfield et al., 1982] and that much higher doses can be given; Wheeler et al. [1982] reported one CR and one PR of five assorted soft-tissue sarcomas using 120 mg/m^2 per dose. If better agents do not emerge soon, it may be appropriate to repeat the adjuvant adriamycin trial in leiomyosarcoma, with a higher dose.

Cervix

Sarcomas of the cervix are exceedingly rare; cell types such as leiomyosarcoma [Jawalekar et al., 1981] can probably be considered with corpus lesions with respect to chemotherapy (see above). Piver et al. [1982] had no response in one patient treated with CYVADIC.

Vulvar Sarcomas

The most common vulvar sarcoma is leiomyosarcoma [Audet-Lapointe et al., 1980]; most of the other soft-tissue sarcoma types have been diagnosed in this location, including such lesions as alveolar soft part sarcoma [Shen et al., 1982] and epithelioid sarcoma [Hall et al., 1980]. DiSaia et al. [1971] reported on 12 patients with sarcoma of the vulva; two (1 leiomyosarcoma and 1 neurofibrosarcoma) benefited from chemotherapy, but a specific protocol was not described.

Vaginal Sarcoma

The major type in this location is embryonal rhabdomyosarcoma (sarcoma botryoides) which is apt to be seen in young children, but rarely has been reported in adults [Lloyd et al., 1983]. In contrast to the adult soft-tissue sarcomas, childhood embryonal rhabdomyosarcoma appears to be relatively responsive to chemotherapy; a multimodality approach with curative intent is indicated [Maurer et al., 1977]. VAC has most been used, in various dose schedules. Piver et al. [1982] used CYVADIC in two patients with advanced disease without response. The general impression is that embryonal rhabdomyosarcoma in different anatomic sites has similar responsiveness [Hays, 1980; Ortner et al., 1982].

Ovary

The most common sarcoma cell type originating in this location is mixed mesodermal sarcoma [Barwik and LiVolsi, 1980]. Hernandez et al. [1977] had one transient response with melphalan and 5FU, one failure on VAC, and one patient given adjuvant adriamycin with inconclusive results. Lele et al. [1980] reviewed the Roswell Park Memorial Institute experience with mixed mesodermal sarcomas of the ovary and noted no consistently useful regimen, only 12% showing a temporary response to actinomycin or adriamycin combinations. The same group did observe a CR in a single case of ovarian angiosarcoma treated with CYVADIC [Piver et al., 1982]. The

GOG protocol 13 (Morrow et al., unpublished observations) included one temporary complete response of six mixed mesodermal tumor patients treated with adriamycin; VAC was not systematically tested but did not appear to be of predictable benefit. A current GOG trial in ovarian sarcomas employs a moderately high dose (75 mg/M^2) of adriamycin; no results are available at present.

Tube

Sarcomas of the tube are usually mixed mesodermal tumors. Hanjani et al. [1980] reported a case where an involved inguinal node regressed on VAC and there was no evidence of disease for 20 months after resection of all resectable gross tumor, but then the patient progressed on adriamycin. Piver et al. [1982] treated one rhabdomyosarcoma of the tube with CY-VADIC and achieved a complete response.

LYMPHOMAS OF THE FEMALE GENITAL TRACT

An even greater rarity than gyn sarcomas are lymphomas of the pelvic structures. Their importance lies not in numbers but in differential diagnosis and in the potential for cure, even when disseminated. Information about classification, staging, and treatment of nodal lymphomas is briefly reviewed on the assumption that it is relevant to pelvic lymphomas.

Classification

The clearest distinction regarding management is between Hodgkin's disease (HD) and "non-Hodgkin's lymphoma" (NHL). Currently, HD is subclassified histologically into lymphocyte predominance, nodular sclerosis, mixed cellularity, and lymphocyte depletion categories. The origin of the malignant cell is in dispute. After radiotherapy, lymphocyte predominance has the best prognosis and lymphocyte depletion the worst. In contrast to this relatively simple system, there are several classifications of NHL, with emphasis variously on histologic patterns, cellular detail, immune phenotype, labelling index, etc. The Rappaport classification of nodular or diffuse architectural effacement of nodes, and cell types including well-differentiated or poorly differentiated lymphocytic, mixed lymphocytic-histiocytic, histiocytic, and undifferentiated lymphomas, is currently used by many pathologists with the recognition that nodular or follicular lymphomas are of B-cell origin and that well-differentited lymphocytic lymphoma is intimately related to chronic lymphocytic leukemia. Diffuse histiocytic lymphoma (DHL), diffuse undifferentiated lymphoma (DUL), and diffuse mixed lymphocytic-histiocytic lymphoma (DML) tend to be more aggressive but are curable in some cases even when disseminated [Fisher et al., 1981; Horwich and Peckham, 1983]. The nodular lymphomas tend to have a more "benign" or indolent course, but paradoxically are less amenable to cure with current therapy. Nodular histiocytic and nodular mixed lymphomas may be curable [Osborne et al., 1980; Ezdinli et al., 1980], but there is controversy about the latter [Glick et al., 1981]. Lukes and Collins [1974] and others [Berard et al., 1981] have attempted to be more precise about classification based on origin of the cells involved, but controversy remains. With the advent of modern immunologic techniques, subclassification of NHL and prognostication can be further refined, hopefully with improvement in results, as more specific treatment is applied.

Staging

Lymphoma staging was developed for nodal Hodgkin's disease, especially in relation to selecting patients for curative radiotherapy. Stage I = one lymph node area involved; stage II = two areas of nodal involvement above or below the diaphragm; stage III = nodal disease above and below the diaphragm; stage IV is extranodal involvement (marrow, liver, skin, lung not contiguous with nodal involvement, etc.). Extranodal stage I = involvement of a single extralymphatic organ or site. The symptom classification is A if there are no relevant symptoms, for example, IA, IIA, etc., whereas B = fever, documented sweats, or weight loss greater than 10% of body weight. B status is generally associated with a worse prognosis, stage for stage. The thrust of staging HD is to determine if a given patient is a candidate primarily for radiotherapy or for chemotherapy. Thus, if a posterior iliac crest needle bone marrow biopsy is positive, the patient is a candiate for combination chemotherapy, and a laparotomy is not needed. If the bone marrow examination (biopsy, not simply aspiration) is negative and intra-abdominal involvement is uncertain, a staging laparotomy is indicated, with node biopsies, splenectomy, and liver biopsies (wedge and needle). However, if a gallium scan, CT scan, and/or sonar scan of the abdomen is convincingly positive, laparotomy is not essential. Lymphangiography was popular in the past, but now has been largely replaced by scanning techniques.

In NHL, the value of detailed staging, and especially staging laparotomy, in the usual case of nodal lymphoma is less clear. If the case appears to be stage I after physical examination, blood counts, a needle bone marrow biopsy, liver function tests, chest x-ray, and sonar or CAT scan, radiotherapy is indicated for cure. However, in diffuse histiocytic lymphoma a high dose of radiation is indicated; if the anatomical location of the lymphoma is likely to produce late effects on normal tissues, for example, radiating the salivary glands with a resultant chronic dry mouth, the risk of an error in non-invasive staging becomes more important. Then, a laparotomy may be indicated first, to exclude occult intra-abdominal disease. If the case is upstaged, combination chemotherapy rather than radiotherapy is given. Gallium scanning may be helpful in staging "aggressive" NHL, but is not usually helpful in well-differentiated lymphocytic lymphoma. In some lymphomas peripheral blood lymphocytes can be identified by marker studies as containing a monoclonal population identical to the phenotype of the nodal malignant cells [Ault, 1979]. Even when there is not an obvious increase of a single cell population, it may be possible to detect a "clonal excess" of kappa- or lambda-bearing cells in the blood by cell-sorter techniques [Ligler et al., 1980]. Further development of such techniques will influence the stage and follow-up of NHL.

Chemotherapy of Hodgkin's Disease

Hodgkin's disease is clearly one of the success stories of cancer chemotherapy. Using MOPP (nitrogen mustard, oncovin, procarbazine, and prednisone) for 6 months, DeVita et al. [1983] achieved a breakthrough in curative treatment of stage IIIB and IV cases. It should be noted, however, that only 50–90% of patients in various series have a remission after initial treatment, and although some patients, especially those who do not relapse immediately, will be able to be cured with retreatment, a substantial fraction, nearly half, do not get cured. The combination of BCNU, vinblastine, cyclophosphamide, prednisone, and procarbazine [Durant et al., 1978] appears to be equal or better with less toxicity and greater ease of administration. Santoro et al. [1982] reported the superiority of a sequence of combinations (MOPP alternating with adriamycin, bleomycin, vinblastine, and dacarbazine) over MOPP alone, although the MOPP arm seemed to be less effective in that trial than expected. Gams et al. [1979] could not confirm the advantage of sequencing, using a different pair of combinations. "Salvage" chemotherapy for relapsed or refractory patients remains a problem for clinical investigation.

The management of IIB and IIIA cases is under investigation; the combination of radiotherapy and chemotherapy is frequently used for these cases but there is increasing interest in chemotherapy alone. It should be mentioned that a higher risk of treatment-induced leukemia has been reported with combined modality therapy [Canellos et al., 1983].

Other active drugs (other than those noted above) in refractory Hodgkin's disease are few. Streptozotocin [Levi et al., 1977] and hexamethylmelamine

[Omura et al.,. 1982] have modest activity; new active agents continue to be sought. Hodgkin's disease presenting in pelvic structures is very rare; Chorlton et al. [1974] mention one case of Hodgkin's disease of the ovary, stage I, retrieved from the files of the Armed Forces Institute of Pathology. That patient died of disease 7 months after diagnosis. The staging procedures and details of treatment are not given, but one suspects that the case may not have had careful staging and modern therapy such as described above.

Gall et al. [1975] cite four cases. Currently such a case, if regarded as extranodal stage I after appropriate staging and adequate resection, might be observed without further treatment but with consideration of a second-look laparotomy a year later. If disease spread was found at initial or secondary evaluation, or if the margins of resection or extent of disease were in question, combination chemotherapy should be given in view of the high cure rate which can be achieved in Hodgkin's disease. In selected well-localized cases, radiotherapy might be used instead, with chemotherapy reserved for recurrence since, at least with nodal HD, chemotherapy may be curative after radiotherapy faiilure [DeVita et al., 1983].

Indolent or Favorable Histology NHL (well-differentiated lymphocytic lymphoma, nodular poorly differentiated lymphocytic lymphoma, and nodular mixed lymphoma)

The majority of patients will respond to alkylating agents and prednisone in a variety of dose schedules. Chlorambucil 0.1 mg/kg per day plus prednisone 100 mg twice a week for 6–12 months is one of the simplest regimens but requires monitoring the white blood count and platelet count every 2–3 weeks and some individualization of chlorambucil dose, depending on hematologic toxicity. Delayed hematologic toxicity from chlorambucil should be anticipated. Fortnightly [Knospe and Loeb, 1980] and monthly [Cadman et al., 1982] pulses of chlorambucil have been advocated with favorable results. Melphalan in monthly 5-day courses could probably be substituted for chlorambucil, but has not been extensively evaluated in lymphomas.

Although remissions can be achieved in many patients with little toxicity, they rarely are sustained; cure has been an elusive goal in the so-called favorable histology cases. Thus, observation of asymptomatic patients for a period of time is still proper [Portlock, 1983]. Once such patients are refractory to corticosteroids and mustard-type alkylating agents, other cytotoxic drugs have so far been of limited value. New drug regimens, interferon [Stiehm et al., 1982], and monoclonal antibody treatment [Ritz and Schlossman, 1982] are being investigated in selected patients.

Unfavorable Histology NHL

To complete the misnomer of current lymphoma terminology, this type of disease, while aggressive, is curable in variable fractions of patients using intensive treatment. In stage I, high-dose radiotherapy should be considered, but many patients present with advanced disease and will require chemotherapy.

Diffuse Histiocytic Lymphoma

Various adriamycin-based combinations such as bleomycin, adriamycin, cyclophosphamide, vincristine, and corticoids with or without methotrexate have produced complete remission in 50–70% of patients; at least a fourth, and possibly 40–50%, appear to be cured [Skarin et al., 1983].

Diffuse Undifferentiated Lymphoma

One of the subsets of diffuse undifferentiated lymphoma is the so-called Burkitt lymphoma which is curable with intensive chemotherapy in at least 50% of cases [Ziegler, 1981]. The ovaries are frequently involved (see below). Undifferentiated non-Burkitt lymphoma is managed like histiocytic lymphoma, with similar results [Skarin et al., 1983].

Diffuse Poorly Differentiated Lymphocytic Lymphoma (DLPD)

This should be distinguished from lymphoblastic lymphoma (see below), which is usually of T-cell origin. DLPD responds to the type of treatment described above—for example, adriamycin, cylophosphamide, prednisone, and vincristine—but sustained remissions are rare [Horwich and Peckham, 1983].

T-Cell Lymphoma

Mycosis fungoides (cutaneous T-cell lymphoma) and lymphoblastic lymphoma are among the T-cell neoplasms which are notable by their relative refractoriness to current drug regimens. Striking responses may be seen initially, but within a few months most patients become refractory to chemotherapy. Further evaluation of standard agents, new drugs, and immunologic approaches is needed [Omura, 1982]. Bone marrow and central nervous system involvement is common in lymphoblastic lymphoma [Streuli et al., 1981]. Recently, a complex multidrug regimen plus radiotherapy has been reported to give promising results in lymphoblastic lymphoma [Levine et al., 1983].

Gyn Non-Hodgkin's Lymphoma

Cervix. Several cases of histiocytic lymphoma of the cervix have been reported [Tunca et al., 1979; Steinfeld, 1979; Wright, 1973]. Castaldo et al.

[1979] reported two cases, one DLPD and one undifferentiated lymphoma. Crips et al. [1982] also reported a cervical lymphoma but the histology was not given. If the disease is confined to the cervix, pelvic radiotherapy should have curative potential [Steinfeld, 1979; Tunca et al., 1979].

Corpus. Gall et al. [1975] cite three cases arising in the corpus and six including their own, where both the corpus and cervix were involved with histiocytic lymphoma. Optimal management is unclear but combination chemotherapy as described above might be considered if there is doubt about extra-uterine extent of the disease.

Vagina. Castaldo et al. [1979] reported three cases, two histiocytic and one undifferentiated. In view of the difficulty of defining the true extent of disease in such cases, multiagent chemotherapy is probably warranted.

Ovary. Rotmensch and Woodruff [1982] reviewed the experience at Johns Hopkins Hospital; of 55 cases, 18 were nodular histiocytic lymphoma, 18 DLPD, six well-differentiated lymphocytic lymphoma, eight mixed lymphoma, four Hodgkin's disease, and one Burkitt lymphoma. Only four (7%) survived. Adjunctive radiotherapy was not clearly helpful. Castaldo et al. [1979] reported three cases (one well-differentiated lymphocytic lymphoma, one DHL, and one Burkitt lymphoma) all of whom died; two had, in retrospect, suboptimal chemotherapy. Chorlton et al. [1974] reported 18 cases of which seven were DLPD and three were histiocytic lymphoma; only one patient survived. Paladugu et al. [1980] also noted that DLPD was the more frequent histology (4 cases) in their series of 11 patients; three cases were histiocytic lymphoma; Burkitt, lymphoblastic, and undifferentiated lymphomas were also seen.

Again, the prognosis was poor. Whether inadequate staging was a factor in the poor results is unclear. Although improved staging (both ovarian staging techniques and lymphoma staging) might demonstrate a better outlook for true stage I cases, there does appear to be an indication for chemotherapy in ovarian lymphoma. As suggested above, the use of regimens that have been successful in nodal lymphomas of specific cell types should be considered. Second-look laparotomy after optimal chemotherapy is not presently recommended; currently available "salvage" therapy is not very effective, so the opportunity to benefit patient management by restaging is limited. Hopefully that will change in the future.

SUMMARY

A brief review of the chemotherapy of soft-tissue sarcomas and lymphomas has been presented, with emphasis on the results that are relevant to gyn sarcomas and lymphomas. The outcome in sarcomas is disappointing, but research in this field is quite active. Before one drowns in the alphabet soup of subclassifications and treatment regimens for malignant lymphomas, it is important to realize that curative therapy exists for certain subtypes. Moreover, the optimal drug regimens appropriate for HD, aggressive lymphomas, and indolent lymphomas are not the same. It would appear that procarbazine and/or vinblastine are very important in HD, and that adriamycin is a major component of combination chemotherapy of aggressive non-Hodgkin's lymphomas. As in other types of cancer, careful staging is also important in juding the indications for and benefit of systemic therapy.

ACKNOWLEDGMENTS

Supported in part by Public Health Service grants CA03013, CA12484, and CA19657 from the National Cancer Institute, National Institutes of Health.

REFERENCES

Audet-LaPointe P, Paquin F, Guerard MJ, Charbonneau A, Methot F, Morand G (1980): Case report: Leiomyosarcoma of the vulva. Gynecol Oncol 10:350–355.

Ault K (1979): Detection of small numbers of monoclonal B lymphocytes in the blood of patients with lymphoma. N Engl J Med 300:1401–1405.

Azizi F, Bitran J, Javehari G, Herbst A (1979): Remission of uterine leiomyosarcomas treated with vincristine, adriamycin, and dimethyl-triazeno-imidazole carboximide. Am J Obstet Gynecol 133:379–381.

Barwick K, LiVolsi V (1980): Malignant mixed mesodermal tumors of the ovary. Am J Surg Pathol 4:37–42.

Berard CW, Greene MH, Jaffe ES, Magrath I, Ziegler J (1981): A multidisciplinary approach to non-Hodgkin's lymphoma. Ann Intern Med 94:218–235.

Blum RH, Corson JM, Wilson RE, Greenberger JS, Canellos GP, Frei E (1980): Successful treatment of metastatic sarcomas with cyclophosphamide, adriamycin, and DTIC (CAD). Cancer 46:1722–1726.

Bodey GP, Rodriguez V, Murphy WK, Burgess MA, Benjamin R (1981): Protected environment–prophylactic antibiotic program for malignant sarcomas. Cancer 47:2422–2429.

Borden EC, Larson P, Ansfield FJ, Bryan GT, Johnson RO, Ramirez G, Wilson WL (1977): Hexamethylmelamine treatment of sarcomas and lymphomas. Med Pediatr Oncol 3:401–406.

Bramwell VHC, Brugarolas A, Mouridsen HT, Cheix F, DeJager R, Van Oosterom AT, Vendrik, CP, Pinedo HM, Sylvester R, DePauw M (1979): EORTC phase II study of cisplatin in Cyvadic-resistant soft tissue sarcoma. Eur J Cancer 15:1511–1513.

Brenner DE, Chang P, Wiernik PH (1981): Doxorubicin and dactinomycin therapy for advanced sarcomas. Cancer Treat Rep 65:231–236.

Brenner J, Magill GB, Sordillo PP, Cheng EW, Yagoda A (1982): Phase II trial of cisplatin (CPDD) in previously treated patients with advanced soft tissue sarcoma. Cancer 50:2031–2033.

Bryant BM, Wiltshaw E (1980): Results of the Royal Marsden Hospital: Second soft tissue sarcoma schedule (STS II) chemotherapy regimen in the management of advanced sarcoma. Cancer Treat Rep 64:689–692.

Buchsbaum HJ, Lifshitz S, Blythe JG (1979): Prophylactic chemotherapy in stages I and II uterine sarcoma. Gynecol Oncol 8:346–348.

Cadman E, Drislane F, Waldron JA, Farber L, Prosnitz L, Bertino JR (1982): High-dose pulse chlorambucil. Effective therapy for rapid remission induction in nodular lymphocytic poorly differentiated lymphoma. Cancer 50:1037–1041.

Canellos GP, Come SE, Skarin AT (1983): Chemotherapy in the treatment of Hodgkin's disease. Semin Hematol 20:1–24.

Castaldo TW, Ballon SC, Lagasse LD, Petrilli ES (1979): Reticuloendothelial neoplasia of the female genital tract. Obstet Gynecol 54:167–170.

Chorlton I, Norris HJ, King FM (1974): Malignant reticuloendothelial disease involving the ovary as a primary manifestation. Cancer 34:397–407.

Creagan ET, Hahn RG, Ahmann DL, Edmonson JH, Bisel HF, Eagan RT (1976): A comparative clinical trial evaluating the combination of adriamycin, DTIC and vincristine, the combination of actinomycin D, cyclophosphamide and vincristine, and a single agent, methyl CCNU, in advanced sarcomas. Cancer Treat Rep 60:1385–1387.

Crisp WE, Surwit EA, Grogan TM, Freedman MF (1982): Malignant pelvic lymphoma. Am J Obstet Gynecol 143:69–74.

DeVita VT, Hubbard SM, Moxley JH (1983): The cure of Hodgkin's disease with drugs. Adv Intern Med 28:277–302.

DiSaia P, Rutledge F, Smith J (1971): Sarcoma of the vulva. Obstet Gynecol 38:180–184.

Durant JR, Gams RA, Velez-Garcia E, Bartolucci A, Wirtschafter D, Dorfman R (1978): BCNU, Velban, cyclophosphamide, procarbazine and prednisone (BVCPP) in advanced Hodgkin's disease. Cancer 42:2101–2110.

Ezdinli EZ, Costello WG, Icli F, Lenhard RE, Johnson GJ, Silverstein M, Berard CW, Bennett JM, Carbone PP (1980): Nodular mixed lymphocytic-histiocytic lymphoma (NM). Cancer 45:261–267.

Fisher RI, Hubbard SM, DeVita VT, Berard CW, Wesley R, Cossman J, Young RC (1981): Factors predicting long-term survival in diffuse mixed, histiocytic, or undifferentiated lymphoma. Blood 58:45–51.

Gall JA, Sartiano G, Deutsch M (1975): Primary reticulum cell sarcoma of the uterus. Oncology 31:157–163.

Gams RA, Durant JR, Omura GA, Bartolucci A (1979): Remission duration and survival in advanced Hodgkin's disease: The influence of bleomycin and alternating non-cross-resistant combination chemotherapy. Blood 54:187A.

Glick JH, Barnes JN, Ezdinli EZ, Berard CW, Orlow EL, Bennett JM (1981): Nodular mixed lymphoma: Results of a randomized trial failing to confirm prolonged disease-free survival with COPP chemotherapy. Blood 58:920–925.

Hall DJ, Grimes MM, Goplerud DR (1980): Epithelioid sarcoma of the vulva. Gynecol Oncol 9:237–246.

Hanjani P, Petersen RO, Bonnell SA (1980): Malignant mixed Mullerian tumor of the Fallopian tube: Report of a case and review of literature. Gynecol Oncol 9:381–393.

Hannigan EV, Freedman RS, Rutledge FN (1983): Adjuvant chemotherapy in early uterine sarcoma. Gynecol Oncol 15:56–64.

Hays DM (1980): Pelvic rhabdomyosarcomas in childhood: Diagnosis and concepts of management reviewed. Cancer 45:1810–1814.
Hernandez W, DiSaia PJ, Morrow CP, Townsend DE (1977): Mixed mesodermal sarcoma of the ovary. Obstet Gynecol 49:59–63.
Horwich A, Peckham M (1983): "Bad risk" non-Hodgkin lymphomas. Semin Hematol 20:35–56.
Jawalekar KS, Zacharopoulou M, McCaffrey RM (1981): Leiomyosarcoma of the cervix uteri. Southern Med J 74:510–511.
Karakousis CP, Holtermann OA, Holyoke ED (1979): Cis-dichlorodiammine-platinum (II) in metastatic soft tissue sarcomas. Cancer Treat Rep 63:2071–2075.
Karakousis CP, Rao U, Carlson M (1980): High-dose methotrexate as secondary chemotherapy in metastatic soft-tissue sarcomas. Cancer 46:1345–1348.
Knospe WH, Loeb V (1980): Biweekly chlorambucil treatment of lymphocytic lymphoma. Cancer Clin Trials 3:329–336.
Lele SB, Piver MS, Barlow JJ (1980): Chemotherapy in management of mixed mesodermal tumors of the ovary. Gynecol Oncol 10:298–302.
Levi JA, Wiernik PH, Diggs CH (1977): Combination chemotherapy of advanced previously treated Hodgkin's disease with streptozotocin, CCNU, adriamycin and bleomycin. Med Pediatr Oncol 3:33–40.
Levine AM, Forman SJ, Meyer PR, Koehler SC, Liebman H, Paganini-Hill A, Pockros A, Lukes RJ, Feinstein DI (1983): Successful therapy of convoluted T-lymphoblastic lymphoma in the adult. Blood 61:92–98.
Ligler FS, Smith RG, Kittman JR, Hernandez JA, Himes JB, Vitteta ES, Uhr JW, Frenkel EP (1980): Detection of tumor cells in the peripheral blood of non-leukemic patients with B-cell lymphoma: Analysis of "clonal excess." Blood 55:792–801.
Lloyd RV, Hajdu SI, Knapper WH (1983): Embryonal rhabdomyosarcoma in adults. Cancer 51:557–565.
Lukes RJ, Collins RD (1974): Immunologic characterization of human malignant lymphoma. Cancer 34:1488–1503.
Lynch G, Magill GB, Sordillo P, Golbey RB (1982): Combination chemotherapy of advanced sarcomas in adults with "CYOMAD" (S7). Cancer 50:1724–1727.
Malkasian GD, Mussey E, Decker DG, Johnson CE (1967): Chemotherapy of gynecologic sarcomas. Cancer Chemother Rep 51:507–516.
Maurer HM, Moon T, Donaldson M, Fernandez C, Gehan EA, Hammond D, Hays DM, Lawrence W, Newton W, Ragab A, Raney B, Soule E, Sutow WW, Tefft M (1977): The intergroup rhabdomyosarcoma study: A preliminary report. Cancer 40:2015–2026.
Mouridsen HT, Bramwell VHC, Lacave J, Metz R, Vendrik C, Hild J, McCreanney J, Sylvester R (1981): Treatment of advanced soft tissue sarcomas with chlorozotocin: A phase II trial of the EORTC soft tissue and bone sarcoma group. Cancer Treat Rep 65:509–511.
Omura GA, Shingleton HM, Creasman WT, Blessing JA, Boronow RC (1978): Chemotherapy of gynecologic cancer with nitrosoureas: A randomized trial of CCNU and methyl-CCNU in cancers of the cervix, corpus, vagina, and vulva. Cancer Treat Rep 62:833–835.
Omura GA, Broun GO, Papps J, Birch R (1981): Phase II study of hexamethylmelamine in refractory Hodgkin's disease, other lymphomas, and chronic lymphocytic leukemia. Cancer Treat Rep 65:1027–1029.
Omura GA (1982): Cytarabine in chronic T-cell neoplasms. Cancer Treat Rep 66:591–592.

Omura GA, Major FJ, Blessing JA, Sedlacek TV, Thigpen JT, Creasman WT, Zaino RJ (1983a): A randomized study of adriamycin with and without dimethyl triazeno imidazole carboxamide in advanced uterine sarcomas. Cancer 52:626–632.
Omura GA, Blessing JA, Major F, Silverberg S (1983b): A randomized trial of adriamycin versus no adjuvant chemotherapy in stage I and II uterine sarcomas. Proc Am Soc Clin Oncol 2, abstract C580.
Ortner A, Weiser G, Haas H, Resch R, Dapunt O (1982): Embryonal rhabdomyosarcoma (botryoid type) of the cervix: A case report and review. Gynecol Oncol 13:115–119.
Osborne CK, Norton L, Young RC, Garvin AJ, Simon RM, Berard CW, Hubbard S, DeVita VT (1980): Nodular histiocytic lymphoma: An aggressive nodular lymphoma with potential for prolonged disease-free survival. Blood 56:98–103.
Paladugu RR, Bearman RM, Rappaport H (1980): Malignant lymphoma with primary manifestation in the gonad. Cancer 45:561–571.
Pinedo HM, Kenis Y (1977): Chemotherapy of advanced soft tissue sarcomas in adults. Cancer Treat Rev 4:67–86.
Piver MS, Barlow JJ, Lele SB, Yazigi R (1979): Adriamycin in localized and metastatic uterine sarcomas. J Surg Oncol 12:263–265.
Piver MS, DeEulis TG, Lele SB, Barlow JJ (1982): Cyclophosphamide, vincristine, adriamycin, and dimethyl-triazeno imidazole carboxamide (CYVADIC) for sarcomas of the female genital tract. Gynecol Oncol 14:319–323.
Poon MC, Durant JR, Norgard MJ, Chang-Poon VY-H (1982): Inflammatory fibrous histiocytoma: An important variant of malignant fibrous histiocytoma highly responsive to chemotherapy. Ann Intern Med 97:858–863.
Portlock CS (1983): "Good risk" non-Hodgkin lymphomas: Approaches to management. Semin Hematol 20:25–34.
Ritz J, Schlossman SF (1982): Utilization of monoclonal antibodies in the treatment of leukemia and lymphoma. Blood 59:1–11.
Rivkin SE, Gottlieb JA, Thigpen T, El Mawla NG, Saiki J, Dixon DO (1980): Methyl CCNU and adriamycin for patients with metastatic sarcomas. Cancer 46:446–451.
Rotmensch J, Woodruff JD (1982): Lymphoma of the ovary: Report of twenty new cases and update of previous series. Am J Obstet Gynecol 143:870–875.
Samson MK, Baker LH, Benjamin RS, Lane M, Plager C (1979); Cis-dichlorodiammineplatinum (II) in advanced soft tissue and bony sarcomas: A Southwest Oncology Group study. Cancer Treat Rep 63:2027–2029.
Santoro A, Bonadonna G, Bonfante V, Valagussa P (1982): Alternating drug combinations in the treatment of advanced Hodgkin's disease. N Eng J Med 306:770–775.
Schoenfeld DA, Rosenbaum C, Horton J, Wolter JM, Falkson G, DeConti RC (1982): A comparison of adriamycin versus vincristine and adriamycin and cyclophosphamide versus vincristine, actinomycin-D, and cyclophosphamide for advanced sarcoma. Cancer 50:2757–2762.
Shen JT, D'ablaing G, Morrow CP (1982): Alveolar soft part sarcoma of the vulva: Report of first case and review of literature. Gynecol Oncol 13:120–128.
Skarin AT, Canellos GP, Rosenthal DS, Case DC, MacIntyre JM, Pinkus GS, Moloney WC, Frei III E (1983): Improved prognosis of diffuse histiocytic and undifferentiated lymphoma by use of high dose methotrexate alternating with standard agents (M-BACOD). J Clin Oncol 1:91–98.
Sordillo PP, Magill GN, Gralla RJ (1981a): Phase II evaluation of Vindesine sulfate in patients with advanced sarcomas. Cancer Treat Rep 65:515–516.

Sordillo PP, Magill GB, Gralla RJ (1981b): Chlorozotocin: Phase II evaluation in patients with advanced sarcomas. Cancer Treat Rep 65:513–514.

Steinfeld AD (1979): Histiocytic lymphoma of the cervix. Gynecol Oncol 8:97–103.

Stiehm ER, Kronenberg LH, Rosenblatt HM, Bryson Y, Merigan TC (1982): Interferon: Immunobiology and clinical significance. Ann Intern Med 96:80–93.

Streuli RA, Kaneko Y, Variakojis D, Kinnealey A, Golomb HM, Rowley JD (1981): Lymphoblastic lymphoma in adults. Cancer 47:2510–2516.

Thigpen T, Shingleton H, Homesley H, Blessing J (1982): Phase II trial of cis-diamminedichloroplatinum (DDP) in treatment of advanced or recurrent mixed mesodermal sarcoma of the uterus. Proc Am Soc Clin Oncol 1:110.

Tunca JC, Reddi PR, Shah SH, Slack ST (1979): Malignant non-Hodgkin's-type lymphoma of the cervix uteri occurring during pregnancy. Gynecol Oncol 7:385–393.

Wheeler RH, Ensminger WD, Thrall JH, Anderson JL (1982): High-dose doxorubicin: An exploration of the dose-response curve in human neoplasia. Cancer Treat Rep 66:493–498.

Wright CJR (1973): Solitary malignant lymphoma of the uterus. Am J Obstet Gynecol 117:114–120.

Yap BS, Baker LH, Sinkovics JG, Rivkin SE, Bottomley R, Thigpen T, Burgess MA, Benjamin RS, Bodey GP (1980): Cyclophosphamide, vincristine, adriamycin, and DTIC (CYVADIC) combination chemotherapy for the treatment of advanced sarcomas. Cancer Treat Rep 64:93–98.

Yap BS, Benjamin RS, Burgess MA, Murphy WK, Sinkovics JG, Bodey GP (1981): A phase II evaluation of methyl CCNU and actinomycin D in the treatment of advanced sarcomas in adults. Cancer 47:2807–2809.

Yazigi R, Piver MS, Barlow JJ (1979): Stage III uterine sarcoma: Case report and literature review. Gynecol Oncol 8:92–96.

Ziegler JL (1981): Burkitt's lymphoma. N Engl J Med 305:735–745.

Chemotherapy of Gestational Trophoblastic Disease

John R. Lurain

Division of Gynecologic Oncology, Brewer Trophoblastic Disease Center, Northwestern University Medical School, Chicago, Illinois 60611

Prior to the use of chemotherapy, results of treatment of gestational trophoblastic disease (choriocarcinoma and invasive mole) were poor. There was a 15% mortality with invasive mole even with early, complete tumor removal [1]. In patients whose choriocarcinoma was thought to be confined to the uterus at the time of surgery, only 41% were cured by hysterectomy [2]. Almost all patients with metastatic disease died [3].

The overall cure rate in the treatment of gestational trophoblastic disease now exceeds 90%. This success is the result of: 1) the inherent sensitivity of trophoblastic tumors to chemotherapy [4]; 2) the effective use of sensitive assays for the tumor marker human chorionic gonadotropin (hCG) [5,6]; 3) referral of patients to specialized treatment centers [6]; 4) identification of high-risk factors which enhance individualization of therapy [5–11]; and 5) aggressive use of combination chemotherapy, irradiation, and occasional surgical intervention in the care of high-risk patients [12,13].

In order to better understand present therapeutic efforts in gestational trophoblastic disease, a brief historical review of the development of the use of chemotherapy in these diseases will be presented. Methods for diagnosis, classification, and follow-up will be discussed briefly. Currently recommended treatment protocols for nonmetastatic and metastatic gestational trophoblastic disease and results of therapy will be reviewed. Newer chemotherapeutic agents and protocols, the use of prophylactic chemotherapy at the time of evacuation of hydatidiform moles, and the long-term effects of chemotherapy will also be discussed.

Chemotherapy of Gynecologic Cancer, pages 231–255

DEVELOPMENT OF CHEMOTHERAPY TREATMENT OF GESTATIONAL TROPHOBLASTIC DISEASE

In 1948 Hertz presented data demonstrating that fetal tissues required large amounts of folic acid to support the estrogen-induced growth of the female genital tract in experimental animals and that this growth could be inhibited by the folic acid antagonist, methotrexate [14]. In 1956 Li et al. first reported complete regression of metastatic trophoblastic disease in three women treated with methotrexate [4].

During the decade that followed, Hertz and his associates at the National Cancer Institute (NCI) systematically studied the effects of chemotherapy on gestational trophoblastic disease (Table I). In 1961 they reported their initial 5-year experience [5]. Twenty-eight of 63 patients (44%) with metastatic disease sustained a complete remission with methotrexate (MTX) therapy alone. Thirteen methotrexate-resistant patients were subsequently treated with vinblastine, yielding an additional two cures (15%) [15]. Twenty-nine deaths occurred, 23 due to disease and six secondary to chemotherapy toxicity. In 1961 these investigators identified actinomycin D (Act D) as a useful agent, producing remissions in six of 13 methotrexate-resistant patients [16].

The second 5-year experience in treating metastatic gestational trophoblastic neoplasms at the NCI using methotrexate and actinomycin D sequentially was reported by Ross et al. in 1965 [6]. Of 50 patients treated, 37 (74%) were placed into lasting remission. In this series, there were no deaths resulting from toxicity. Responses to either methotrexate or actinomycin D used as primary agents were comparable and remission rates appeared to be independent of the sequence in which the agents were given. Li's triple therapy for treatment of testicular cancer, consisting of a combination of methotrexate, actinomycin D, and an alkylating agent (MAC), was used in

TABLE I. Response of Trophoblastic Disease to Chemotherapy—National Cancer Institute 1956–1966

Extent of disease	Agent(s) used	No. patients	Complete remissions (%)	Deaths	
				Disease	Drug
Metastatic	MTX	63	30 (47)	23	6
Metastatic	MTX/Act D	75	56 (74)	9	0
	MAC	10	2 (20)	5	3
Nonmetastatic	MTX	58	54 (93)[a]	1	0

[a]Three patients with nonmetastatic disease resistant to MTX later entered remission with either Act D (1) or hysterectomy (2).
Modified from Hammond CB, Parker RT: Obstet Gynecol 35:132, 1970.

patients with trophoblastic disease resistant to single-agent chemotherapy, but remissions were few and toxicity was great [6,17].

During the last 5 years of the NCI study, 58 patients with nonmetastatic trophoblastic disease were treated with chemotherapy [18]. Fifty-four of these patients (93%) were placed into sustained remission with methotrexate alone. Two additional patients were cured with hysterectomy and one patient required actinomycin D before entering remission. One patient died after developing metastatic disease during therapy. The overall cure rate in this group therefore exceeded 98%, proving that disease localized to the uterus could usually be eradicated without hysterectomy, thereby preserving reproductive potential.

The investigations at the NCI made many important contributions to the treatment of trophoblastic disease and to cancer chemotherapy in general. First, they proved that metastatic as well as nonmetastatic cancer could be cured by drugs. Second, they established that high-dose pulse chemotherapy was more effective than a low daily dosage. Third, they demonstrated that by accurately measuring the tumor marker hCG, chemotherapy treatment response could be effectively monitored. Hertz and his colleagues also emphasized that the successful response of gestational trophoblastic disease to chemotherapy was dependent upon four factors: 1) duration of disease prior to initiation of chemotherapy; 2) height of the pretreatment hCG titer; 3) proper administration of the drugs; and 4) absence of central nervous system or hepatic metastases [5,6].

Other authors reported on the treatment of trophoblastic disease in the early 1960s using different chemotherapeutic agents or combinations of agents. Sung et al. (1963) reported on the use of 6-mercaptopurine (6-MP) and surgery [19]. Remission was achieved in 52 of 93 patients (56%) treated, but toxicity was high. Bagshawe (1963) used 6-MP combined with methotrexate to treat 23 patients with trophoblastic disease [20]. Seventeen complete remissions were obtained (74%). Moderately severe toxicity was encountered and patients who were resistant to MTX-6-MP were also resistant to Act D. There seemed to be no advantage of 6-MP over MTX or Act D, and toxicity was significantly greater. Bagshawe and Wilde (1964) reported using methotrexate with citrovorum factor (folinic acid) rescue (MTX-CF) in gestational trophoblastic disease [21]. They found this to have comparable effectiveness to MTX in conventional dosage while limiting systemic toxicity. Karnofsky et al. (1964) found the alkylating agent 6-diazo-5-oxo-L-norleucine (DON) to have activity in trophoblastic disease [22]. In 1964 Brewer et al. reported on the use of sequential MTX, Act D, and MAC in 28 patients with gestational trophoblastic disease, yielding a 73%

remission rate, thereby confirming the value of sequential therapy as championed at the NCI [23].

Other chemotherapeutic agents were subsequently found to be effective in gestational trophoblastic disease. Song reported excellent results with 5-fluorouracil (5FU) and Kengshengmycin, an antitumor antibiotic similar to actinomycin D, either alone, alternately, or in combination. The mortality from choriocarcinoma was reduced from 89.2% before 1958 to 21.4% during the period 1973–1975 [24]. Yim et al. treated five patients with bleomycin as primary treatment for gestational trophoblastic disease. All patients showed an initial good response, and three went into complete remission with bleomycin alone. They suggested that bleomycin should not replace methotrexate or actinomycin D as first-line drugs, but that it may be useful when used in combination chemotherapy regimens for patients who are resistant to conventional drugs or for high-risk patients [25].

DIAGNOSIS, CLASSIFICATION, AND FOLLOW-UP

Gestational trophoblastic disease is diagnosed by rising or plateauing hCG titers following evacuation of a hydatidiform mole, a histopathologic diagnosis of invasive mole or choriocarcinoma, or persistent elevation of hCG and/or demonstration of metastases in conjunction with an elevated hCG following any pregnancy event. Once the diagnosis of malignant trophoblastic disease has been made, it is necessary to determine the extent of disease. After a thorough general history and physical and pelvic examination, the following clinical studies should be obtained: chest x-ray (CT scan of lungs if negative), intravenous pyelogram, radionuclide or CT liver scan, CT brain scan, complete blood count with differential, platelet count, serum chemistries including liver and renal function studies, and a quantitative serum hCG. Pelvic ultrasound may also be useful to determine intrauterine or extrauterine pelvic disease.

After these initial studies, patients are categorized as having nonmetastatic or metastatic gestational trophoblastic disease. Patients with metastatic gestational trophoblastic disease are further classified as being at high risk based on the presence of one or more of the following: 1) immediate pretreatment hCG titer in excess of 100,000 IU/24 h urine or 40,000 mIU/ml serum (β-subunit assay); 2) time greater than 4 months from antecedent pregnancy event or onset of symptoms to treatment; 3) metastases to sites other than the lungs and/or vagina; 4) antecedent term gestation; or 5) prior unsuccessful chemotherapy [13]. On the basis of this classification, treatment is then carried out accordingly.

During treatment, patients are followed with complete blood, differential, and platelet counts every other day. Between treatments, hematologic profiles are obtained weekly. Chemistry profiles, chest x-rays, and physical examinations are performed routinely at approximately 2-week intervals before each course of therapy. Studies with prior abnormal results are followed at appropriate intervals. Response to treatment is determined by hCG assays, change in size or disappearance of existing metastases, or appearance of new lesions. Human chorionic gonadotropin titers should be obtained before each course of chemotherapy and the result available prior to administering therapy.

Complete remission is diagnosed after three consecutive weekly hCG levels are within normal range and there is no clinical or radiologic evidence of disease. An additional two courses of chemotherapy are usually given after the first normal hCG titer to decrease the incidence of relapse [13]. Following remission, hCG titers are obtained every 2 weeks for 6 weeks, monthly for 6 months, every other month for the remainder of the first year, and at 6-month intervals indefinitely thereafter. Physical examinations are performed and chest x-rays taken at 6- to 12-month intervals.

Pregnancy is prohibited for 1 year following remission. Barrier methods of contraception rather than oral contraceptives are recommended during treatment, at least until the hCG reaches normal range, and usually during the follow-up period because of the possible stimulating effects of estrogen/progestin combinations on trophoblastic proliferation [26,27]. When a patient does become pregnant following therapy for trophoblastic disease, a pelvic ultrasound is recommended in the first trimester to confirm a normal gestation, since these patients are at increased risk for another gestational trophoblastic disease event [28,29]. Also, the products of conception or placentas from future pregnancies should be carefully examined histopathologically and an hCG titer obtained 6 weeks after pregnancy termination.

NONMETASTATIC TROPHOBLASTIC DISEASE

Nonmetastatic gestational trophoblastic disease—that is, disease apparently confined to the uterus without evidence of distant metastases—is diagnosed most frequently during follow-up after evacuation of a hydatidiform mole. Approximately 20% of patients with hydatidiform mole will require treatment after evacuation, and 85% of these patients will have nonmetastatic disease [30–32]. The diagnosis of persistent trophoblastic disease is almost always made by the demonstration of a rise or plateau in hCG levels after molar evacuation. Occasionally the diagnosis is made following other types of pregnancy, usually by the finding of abnormal trophoblastic tissue at the time of curettage for abnormal uterine bleeding in conjunction with an elevated gonadotropin level. Studies to determine the extent of disease, as noted above, should be carried out once the diagnosis of trophoblastic disease is made. When no evidence of metastases is found, it is then important to ascertain whether the patient desires further reproduction.

If the patient with nonmetastatic gestational trophoblastic disease no longer wishes to preserve her fertility, hysterectomy may be advised as primary therapy. Adjuvant single-agent chemotherapy at the time of operation is indicated in order 1) to eradicate any occult metastases that may be present at the time of surgery, 2) to reduce the likelihood of viable tumor dissemination at surgery, and 3) to maintain cytotoxic levels of chemotherapy in tissues and plasma in the event viable tumor cells are disseminated at the time of hysterectomy [33]. Several series support the beneficial results of this practice. Hammond et al. reported that initial hysterectomy for nonmetastatic disease significantly reduced the number of courses of chemotherapy and the duration of treatment when compared to initial treatment with chemotherapy alone [12]. Goldstein and Berkowitz managed 19 patients with nonmetastatic disease with primary hysterectomy and one course of adjuvant chemotherapy; all 19 attained complete sustained remission with no further therapy [34]. Hysterectomy is generally performed midway through the course of the chemotherapy protocol. No increase in postoperative morbidity has been reported.

When patients with nonmetastatic gestational trophoblastic disease wish to preserve their fertility, single-agent chemotherapy is the treatment of choice (Table II). Several different protocols have been used, all yielding excellent and comparable remission rates [7,8,10–13,18]. Methotrexate 20–25 mg IM or IV daily for 5 days per treatment course has traditionally been the treatment of choice [18]. Actinomycin D 10–13 μg/kg IV daily for 5 days per course has alternately been used and is the appropriate therapeutic

TABLE II. Chemotherapy for Nonmetastatic and Low-Risk Metastatic Gestational Trophoblastic Disease

1)	Methotrexate 20–25 mg IV or IM q.d. × 5 d; repeat every 12–14 d (7–9 day window)
2)	Actinomycin D 10–13 μg/kg IV q.d. × 5 d; repeat every 12–14 d (7–9 day window)
3)	Methotrexate 1 mg/kg IM days 1, 3, 5, 7; Folinic acid 0.1 mg/kg IM days 2, 4, 6, 8; repeat every 15–18 d (7–10 day window)

regimen for patients with liver or renal disease contraindicating the use of methotrexate [16,35]. Courses of chemotherapy are repeated as often as toxicity permits, usually every 12–14 days (7- to 9-day window). Chemotherapy is changed to the alternate agent if the hCG titer plateaus or rises after two chemotherapy courses or if toxicity precludes an adequate dose or frequency of treatment.

No course of chemotherapy should be started if the white blood cell count is below 3,000/ml or the platelet count is below 100,000/ml. A single dose of methotrexate should not exceed 0.4 mg/kg/day and the dose of actinomycin D should not be greater than 13 μg/kg/day. Additionally, actinomycin D should be administered as an injection over 5–10 min through a well-running intravenous infusion since extravascular extravasation results in extensive tissue necrosis and slough.

The most common toxic reactions to these drugs are oropharyngeal ulcerations (stomatitis) as well as ulceration of the esophagus, stomach, and small and large bowel. Topical anesthetics combined with antibiotics and systemic analgesics provide some relief from these complications, which usually do not appear until several days after completion of a treatment course. These manifestations usually persist for only a short time, but must be resolved before another course of chemotherapy is initiated. Other toxic side effects include hair loss (usually minimal with single-agent therapy); conjunctivitis, best managed by methylcellulose drops; pleuritic or peritoneal pain due to mesothelial irritation from the agents, which should be treated with systemic analgesics; and vulvovaginitis secondary to monilia or ulcerations similar to those occurring in the oral cavity, which can be treated with topical preparations. Less common toxic reactions are skin rash, gastrointestinal hemorrhage secondary to ulcerations and thrombocytopenia, and significant leukopenia with subsequent infection.

More recently Goldstein et al. have advocated the use of slightly higher doses of methotrexate combined with folinic acid (citrovorum factor, CF) rescue for the treatment of nonmetastatic gestational trophoblastic disease [36]. Methotrexate is administered in a dose of 1.0–1.5 mg/kg IM every other day for four doses with folinic acid given IM at a dosage of 0.1–0.15 mg/kg 24 h after each dose of methotrexate. Subsequent courses of MTX-CF are administered if the hCG titer does not fall by 1 log within 18 days of the previous treatment, if the hCG level plateaus for more than 2 consecutive weeks, or if the hCG titer becomes reelevated after attaining a normal level.

Using this protocol, Berkowitz and Goldstein demonstrated a 95% remission rate in 94 patients with nonmetastatic trophoblastic tumors, with 81%

of these patients requiring only one course of MTX-CF [37]. Resistance to MTX-CF was observed in five patients; four of these subsequently achieved sustained remission following one or two courses of actinomycin D, and one patient who was also resistant to actinomycin D attained remission following hysterectomy. Granulocytopenia, thrombocytopenia, and hepatotoxicity were observed in only 6.6%, 2.8%, and 9.4% of patients, respectively. There was significantly less toxicity, especially stomatitis, than noted with the previously described 5-day, conventional dosage regimens.

Investigators at the Southeastern Regional Trophoblastic Disease Center compared the results of treatment of patients with nonmetastatic gestational trophoblastic disease with methotrexate alone versus methotrexate plus folinic acid [38]. Of 39 women treated with methotrexate alone, 7.7% developed methotrexate-resistant disease requiring a change in chemotherapy. In contrast, 27.5% of 29 patients treated with methotrexate–folinic acid required a change in chemotherapy to achieve remission. Ultimately, remission was achieved in all patients. Methotrexate–folinic acid was found to be consistently less toxic than methotrexate alone. The authors recommended that the methotrexate–folinic acid regimen be used in treatment of nonmetastatic disease because of its decreased toxicity but with the awareness of an increased need for a change in chemotherapy to achieve remission.

Smith has advocated alternating courses of methotrexate and actinomycin D given as described above [39]. He feels that the sensitivity of the tumor to both agents permits a maximum amount of medication to be given in a minimum amount of time, usually before resistance to the drug(s) develops. This alternating therapy also takes advantage of the different mechanisms of action of the two drugs and their slightly different toxicity. Using this protocol to treat 31 patients with nonmetastatic disease, all were cured. Fewer courses of chemotherapy and a shorter duration of treatment were noted with alternating compared to sequential chemotherapy.

A small percentage of patients with nonmetastatic gestational trophoblastic disease fail to achieve complete remission with systemic chemotherapy as outlined above. Pelvic arteriography, computed tomography, or ultrasonography may demonstrate a focus of trophoblastic disease within the myometrium. Under these circumstances, hysterectomy may be performed as definitive treatment [12,18,37]. When a patient with nonmetastatic disease resistant to chemotherapy desires to perserve her fertility, conservative operative treatment or pelvic arterial infusion chemotherapy may be considered. Wilson et al. reported on the local uterine resection of invasive trophoblastic tumors in five patients; all five achieved complete sustained remissions with no further treatment, and one patient had two subsequent term pregnancies [40]. Maroulis et al. performed pelvic arterial infusion chemotherapy with methotrexate or actinomycin D in five patients whose disease was resistant to systemic chemotherapy. Two of these were cured; three patients who were not cured by infusion subsequently underwent hysterectomy and entered remission [41].

Currently, cure is anticipated in essentially all patients with nonmetastatic gestational trophoblastic disease (Table III). In 1967 the group from NCI reported that all but one of 58 patients with nonmetastatic disease (98%) achieved cure: 54 with methotrexate alone, two with the addition of hysterectomy, and one with subsequent actinomycin D therapy [18]. Hammond et al. reported curing all 139 patients treated at their center for nonmetastatic gestational trophoblastic disease [12]. Of these patients, 122 were initially treated with chemotherapy alone and remission was achieved in 106 (87%). Of the 16 patients (13%) who failed to achieve remission with chemotherapy alone, nine underwent secondary hysterectomy, three were cured following pelvic arterial infusion chemotherapy, and four in whom arterial infusion failed subsequently had hysterectomy. Seventeen of the 139 patients underwent initial elective hysterectomy at the time of the institution of systemic chemotherapy, and all were cured. At the New England Trophoblastic Disease Center 179 patients with nonmetastatic disease were treated with single-agent chemotherapy between 1965 and 1979 [34]. Complete sustained remission was induced in 174 patients (97%) with sequential single-agent chemotherapy. Of the five patients (3%) who were resistant to single-agent therapy, all attained remission with further combination chemotherapy (2), infusion chemotherapy (1), or surgical intervention (2). At the John I. Brewer Trophoblastic Disease Center in Chicago, we treated 225 patients with nonmetastatic gestational trophoblastic disease between 1962 and 1982. One hundred ninety-nine patients (88%) were treated initially with chemotherapy only. Of these patients, 172 (86%) were cured by the

TABLE III. Remissions in Nonmetastatic Gestational Trophoblastic Disease

Author	Year	No. patients	Remissions	
			Patients	Percent
Hammond et al. [18]	1967	58	57	98
Brewer et al. [7]	1971	80	80	100
Jones and Lewis [10]	1974	18	18	100
Goldstein [8]	1972	49	49	100
Hammond et al. [12]	1980	139	139	100
Lurain et al. [13]	1982	200	200	100
Goldstein and Berkowitz [34]	1982	179	179	100

initial chemotherapy regimen; 21 (10.6%) received secondary chemotherapy with either actinomycin D (17), methotrexate (3), or MAC (1) to achieve remission; and only 6 (3%) required hysterectomy. An additional 26 patients (11.6%) were treated primarily by hysterectomy, usually combined and adjuvant chemotherapy. All patients in this series were cured. Significant chemotherapy toxicity occurred in only 14 patients (6.3%), the most common side effect being severe stomatitis.

METASTATIC TROPHOBLASTIC DISEASE

Hertz and co-workers at the NCI first demonstrated the efficacy of chemotherapy in the treatment of metastatic gestational trophoblastic disease [5,6]. In their series, complete remission was obtained in 47% of patients with methotrexate alone [5] and in 74% of patients treated with both methotrexate and actinomycin D sequentially [6]. These investigators also recognized that a successful outcome to therapy was dependent to a large extent on duration of disease, height of the pretreatment hCG titer, presence or absence of brain or liver metastases, and expertise in the use of the drugs. Over 95% of patients who were diagnosed early and treated vigorously were cured, whereas patients who were treated later with more extensive disease had only a 36% remission rate. This observation led to the recognition of the previously listed factors which are significant in determining prognosis and therefore in categorizing patients as at higher risk for treatment failure. Bagshawe has devised a comprehensive scoring system in which factors affecting prognosis are assigned numerical values which when added together are used to divide patients into low-, medium-, and high-risk categories (Table IV)[11].

Patients with high-risk metastatic disease are now treated more aggressively with initial combination chemotherapy with or without adjuvant radiation therapy or surgery. The benefit of this approach was first noted at the John I. Brewer Trophoblastic Disease Center in 1968. Patients with high-risk disease who were initially treated with MAC had a survival of 65%, whereas the rate for similar patients who were treated initially with a single-agent followed by MAC as secondary chemotherapy was 39% [13]. Hammond et al. [9] in 1973 reported on the results of therapy in 91 patients with metastatic gestational trophoblastic disease. Seventy-one "good prognosis" patients were treated initially with single-agent chemotherapy with a 98.6% survival. Of 17 "poor prognosis" patients, seven received initial single-agent chemotherapy followed by MAC combination chemotherapy if resistance developed, and ten were initially treated with MAC combination

TABLE IV. Scoring System Based on Prognostic Factors in Gestational Trophoblastic Disease

	Score			
Risk factors	0	10	20	40
Age (years)	< 39	> 39		
Parity	1, 2, > 4	3 or 4		
Antecedent pregnancy	Mole	Abortion	Term	
Pregnancy event to treatment interval (mo)	< 4	4–7	7–12	> 12
hCG (IU/L)	$< 10^3$	10^3–10^4	10^4–10^5	$> 10^5$
ABO blood group (female × male)	A × A × B × A B	O × O A × O	B × A B ×	
No. metastases	Nil	1–4	4–8	> 8
Site of metastases	Not detected Lungs Vagina	Spleen Kidney	GI tract Liver	Brain
Largest tumor mass (cm)	< 3	3–5	> 5	
Lymphocytic infiltration	Marked	Moderate or unknown	Slight	
Immune status	Reactive	Unknown	Unreactive	
Previous chemotherapy	Nil	Unknown	Single drug	Two or more drugs

Scores for individual risk factors are added and risk group determined by the total score as follows: low risk, ⩽50; medium risk, 60–90; high risk, >90.
Modified from Bagshawe KD: Cancer 38:1373, 1976.

chemotherapy. Only one of seven patients (14%) treated with single-agent chemotherapy followed by MAC survived compared to seven of ten patients (70%) treated initially with MAC. Others have subsesquently confirmed the value of initial combination chemotherapy in treating patients with high-risk metastatic gestational trophoblastic disease [8,10,11]. The added toxicity of such combination chemotherapy, however, does not appear to warrant its use in patients with less extensive metastatic disease, since the survival rate in this group can be anticipated to approach 100% with the use of single-agent chemotherapy.

Low-Risk Metastatic Disease

Patients categorized into the low-risk group should be treated with single-agent chemotherapy with methotrexate or actinomycin D as described in the section on nonmetastatic trophoblastic disease (Table II). Selection of the initial agent should be based on indexes of hepatic and renal function, avoiding methotrexate if there is an abnormality in either of these systems. At our center we prefer to begin treatment with methotrexate unless contraindicated, and administer the drugs sequentially; that is, when resistance to the first drug occurs, the second drug is begun. Patients who develop resistance to sequential single-agent chemotherapy are then treated with combination chemotherapy as for high-risk disease.

Several studies have demonstrated the high curability of low-risk metastatic gestational trophoblastic disease when appropriate therapy is administered (Table V). Ross and co-workers were the first investigators to identify the highly favorable prognosis in this group of patients, curing 20 of 21 patients (95%) with relatively nontoxic sequential methotrexate and actinomycin D chemotherapy [6]. Subsequent reports from Brewer [7], Hammond [9,12], Goldstein [8,34], Bagshawe [11], Jones and Lewis [10,42], and Lurain [13] have documented virtually 100% cures with low-risk metastatic disease. It is apparent from some of these studies, however, that 40–50% of patients will develop resistance to the first chemotherapeutic agent and require alternate treatment [8,9,41]. It is therefore very important to carefully monitor patients undergoing treatment for evidence of drug resistance (plateau or rise in hCG titer and/or the development of new metastases) so that a change to a second agent can be made at the earliest possible time. Interestingly, it appears that combination chemotherapy with MAC after failure of sequential single-agent chemotherapy is curative in many patients with low-risk metastatic disease, unlike the case in high-risk patients

TABLE V. Remissions in Metastatic Gestational Trophoblastic Disease

		Remissions/total patients (%)		
Author	Year	Total	Low-risk	High-risk
Ross et al. [6]	1965	37/50 (74%)	20/21 (95%)	17/29 (59%)
Brewer et al. [7]	1971	62/71 (87%)		
Goldstein [8]	1972	31/38 (82%)	29/29 (100%)	2/9 (22%)
Hammond et al. [9]	1973	78/88 (89%)	70/71 (99%)	8/17 (47%)
Jones and Lewis [10]	1974	18/21 (86%)	6/6 (100%)	12/15 (80%)
Hammond et al. [12]	1980	97/118 (82%)	55/55 (100%)	42/63 (67%)
Goldstein and Berkowitz [34]	1982		95/95 (100%)	
Lurain et al. [13]	1982	144/174 (83%)	69/69 (100%)	75/105 (71%)
Begent and Bagshawe [44]	1982			59/72 (82%)

[9,12,34,42]. Approximately 10–15% of patients treated for low-risk metastatic disease with sequential single-agent chemotherapy in these series required combination chemotherapy with or without surgery to achieve complete remission.

Surgery may be necessary to eradicate persistent disease in the uterus if all evidence of metastatic disease has disappeared and the hCG remains elevated despite repeated courses of chemotherapy. This occurred in 12.5% (5/40) of patients treated initially with chemotherapy only in the report of Hammond et al. [12]. These same authors initially treated 15 other patients with low-risk metastatic disease with hysterectomy done coincident with the institution of chemotherapy. Remission occurred in all 15 patients with a shorter duration of treatment and fewer courses of chemotherapy than in those patients treated initially with chemotherapy alone.

High-Risk Metastatic Disease

In patients categorized as having high-risk metastatic gestational trophoblastic disease based on the aforementioned prognostic factors, initial treatment should be combination chemotherapy. Until recently, the primary multidrug regimen used as initial therapy in these patients has been MAC, consisting of methotrexate 15 mg IV or IM, actinomycin D 0.5 mg IV, and cyclophosphamide 3 mg/kg IV or chlorambucil 10 mg PO, each drug given daily for 5 days per course (Table VI). Goldstein has modified this triple therapy slightly to include methotrexate with folinic acid rescue instead of conventional-dose methotrexate [34]. The interval between courses should be 9 to 14 days. After 3–4 courses of such combination chemotherapy, treatment may need to be changed to single-agent chemotherapy because of the cumulative toxicity and the inability to treat the patient as often as desired.

With the use of initial MAC chemotherapy in the treatment of high-risk patients, reported cure rates range from 67% to 80% (Table V) [9,10,12,13].

TABLE VI. Methotrexate, Actinomycin D, and Cyclophosphamide (MAC) Chemotherapy for High-Risk Gestational Trophoblastic Disease

Regimen	Schedule
(1) Methotrexate 15 mg IV or IM Actinomycin D 0.5 mg IV Cyclophosphamide 3 mg/kg IV or chlorambucil 10 mg PO	q.d. × 5 d
(2) Methotrexate 1.0 mg/kg IM days 1, 3, 5, 7 Folinic acid 0.1 mg/kg IM days 2, 4, 6, 8 Actinomycin D 12 μg/kg IV days 1–5 Cyclophosphamide 3 mg/kg IV days 1–5	

Hammond and colleagues originally reported curing seven of ten high-risk patients (70%) when MAC was used as initial chemotherapy [9]. They similarly treated a total of 63 high-risk patients from 1966 to 1979, achieving cure in 42 (67%) [12]. Jones and Lewis obtained an 80% remission rate in 15 high-risk patients treated with MAC [10]. All three deaths occurred in patients with brain and/or liver metastases and all patients who were at high risk because of high hCG level or prolonged duration of disease only were cured. In 1982, Lurain et al. reported the treatment of 105 high-risk patients, 75 (71%) of whom were cured, usually employing MAC chemotherapy [13].

Several other multidrug chemotherapy regimens have been proposed by Bagshawe for treatment of high-risk patients [11,43,44]. The regimen that has proved most useful has been the seven-drug CHAMOCA protocol, employing hydroxyurea, actinomycin D, methotrexate with folinic acid rescue, cyclophosphamide, vincristine (Oncovin), and doxorubicin (Adriamycin) (Table VII). Most of the agents used in this protocol have proven activity in gestational trophoblastic disease, they have different mechanisms of action to minimize drug resistance, and no two agents have the same major organ-specific toxicity. Methotrexate is administered in a high dosage

TABLE VII. Modified Bagshawe Regimen (CHAMOCA) for High-Risk Metastatic Gestational Trophoblastic Disease

Day 1		Hydroxyurea 500 mg PO q.i.d.
		Actinomycin D 0.2 mg IV
Day 2	0700	Vincristine 1 mg/m^2 IV
	1900	Methotrexate 100 mg/m^2 IV push
		Methotrexate 200 mg/m^2 IV over 12 h
		Actinomycin D 0.2 mg IV
Day 3	1900	Actinomycin D 0.2 mg IV
		Cyclophosphamide 500 mg/m^2 IV
		Folinic acid 14 mg IM
Day 4	0100	Folinic acid 14 mg IM
	0700	Folinic acid 14 mg IM
	1300	Folinic acid 14 mg IM
	1900	Folinic acid 14 mg IM
		Actinomycin D 0.5 mg IV
Day 5	0100	Folinic acid 14 mg IM
	1900	Actinomycin 0.5 mg IV
Day 6	No treatment	
Day 7	No treatment	
Day 8		Cyclophosphamide 300 mg/m^2 IV[a]
		Doxorubicin 30 mg/m^2 IV[a]

[a]Check WBC and platelets before giving.

with folinic acid rescue, which decreases the hemopoietic and gastrointestinal toxicity while providing for a high serum concentration of methotrexate, which may facilitate drug passage across the blood-brain barrier. Actinomycin D and cyclophosphamide are known to be effective in trophoblastic disease. Adriamycin, although active in many gynecologic malignancies, has not been shown to have an effect in gestational trophoblastic disease. Vincristine, a phase-specific mitotic inhibitor, is utilized to increase the cellular uptake of the methotrexate; also, the closely related drug vinblastine has proven effectiveness in methotrexate-resistant trophoblastic disease. Hydroxyurea is an antimetabolic, phase-specific agent with demonstrated modest activity against gestational trophoblastic disease. It is utilized on the first day of the protocol to synchronize the tumor's cells in the S-phase of the cell cycle for the methotrexate that follows. Courses of this regimen are repeated on the ninth day after completion of the prior course if toxicity permits, using the CHAMOCA regimen primarily in treating 72 high-risk patients over a 5-year period. Begent and Bagshawe reported an 82% remission rate [44]. Causes of death in 13 patients were initial extent of disease (6), drug resistance (5), infection (1), and leukemia (1).

If central nervous system metastases are present, whole-brain irradiation (3,000–3,600 rads in 10–12 ×300 rad fractions) is given simultaneously with the initiation of combination chemotherapy. In 1968, Brace reported on 21 patients with brain metastases who were treated with whole-brain irradiation (2,000 rads) in addition to chemotherapy at the NCI. Five patients survived and several others who died had no evidence of brain metastases at autopsy [45]. Since this report, most patients with brain metastases have been treated with adjuvant whole-brain irradiation. Weed et al. [46,47] at the Southeastern Regional Trophoblastic Disease Center treated 23 patients with brain metastases with brain irradiation and chemotherapy. Seven of 11 patients (64%) who presented initially with evidence of brain lesions were successfully treated. Only three of 12 patients (25%) survived who developed brain lesions while undergoing systemic chemotherapy or while in remission. Lurain et al. [13] at the Brewer Trophoblastic Disease Center reported on 20 patients who received whole-brain radiotherapy for metastases in addition to chemotherapy: 16 as part of their initial treatment for trophoblastic disease, and four for metastases that appeared during chemotherapy. Twelve of these patients (60%) experienced complete resolution of their brain tumors, but only eight of the 16 patients who had undergone brain irradiation as initial treatment entered permanent remission.

Bagshawe recommends intrathecal methotrexate for CNS lesions and as prophylaxis for all patients with pulmonary metastases or high-risk disease

[11,44]. Intrathecal methotrexate 12.5 mg is given with each course of chemotherapy that does not include a high dose (> 1 g/m^2) of methotrexate. When brain metastases are detected on presentation, the dosage of methotrexate on day 2 of the CHAMOCA regimen is increased to 1 g/m^2 in conjunction with folinic acid 30 mg every 12 h for 3 days starting 32 h after the beginning of the infusion. Seven of 12 patients (58%) with brain metastases achieved sustained complete remission, and no patients developed cerebral metastases during treatment when these measures were employed. Ausman et al. [48], utilizing a monkey brain tumor model with transplanted choriocarcinoma, have demonstrated, however, a significant increase in the permeability of the blood-brain barrier in the presence of tumor. This implies that any water-soluble drug could be expected to exchange readily between the blood and tumor tissue as long as a constant drug concentration was maintained in plasma, lending support to the use of prolonged intravenous infusional chemotherapy rather than bolus therapy, and negating the need for intrathecal therapy in patients with brain metastases.

Liver metastases from choriocarcinoma are particularly ominous, as the reported survival in patients with hepatic lesions ranges from 0% to 40% [13,24,49]. Most patients with liver metastases have extensive disease when they present for treatment and this primarily is the reason for treatment failure. These patients are at significant risk from serious hepatic bleeding, especially during the first course of chemotherapy. Some authors have recommended whole-liver irradiation to 2,000 rads over 2 weeks combined with systemic chemotherapy if metastases are present [9,10,12,49]. Concomitant whole-liver irradiation may reduce the morbidity and mortality from hemorrhage as it does with brain metastases, but this concept cannot be supported by the literature. The technique of selective hepatic artery occlusion by means of detachable silicone balloons described by Grumbine et al. has been shown to be effective in controlling hemorrhage from hepatic metastases from choriocarcinoma [50]. Some authors have recommended hepatic artery infusion chemotherapy, but no results of this technique have been reported. [24].

CHEMOTHERAPY OF RESISTANT TROPHOBLASTIC DISEASE

Despite the success of chemotherapy in curing over 90% of patients with gestational trophoblastic disease, approximately 20–30% of patients who present with metastatic, high-risk disease still die. Therefore, there is a significant group of patients who fail to respond to present treatment methods. Failure to cure patients with gestational trophoblastic disease can mainly be attributed to the presence of extensive disease at the time of initial treatment, lack of initial, appropriately aggressive treatment in high-risk patients, and failure of presently used chemotherapy protocols to control advanced disease.

Secondary chemotherapy in patients with gestational trophoblastic disease yields poor results [13,51,52]. The complete response rate to MAC when used after failure of single-agent therapy is about 17% [8,9,13]. At the Brewer Trophoblastic Disease Center, we have been unable to achieve any complete remissions with other second-line chemotherapy regimens including Bagshawe's multiagent protocol (CHAMOCA) or the combination of vinblastine, bleomycin, and cis-platinum, although significant partial responses (> 50% decrease in hCG level) were obtained with these combinations [13]. Other drugs which were tried as secondary or tertiary treatment included doxorubicin, dacarbazine (DTIC), L-asparaginase, vinblastine, bleomycin, high-dose methotrexate with citrovorum factor rescue, and VP 16-213 (Etoposide). Of these agents, only bleomycin and VP 16-213 produced any partial responses. Bagshawe reported that the drugs vincristine, vinblastine, nitrogen mustard, daunorubicin, procarbazine, bleomycin, cytosine arabinoside, and asparaginase did not show useful evidence of antitumor activity when used alone in patients who had become resistant to methotrexate [52].

Weed and colleagues [53] used the CHAMOCA protocol to treat 16 patients who had received prior chemotherapy. Eight of the 16 (50%) were alive without evidence of disease for more than 12 months after first achieving normal hCG titers. This relatively high remission rate in patients who had failed on previous chemotherapy is encouraging. An alternate regimen has been suggested for patients who are responsive to the CHAMOCA protocol but who have chronic bone marrow suppression, precluding adequate treatment (Table VIII)[54]. Bleomycin and cis-platinum, which cause little marrow suppression, are substituted for actinomycin D and cyclophosphamide in this regimen.

Cis-platinum and VP 16-213 are the most active new agents for the treatment of resistent trophoblastic disease. The most experience in using cis-platinum in gestational choriocarcinoma has been reported by Newlands and Bagshawe [55,56]. In their series, cis-platinum appeared to be most effective when combined with vincristine and methotrexate. On day 1 vincristine 1.0 mg/m^2 was given intravenously at 10:00 a.m. followed by methotrexate 100 mg/m^2 IV push and 200 mg/m^2 IV over 12 h. Folinic acid 15 mg IM was given 24 h after the start of the methotrexate infusion and continued every 12 h for four doses. On day 4 cis-platinum 120 mg/m^2

TABLE VIII. Alternate Chemotherapy for Marrow Suppression in High-Risk Metastatic Gestational Trophoblastic Disease

Day 1		Hydroxyurea 500 mg PO q.i.d.
		Cis-platinum 50 mg/m^2 IV
Day 2	0700	Vincristine 1 mg/m^2 IV
	1900	Methotrexate 100 mg/m^2 IV push
		Methotrexate 200 mg/m^2 IV over 12 h
Day 3	1900	Folinic acid 14 mg IM
Day 4	0100	Folinic acid 14 mg IM
	0700	Folinic acid 14 mg IM
	1300	Folinic acid 14 mg IM
	1900	Folinic acid 14 mg IM
Days 1–4		Bleomycin 15 U/24 h (continuous IV infusion)

From Surwit EA: Semin Oncol 9:204, 1982.

was given IV with hydration and mannitol diuresis. This regimen was usually repeated every 3–4 weeks. The side effects of this combination are principally related to the cis-platinum which induces nausea and vomiting in most patients, occasional transient increases in blood urea nitrogen and creatinine, rare high-frequency hearing loss, hypocalcemia and hypermagnesemia, and thrombocytopenia and anemia. The response rate (greater than 50% decrease in hCG following a single course of chemotherapy) was 62% in 24 patients. Some of these patients were off treatment and in complete remission for up to 37 months. Surwit and Hammond [49] and Schlaerth et al. [57] each reported two patients in remission after treatment with a vinblastine, bleomycin, cis-platinum protocol. Others have also noted responses to cis-platinum–containing combinations [58,59].

More recently, Newlands and Bagshawe have reported on the use of VP 16-213 in patients with drug-resistant choriocarcinoma [55,60]. VP 16-213 is a semisynthetic derivative of podophyllotoxin. It is clinically well tolerated, causing minimal nausea and vomiting in most patients. Temporary alopecia occurs in some patients. Myelosuppression involving both leukopenia and thrombocytopenia is moderate and reversible over a period of 10–20 days. VP 16-213 was used in a dose of 100 mg/m^2 IV diluted in 200 ml of saline given over a 30-min infusion for 5 consecutive days. Courses were repeated usually every 3 weeks. Of the 55 patients with drug-resistant choriocarcinoma who were treated with VP 16-213 as a single agent, 37 were evaluable for response. Twenty-one patients (57%) had a greater than 50% decrease in hCG titer following one course of this agent. VP 16-213 has also been used in combination with methotrexate and vincristine or bleomycin and cis-platinum (Table IX) [54,60]. The use of regimens employing these new

TABLE IX. Alternate Chemotherapy for Primary Drug Resistance in High-Risk Metastatic Trophoblastic Disease

Day 1	Cis-platinum 50 mg/m^2 IV
Days 1–4	Bleomycin 15 U/24 h (continuous IV infusion)
Days 1–4	VP 16-213 100 mg/m^2 IV

From Surwit EA: Semin Oncol 9:201, 1982.

agents as primary treatment for high-risk metastatic disease needs further study.

Continued efforts toward improved follow-up of hydatidiform moles and a greater awareness of the possibility of choriocarcinoma associated with other types of pregnancy will hopefully lead to fewer patients presenting with advanced disease. Referral of high-risk patients to trophoblastic disease centers or gynecologic oncologists for treatment should result in appropriate initial treatment. Finally, new effective chemotherapeutic protocols which limit drug resistance while at the same time maintaining a low rate of morbidity and mortality from drug toxicity need to be developed for use in high-risk patients.

PROPHYLACTIC CHEMOTHERAPY FOR HYDATIDIFORM MOLE

It has been observed that the prophylactic administration of either actinomycin D or methotrexate to patients at the time of termination of a molar pregnancy is associated with a reduced rate of development of trophoblastic sequelae (invasive mole or choriocarcinoma). Goldstein [61] in 1974 reported on the results of a prospective study utilizing prophylactic actinomycin D 12 μg/kg/day IV for 5 days starting 3 days prior to molar evacuation in a group of 100 patients compared to a comparable group of 100 patients with molar pregnancy evacuated without prophylactic chemotherapy. Proliferative trophoblastic sequelae occurred in two patients in the treated group, in contrast to 16 patients in the untreated group, including four with metastatic disease ($P < 0.01$).

Fasoli et al. [62] recently reported on the use of methotrexate 10 mg/day PO for 5 days every 3 weeks for three cycles starting immediately after evacuation of hydatidiform mole. Of 104 patients who received this prophylactic chemotherapy, three (3%) developed persistent trophoblastic disease. This is significantly fewer than the 23 (9%) who developed trophoblastic sequelae of the 250 untreated patients ($P < 0.05$). Among high-risk patients, prophylactic chemotherapy appeared to reduce by more than seven times the risk of persistent disease. Also, no patients receiving prophylactic chemotherapy developed metastatic disease.

Several arguments have been advanced against the use of prophylactic chemotherapy. First, none of the regimens described prevents the development of trophoblastic sequelae in all patients treated, and even metastatic disease has been reported in patients receiving prophylactic therapy. Second, most patients with hydatidiform mole are cured by evacuation alone. If all patients with molar pregnancy were treated with prophylactic chemotherapy, 80% or more would be treated unnecessarily. While long-term effects of systemic chemotherapy have been minimal to date, the cytotoxic agents used are teratogens, and mutagenic changes may therefore occur which could effect the long-term prognosis of such patients. Third, severe drug reactions, although rare, do occur, and deaths have been reported following a single course of chemotherapy. This may even be more likely to occur in patients receiving prophylactic chemotherapy in a setting which might not be optimal for control or treatment of toxicity. Fourth, the administration of prophylactic chemotherapy may provide a false sense of security, with a resultant inadequate follow-up with serial hCG assays to assure complete regression. Finally, essentially all patients who are followed with hCG titers following evacuation of a hydatidiform mole and found to have rising or plateauing hCG levels with or without metastases can be cured with chemotherapy. Therefore, it seems that despite the demonstrated effectiveness and safety of prophylactic chemotherapy at the time of molar evacuation, its use should be limited at present to special situations where the risk of developing invasive mole or choriocarcinoma is greater than normal or where adequate gonadotropin follow-up is not possible.

LONG-TERM FOLLOW-UP AFTER CHEMOTHERAPY FOR GESTATIONAL TROPHOBLASTIC DISEASE

Reproductive Performance

The successful treatment of gestational trophoblastic disease with chemotherapy has resulted in an increasing number of women whose reproductive potential has been retained despite exposure to drugs that have teratogenic potential. A large number of successful pregnancies have been reported in this group of patients [34,63,64]. In general, those patients experienced no increase in abortions, stillbirths, congenital anomalies, prematurity, or major obstetrical complications. Goldstein and Berkowitz [34] reported a slightly increased risk of spontaneous abortion (20%), and Van Thiel et al. [65] found an increased incidence of partial placenta accreta in subsequent pregnancies in their series. At the Brewer Trophoblastic Disease Center from 1962 to 1982, 176 pregnancies occurred in 112 of the 193 patients who were treated with chemotherapy alone for nonmetastatic gestational trophoblastic disease. Of the 176 pregnancies, there were 128 (72.7%) term deliveries, four (2.3%) premature deliveries, 28 (15.9%) spontaneous abortions, 15 (8.5%) therapeutic abortions, and one (0.6%) hydatidiform mole. Major congenital malformations occurred in only one (0.8%) of the 132 term or premature births and there were four (3.0%) major obstetrical complications. There has been no evidence for reactivation of disease due to a subsequent pregnancy. Patients who have had one trophoblastic disease episode are at greater risk for the development of a second episode in a subsequent pregnancy, but this is unrelated to whether or not they had received chemotherapy [28,29]. Patients are advised to delay conception for 1 year from cessation of chemotherapy. This not only allows uninterrupted hCG follow-up to assure cure, but may permit mature ova, damaged by exposure to cytotoxic drugs, to be eliminated, thus allowing more immature oocytes to produce gametes for subsequent fertilization.

Secondary Malignancies

Because many anticancer drugs are known carcinogens, there is concern that the chemotherapy used to induce long-term remissions or cures of one cancer may induce second malignancies. There have been no reports, however, of increased susceptibility to the development of other malignancies after successful chemotherapy of trophoblastic disease [66,67]. Rustin et al. investigated the incidence of second tumors after cytotoxic chemotherapy in 457 long-term survivors treated for gestational trophoblastic disease between 1958 and 1978 [67]. Treatment was given according to regular intermittent schedules over a mean period of 4 months. Methotrexate was given to all but two patients, and 261 (57%) also received other cytotoxic agents, including actinomycin D, cyclophosphamide, vincristine, 6-mercaptopurine, and 6-azauridine. After a mean period of 7.8 years since the beginning of treatment and a total of 3,522 patient-years of risk, only two second neoplasms had developed (one acute leukemia and one carcinoma of the breast). This is less than the expected number of cases (3.5) and suggests that methotrexate as used in the treatment of gestational trophoblastic disease is not carcinogenic.

REFERENCES

1. Greene RR: Chorioadenoma destruens. Ann NY Acad Sci 80:143, 1959.

2. Brewer JI, Smith RT, Pratt GB: Choriocarcinoma. Absolute 5-year survival rates of 122 patients treated by hysterectomy. Am J Obstet Gynecol 85:841, 1963.
3. Park WW, Lees JC: Choriocarcinoma: General review and analysis of 516 cases. Arch Pathol 49:73, 1950.
4. Li MD, Hertz R, Spencer DB: Effects of methotrexate therapy upon choriocarcinoma and chorioadenoma. Proc Soc Exp Biol Med 93:361, 1956.
5. Hertz R, Lewis J Jr, Lipsett MB: Five years experience with chemotherapy of metastatic choriocarcinoma and related trophoblastic tumors in women. Am J Obstet Gynecol 82:631, 1961.
6. Ross GT, Goldstein DP, Hertz R, Lipsett MB, Odell WD: Sequential use of methotrexate and actinomycin D in the treatment of metastatic choriocarcinoma and related trophoblastic diseases in women. Am J Obstet Gynecol 93:223, 1965.
7. Brewer JI, Eckman TR, Dolkart RE, Torok EE, Webster A: Gestational trophoblastic disease. A comparative study of the results of therapy in patients with invasive mole and with choriocarcinoma. Am J Obstet Gynecol 109:335, 1971.
8. Goldstein DP: The chemotherapy of gestational trophoblastic disease. Principles of clinical management. JAMA 220:209, 1972.
9. Hammond CB, Borchert LG, Tyrey L, Creasman WT, Parker RT: Treatment of metastatic trophoblastic disease: Good and poor prognosis. Am J Obstet Gynecol 115:451, 1973.
10. Jones WB, Lewis JL Jr: Treatment of gestational trophoblastic disease. Am J Obstet Gynecol 120:14, 1974.
11. Bagshawe KD: Risk and prognostic factors in trophoblastic neoplasia. Cancer 38:1373, 1976.
12. Hammond CB, Weed JC Jr, Currie JL: The role of operation in the current therapy of gestational trophoblastic disease. Am J Obstet Gynecol 136:844, 1980.
13. Lurain JR, Brewer JI, Torok EE, Halpern B: Gestational trophoblastic disease. Treatment results at the Brewer Trophoblastic Disease Center. Obstet Gynecol 60:354, 1982.
14. Hertz R: Interference with estrogen-induced tissue growth in the chick genital tract by a folic acid antagonist. Science 107:300, 1948.
15. Hertz R, Lipsett MB, Moy RH: Effect of vincaleukoblastine on metastatic choriocarcinoma and related trophoblastic tumors in women. Cancer Res 20:1050, 1960.
16. Ross GT, Stolbach LL, Hertz R: Actinomycin D in the treatment of methotrexate-resistant trophoblastic disease in women. Cancer Res 22:1015, 1962.
17. Li MC, Whitmore WF Jr, Golbey R, Grabstald H: Effects of combined drug therapy on metastatic cancer of the testis. JAMA 174:1291, 1960.
18. Hammond CB, Hertz R, Ross GT, Lipsett MB, Odell WD: Primary chemotherapy for nonmetastatic gestational trophoblastic neoplasms. Am J Obstet Gynecol 98:71, 1967.
19. Sung H-C, Wu P-C, Ho T-H: Treatment of choriocarcinoma and chorioadenoma destruens with 6-mercaptopurine and surgery. Chin Med J 82:24, 1963.
20. Bagshawe KD: Trophoblastic tumors. Chemotherapy and developments. Br Med J 2:1303, 1963.
21. Bagshawe KD, Wilde CE: Infusion therapy for pelvic trophoblastic tumors. J Obstet Gynaecol Br Commonw 71:565, 1964.
22. Karnofsky DA, Golbey RB, Li MC: Remissions induced in patients with trophoblastic tumors by 6-diazo-5-oxo-L-norleucine (DON). Am J Cancer Res 5:33, 1964.
23. Brewer JI, Gerbie AB, Dolkart RE, Skom JH, Nagle RG, Torok EE: Chemotherapy of trophoblastic diseases. Am J Obstet Gynecol 90:566, 1964.

24. Song H, Zia Z, Wu B, Wang Y: Twenty years' experience in chemotherapy of choriocarcinoma and malignant mole. Chin Med J 92:677, 1979.
25. Yim CM, Wong LC, Ma HK: Clinical trial of bleomycin in the treatment of gestational trophoblastic disease. Gynecol Oncol 8:296, 1979.
26. Lajos L, Gorcs J, Szekely J, Csaba I, Domany S: The immunologic and endocrinologic basis of successful transplantation of human trophoblast. Am J Obstet Gynecol 89:595, 1964.
27. Stone M, Bagshawe KD: An analysis of the influences of maternal age, gestational age, contraceptive method, and the mode of primary treatment of patients with hydatidiform moles on the incidence of subsequent chemotherapy. Br J Obstet Gynaecol 86:782, 1979.
28. Sand PK, Lurain JR, Brewer JI: Repeat gestational trophoblastic disease. Obstet Gynecol (in press).
29. Federschneider JM, Goldstein DP, Berkowitz RS, Marean AR, Bernstein MR: Natural history of recurrent molar pregnancy. Obstet Gynecol 55:457, 1980.
30. Curry SL, Hammond CB, Tyrey L, Creasman WT, Parker RT: Hydatidiform mole: Diagnosis, management and long-term follow-up of 347 patients. Obstet Gynecol 45:1, 1975.
31. Morrow CP, Kletsky OA, DiSaia PJ, Townsend DE, Mishell DR, Nakamura RM: Clinical and laboratory correlates of molar pregnancy and trophoblastic disease. Am J Obstet Gynecol 128:424, 1977.
32. Lurain JR, Brewer JI, Torok EE, Halpern B: Natural history of hydatidiform mole after primary evacuation. Am J Obstet Gynecol 145:591, 1983.
33. Lewis J Jr, Gore H, Hertig AT, Goss DA: Treatment of trophoblastic disease. With rationale for the use of adjuvant chemotherapy at the time of indicated operation. Am J Obstet Gynecol 96:710, 1966.
34. Goldstein DP, Berkowitz RS: Nonmetastatic and low-risk metastatic gestational trophoblastic neoplasms. Semin Oncol 9:191, 1982.
35. Osathanondh R, Goldstein DP, Pastorfide GB: Actinomycin D as the primary agent for gestational trophoblastic disease. Cancer 36:863, 1975.
36. Goldstein DP, Saracco P, Osathanondh R, Goldstein PR, Marean AR, Bernstein MR: Methotrexate with citrovorum factor rescue for gestational trophoblastic neoplasms. Obstet Gynecol 51:93, 1978.
37. Berkowitz RS, Goldstein DP, Bernstein MR: Methotrexate with citrovorum factor rescue as primary therapy for gestational trophoblastic disease. Cancer 50:2024, 1982.
38. Smith EB, Weed JC Jr, Tyrey L, Hammond CB: Treatment of nonmetastatic gestational trophoblastic disease: Results of methotrexate alone versus methotrexate–folinic acid. Am J Obstet Gynecol 144:88, 1982.
39. Smith JP: Chemotherapy in gynecologic cancer. Malignant trophoblastic tumors. Clin Obstet Gynecol 18:113, 1975.
40. Wilson RB, Beecham CT, Symmonds RE: Conservative surgical management of chorioadenoma destruens. Obstet Gynecol 26:814, 1965.
41. Maroulis GB, Hammond CB, Johnsrude IS, Weed JC Jr, Parker RT: Arteriography and infusional chemotherapy in localized trophoblastic disease. Obstet Gynecol 45:397, 1975.
42. Jones WB: Management of low-risk metastatic gestational trophoblastic disease. J Reprod Med 26:213, 1981.
43. Bagshawe KD: Treatment of trophoblastic tumors. Recent Results Cancer Res 62:192. 1977.

44. Begent RHJ, Bagshawe KD: The management of high-risk choriocarcinoma. Semin Oncol 9:198, 1982.
45. Brace KC: The role of irradiation in the treatment of metastatic trophoblastic disease. Radiology 91:540, 1968.
46. Weed JC Jr, Hammond CB: Cerebral metastatic choriocarcinoma: Intensive therapy and prognosis. Obstet Gynecol 55:89, 1980.
47. Weed JC Jr, Woodward KT, Hammond CB: Choriocarcinoma metastatic to the brain: Therapy and prognosis. Semin Oncol 9:208, 1982.
48. Ausman JI, Levin VA, Brown WE, et al: Brain tumor chemotherapy. J Neurosurg 46:155, 1977.
49. Surwit EA, Hammond CB: Treatment of metastatic trophoblastic disease with poor prognosis. Obstet Gynecol 55:565, 1980.
50. Grumbine FC, Rosenshein NB, Brereton HD, Kaufman SL: Management of liver metastases from gestational trophoblastic neoplasia. Am J Obstet Gynecol 137:959, 1980.
51. Lurain JR, Brewer JI, Mazur MT, Torok EE: Fatal gestational trophoblastic disease: An analysis of treatment failures. Am J Obstet Gynecol 144:391, 1982.
52. Bagshawe KD: Trophoblastic disease. Adv Obstet Gynaecol 19:225, 1978.
53. Weed JC Jr, Barnard DE, Currie JL, Clayton LA, Hammond CB: Chemotherapy with the modified Bagshawe protocol for poor prognosis metastatic trophoblastic disease. Obstet Gynecol 59:377, 1982.
54. Surwit EA: The management of poor prognosis trophoblastic disease. Semin Oncol 9:204, 1982.
55. Newlands ES, Bagshawe KD: Activity of high-dose cis-platinum in combination with vincristine and methotrexate in drug-resistant gestational choriocarcinoma. Br J Cancer 40:943, 1979.
56. Newlands ES: New chemotherapeutic agents in the management of gestational trophoblastic disease. Semin Oncol 9:239, 1982.
57. Schlaerth JB, Morrow CP, DePetrillo AD: Sustained remission of choriocarcinoma with cis-platinum, vinblastine and bleomycin after failure of conventional combination drug therapy. Am J Obstet Gynecol 136:983, 1980.
58. Goldstein DP: Case records of the Massachusetts General Hospital. N Engl J Med 296:926, 1977.
59. Lurain JR, Piver MS: Metastatic gestational trophoblastic disease. Secondary chemotherapy. NY State J Med 80:234, 1980.
60. Newlands ES, Bagshawe KD: Anti-tumor activity of the epipodophyllin derivative VP 16-213 (Etoposide: NSC-141540) in gestational choriocarcinoma. Eur J Cancer 16:401, 1980.
61. Goldstein DP: Prevention of gestational trophoblastic disease by use of actinomycin D in molar pregnancies. Obstet Gynecol 43:475, 1974.
62. Fasoli M, Ratti E, Franceschi S, LaVecchia C, Pecorelli S, Mangioni C: Management of gestational trophoblastic disease: Results of a cooperative study. Obstet Gynecol 60:205, 1982.
63. Ross GT: Congenital anomalies among children born of mothers receiving chemotherapy for gestational trophoblastic neoplasms. Cancer 37:1043, 1976.
64. Walden PAM, Bagshawe KD: Pregnancies after chemotherapy for gestational trophoblastic tumors. Lancet 2:1241, 1979.
65. Van Thiel DH, Grodin JM, Ross GT, Lipsett MB: Partial placenta accreta in pregnancies following chemotherapy for gestational trophoblastic disease. Am J Obstet Gynecol 112:54, 1972.

66. Lewis JL Jr: Treatment of metastatic gestational trophoblastic neoplasms. A brief review of developments in the years 1968 to 1978. Am J Obstet Gynecol 136:163, 1980.
67. Rustin GJS, Rustin F, Dent J, Booth M, Salt S, Bagshawe KD: No increase in second tumors after cytotoxic chemotherapy for gestational trophoblastic tumors. N Engl J Med 308:473, 1983.

Chemotherapy of Breast Cancer

Lawrence S. Perlow and James F. Holland

Department of Neoplastic Diseases, Mount Sinai School of Medicine of the City University of New York, New York, New York 10029

It is estimated that in 1983 invasive breast cancer will be diagnosed in 114,000 women, and that 37,000 of these women will die of their disease [1]. At present, the recurrence of breast cancer following primary therapy of the tumor is nearly always associated with eventual death from the tumor. Currently available opportunities exist to provide important palliation to the majority of these women. Efforts are in progress to prevent recurrent disease and to cure it when it does occur.

The influence of endocrine factors on the development of breast cancer [2] is implicit in the normal functions of the breast. Treatment of breast cancer by hormonal manipulation of the endocrine environment, chemotherapy, immunotherapy, and adjuvant therapy will be discussed in that order. Clinical results from controlled trials will be emphasized, when available, since they represent the final focus of the multidisciplinary efforts to cure breast cancer.

ENDOCRINE THERAPY

Receptors

Manipulation of the endocrine environment in women with recurrent or advanced primary breast cancer has become more successful during the past decade since the use of receptor assays allows physicians to focus therapy on those most likely to respond. Among the one-half to two-thirds of patients shown to have levels of estrogen receptor protein commonly associated with response, numerous reports document tumor regression in the

Chemotherapy of Gynecologic Cancer, pages 257–299

range of 50–70% from a variety of endocrine treatments [3–9]. In the absence of threshold levels of estrogen receptors, response rates are consistently under 15% [5,6,10–12]. High levels of estrogen receptor, greater than 50–100 fmol/mg protein, are associated with even more frequent responses. In one series, responses occurred in 42% when the receptor level was 3–100 fmol/mg protein and in 64% when it was greater than 100 fmol/mg protein [3]. A response rate of 45% among patients with receptor levels above 20 fmol/mg protein improved to 80% when only levels above 200 fmol/mg were considered [10]. The failure of up to 50% of estrogen receptor–positive patients to respond to hormonal treatment may well be due to a defective transport mechanism for translocation of the receptor-steroid complex to the nucleus [11,13].

An intact estrogen receptor system appears to be required for the production of progesterone receptor proteins. Despite contrary reports [6], preponderant data indicate that the presence of progesterone receptors indicates greater sensitivity to endocrine maneuvers in general [3,5,12,14,17]. Bloom et al. found that 77% of ER +/PR + patients responded to adrenalectomy, adrenalectomy plus oophorectomy, or tamoxifen compared to 21% of ER +/PR − [15]. Only about 4–6% of patients are found to be ER −/PR + [15,16]. These appear to represent false-negative ER determinations caused by inhibition of binding in the assay by estrogenic compounds in the cystosol [16]. Although the small numbers of these patients make analysis difficult, their response appears intermediate between ER +/PR + and ER −/PR−.

The optimum time to obtain tissue for receptor analysis is immediately prior to the proposed hormone treatment. However, because of the inaccessibility and small size of some metastases, as well as a desire to avoid removal of the sole site of measurable disease, this often is not possible. Concordance between two consecutive receptor biopsies was found in 88% of cases in the absence of intervening therapy [18]. This was especially true when the initial biopsy was receptor-negative. The greater effect of hormonal therapy compared to chemotherapy in causing a reduction in the ER content of tissue obtained at subsequent relapse was shown in a group of 26 patients [18]. Among 12 women treated with hormonal therapy, the receptor level fell from 199 fmol/mg protein to 57 fmol/mg. The fall in 14 chemotherapeutically treated women was from 128 to 110 fmol/mg protein. Such a result might have been anticipated since the unretarded growth of receptor-negative tumor cells would account for many relapses in patients treated with hormonal therapy. Simultaneous progesterone receptor measurements from multiple biopsy sites were found to be concordant 89% of the time

[19]. When sequential biopsies were performed in the absence of treatment there was a 27% discordance, with chemotherapy plus endocrine therapy 50%, and with endocrine therapy alone 70%. In only 9% of cases did a PR − biopsy evolve to become PR +.

Endocrine Ablation

Endocrine ablation was the first treatment used in premenopausal patients. In a series of 177 mainly premenopausal women treated before the advent of receptor assays, 48% achieved at least a 25% reduction in tumor size [20]. The results were equal whether surgery or radiotherapy was used to remove ovarian function, although response was often delayed by several months in the radiotherapy group. The median duration of the response was 12 months.

Adrenalectomy has been used to remove the adrenal secretion of sex steroids and androstenedione, a steroid that can be converted by peripheral tissues to estrogens. A 33% regression rate, lasting a minimum of 6 months, was found in 64 patients, with a 60% response rate in prior oophorectomy responders [21]. In a larger series, 40% of those responding to castration subsequently responded to adrenalectomy compared to 17% of oophorectomy nonresponders for a total response rate of 31% [22], indicating a low yield of adrenalectomy in oophorectomy nonresponders. Simultaneous oophorectomy and adrenalectomy resulted in a 33.7% response rate [22]. While the results of adrenalectomy are of value, major surgery is involved, often with women in poor physical condition, leading to its decline in popularity.

The development of the transphenoidal approach has made hypophysectomy a safer procedure than when craniotomy was used. There was a 42% partial response rate in 199 patients preselected to exclude nonresponders to oophorectomy [23]. Chronic requirements for thyroid hormone, adrenocortical steroids, and possible antidiuretic hormone along with the cost of the procedure and potential morbidity are serious disadvantages. The increasing use of aminoglutethimide and tamoxifen, to be discussed later, have also diminished the resort to this procedure.

Estrogens

Additive hormonal therapy has been applied with good palliative success. In a retrospective study of 944 women by the American Medical Association, diethylstilbesterol (DES) produced 36.8% responses and was superior to testosterone, which had a 21.4% response rate [24]. Kennedy [25] substantiated these data in comparing the two treatments in 59 postmenopausal women. He found 30% responses for DES and only 10% for the androgen [25]. In 483 women studied by the Cooperative Breast Cancer Group from 1961 to 1963, response rates of 16% with DES and 10% with testosterone proprionate were found [25a]. The usual dose of DES is 5 mg t.i.d. A randomized double-blind study involving 523 postmenopausal women evaluated dosages of 1.5, 15, 150, and 1,500 mg daily [26]. Response rates were 10%, 15%, 17%, and 21%, respectively. Although the difference in response rates was significant, toxicity was higher with larger doses. The authors provided a retrospective mathematical model predicting the best dosage based on age from menopause and dominant site of disease, but this has not been proved prospectively. Side effects of DES include gastrointestinal disturbance, edema, uterine bleeding, and urinary urgency [27]. Hypercalcemia in the presence of bone disease is less common, occurring in under 5% of cases [26].

Androgens

Androgen therapy, associated with lower response rates than DES, has also been compared to tamoxifen [28]. In a prospective crossover study in 79 postmenopausal women, the response rate to fluoxymesterone as a first drug was 19% compared to 30% for tamoxifen. Responses to tamoxifen were longer, and survival was significantly better in the group that received tamoxifen as initial therapy. Equivalence was found in the treatment of bone metastases. The Eastern Cooperative Oncology Group found that the addition of fluoxymesterone to chemotherapy improved marrow tolerance and allowed for higher chemotherapy doses [29]. Largely because of their marrow-stimulating effect, efficacy in the treatment of bone metastases, and their value in providing subjective overall improvement, androgens will continue to play a role in a minority of patients.

Tamoxifen

The antiestrogen tamoxifen is a compound with weak estrogenic activity that is able to antagonize the actions of estrogen on breast tissue, probably by competitive binding to the estrogen receptor protein. Although used mainly in postmenopausal patients, there are a few studies of the use of tamoxifen in premenopausal women. Using doses of 40–120 mg per day, Manni achieved an objective response rate in 5/11 cases with a median duration of response of over 19 months [30]. It was not necessary to suppress the menses completely to achieve an antitumor effect. Elevated levels of gonadotropins and of estrogens were found during tamoxifen treatment. This suggested the need for later oophorectomy or higher doses of tamoxifen following relapse on the initial tamoxifen schedule. Forty-two premenopausal patients studied by Pritchard were treated with 20 mg b.i.d. of tamoxifen with 32% responses and a median duration of response of at least 10 months [31]. Response was 5/11 for estrogen receptor–positive patients and 0/8 for estrogen receptor–negative patients. Among eight responders who relapsed, there were five secondary responses to oophorectomy, whereas none were seen in 13 patients who did not respond to tamoxifen. The Southwest Oncology Group (SWOG) obtained a similar response rate of 37% in 38 premenopausal women with a dose of 10 mg b.i.d., but obtained no secondary responses to oophorectomy [32]. This difference from the secondary responses reported by Pritchard is unexplained. The lower doses of tamoxifen used in the SWOG study may account for the 5/22 response rate to oophorectomy among women who had no response to tamoxifen in this study. Evidence is accumulating that premenopausal women may have response rates to tamoxifen approaching those of postmenopausal women. Uncertainty remains as to the clinical importance and management of the secondary rise in estrogens.

In postmenopausal women, tamoxifen has increasingly been used in place of DES as the first hormonal treatment. At a dose of tamoxifen 10 mg b.i.d. 33% responses were seen compared to 41% with DES at 5 mg t.i.d. [27]. The responses lasted about 5 months in each group. While tamoxifen was substantially more expensive, the authors concluded that it was the preferable agent because of a much lower incidence of toxicity. Beex has reported tamoxifen to be preferable to ethinyl estradiol because of equal efficacy and less toxicity [33]. Although no clear dose-response curve for tamoxifen was described in a review of clinical trials in Europe and the United States [34], there is a report of response in a few patients at 20 mg b.i.d. who did not respond to 10 mg b.i.d. [35]. Since blood levels do not reach steady-state until 16 weeks of chronic dosing, there are theoretical reasons to believe that a loading dose could be of value [36]. The prolonged serum half-life suggests that at least a month should elapse following tamoxifen treatment before performing an estrogen receptor measurement on a biopsy.

Aminoglutethimide

The opportunity to suppress adrenal function without the need for surgery followed recognition that aminoglutethimide, an anticonvulsant, inhibited steroidogenesis as well as blocking peripheral aromatization of androstenedione to estrone. One hundred twenty-nine women were studied with responses occurring in 37% of unselected cases and 49% of estrogen receptor-positive women [36a]. In a group with more liver and other visceral metastatic disease, a lower response rate of 16% was observed [37]. A randomized trial showed that medical and surgical adrenalectomy could achieve similar results (53% and 45%, respectively) [38]. The same group found aminoglutethimide to be equivalent to tamoxifen [39]. The recommended starting dose of 250 mg PO b.i.d for 2 weeks and then 250 mg q.i.d. The corticosteroid replacement should be hydrocortisone 40 mg daily, since the authors found that dexamethasone is rapidly metabolized in the presence of aminoglutethimide and the resulting increased levels of ACTH can overcome the adrenal block. Toxicity consists of lethargy which lasts 4–6 weeks with a maculopapular skin rash occurring 30% of the time, often during the second week and lasting 5 days. Neither of these should require cessation of therapy. Nagel has used 1,500 mg a day of medroxyprogesterone acetate as a further antitumor agent in place of hydrocortisone in 45 women receiving aminoglutethimide, with successful prevention of hypoadrenalism [40].

Progestins

Progestational agents have been tested over a wide dose range. During a 10-year period, Alexieva-Figusch treated 227 postmenopausal women of whom 160 were evaluable. At doses of megestrol acetate 60–180 mg per day, there was a 30% objective remission rate, including prior hormone responders [41]. In new cases, 24% responded. One month of daily treatment with a very high dose of 1,500 mg of medroxyprogesterone acetate (MPA) given intramuscularly led to a 43% response rate in 44 patients [42]. Toxicity was high with one-third of women experiencing gluteal abscesses and one-fourth developing moon facies. The local complications have been eliminated by giving MPA as an oral dose of 400 mg t.i.d. with similar efficacy [43]. A dose of 1,500 mg PO daily was noted to suppress endogenous cortisol production almost completely in 23 of 23 patients [43a]. When 51 women with advanced breast cancer were treated with 1,500 mg PO MPA daily or 500 mg IM 5 days a week, there were five complete and seven partial remissions. After a remission of breast cancer from MPA treatment, if a patient developed hyperprolactinemia (> 1,000 IU/liter), it was always accompanied by clinical relapse. The observation that the progesterone receptor is produced in response to estrogens has led to the sequencing of ethinyl estradiol and MPA with a 31% response rate in 19 refractory heavily pretreated patients [43b].

GnRH Analogues

Several compounds have been used to decrease gonadotropin release and thereby ultimately inhibit estrogen production. These GnRH and LHRH analogues have a spectrum of agonistic/antagonistic properties at the pituitary level. They may also exert effects at extrapituitary loci [44]. Leuprolide, a synthetic gonadotropin-releasing hormone analogue has been reported to have produced 12 brief remissions without toxicity when tested in 31 postmenopausal women with advanced breast cancer [44a]. Buserelin, a luteinizing-hormone–releasing hormone analogue, given in doses sufficient to suppress LH release, caused remissions in two of four premenopausal women [44] without significant adverse effects. Danazol, an attenuated androgen which is an inhibitor of LH and FSH release, was without benefit in 15 women, however [45]. Nagel has correlated a high prolactin level with aggressive disease and with poor response to chemotherapy using cyclophosphamide-methotrexate-5FU or vincristine-doxorubicin-cyclophosphamide (27.5% response with high prolactin [> 1,000 IU/liter] but 63% for the group as a whole) [46]. In women with elevated prolactin levels the addition of bromocryptine to a failed chemotherapy regimen which was continued resulted in 12/22 responses. Prolactin levels in all 22 women returned to low levels.

SINGLE-AGENT CHEMOTHERAPY

While the presence of estrogen and progesterone receptors has enabled physicians to predict reliably the response of patients to endocrine treatment, similar prognostication is more elusive with chemotherapy. Despite lack of universal agreement [49], it is generally felt that soft tissue–dominant disease responds more often to chemotherapy than bone- or visceral-dominant tumor [47,48]. In a study of 619 women by Swenerton, the factors predicting a response to chemotherapy were minimal prior to radiotherapy, good performance status, absent weight loss, normal hematologic and liver function, and less overall extent of disease [49]. Of note was the absence of predictive value of age, menopausal status or particular site of dominant disease. A longer disease-free interval, perhaps reflecting a tumor with a slower natural history, predicted a longer survival, but not a different response rate [49]. Bone disease was also associated with a longer survival. A multivariate analysis of the data of doxorubicin-cyclophosphamide combinations was performed by Nash [50]. Absence of liver involvement and age between 40 and 49 were most favorable for response. Duration of response was greatest for those over 50 without lung involvement. Finally, survival correlated best with age over 50 and two or fewer sites of disease. It may be that the differences in these studies using doxorubicin plus cyclophosphamide indicate that many of the factors previously felt important as predictors are not really so. Tormey has speculated that each drug or regimen may be influenced by different predictive pretreatment variables [51].

The response to prior hormonal therapy does not seem predictive of response to chemotherapy [52–54]. However, in two of the studies, there was a much longer duration of response and survival time in the previously hormone-responsive patients [52,53]. This may also reflect a more differentiated tumor with a slower natural growth rate.

The utility of the estrogen receptor level as a predictive tool for chemotherapy was suggested by Lippman, who noted a 12% response rate in receptor-positive women and a 76% response rate in receptor-negative patients [55]. Contradictory data have been preponderant, however, with a few studies obtaining opposite results [9,56–58] and most finding no important differences [8,59,60]. When taken together, the influence of receptor proteins on response to chemotherapeutic drug regimens now in use appears to be negligible.

For those tumors now considered curable with chemotherapy, the initial inroads were made by the development and application of single-drug treatments able to effect demonstrable killing of tumor cells. Cytotoxic agents with a wide variety of mechanisms of action have been shown reproducibly to reduce measurable breast cancer, usually in about 10–30% of cases. Along with the hormonal treatments described, these cytotoxic drugs comprise the foundation upon which more elaborate and successful programs for breast cancer regimens are built.

Response Criteria

By accepted custom in the past 25 years, a reduction of 50% in the sums of the products of the perpendicular diameters of all measurable lesions in the absence of new or significantly advancing old lesions is required for an objective partial response. Even when this is specified, it does not relate directly to killing effect on clonogenic tumor cells nor to tissues where healing is required to determine therapeutic effect [61]. Caution is required concerning the definitions of response to chemotherapy in individual sites, such as bone. Similarly, lymphangitic lung disease is hard to quantify. Subtle differences in the rigidity of criteria in these areas may substantially influence reported results. Because of differences in patient characteristics, it is wise to compare results from different observers, from different institutions, and results from different times in a general way only. Small changes in stipulated dosage, schedule, or in dose modification for toxicity may account, in large part, for the wide range of results reported for each drug or combination.

Alkylating Agents

Cyclophosphamide is the most commonly used alkylating agent in the treatment of advanced breast cancer. It can be administered orally or parenterally and has been tested in many dose schedules with a response rate of 20–35% [62]. The use of moderate oral doses (60–120 mg/m^2/day) seems to be as effective as larger intermittent parenteral doses [62–64]. Although this may be true for clinical control, it does not kill as many cells as larger single doses; the strategy for eventual curative treatment may be different [65]. Among the alkylating agents, cyclophosphamide has the unique toxicity of hemorrhagic cystitis, which is time- and dose-related, in a small percentage of cases.

The efficacy of the other alkylating agents has been much less extensively studied. Chlorambucil is reported to have 19% activity in 52 patients treated at 0.2 mg/kg/day for 42 days, with two complete responses [66]. Thiotepa is available only for parenteral use. Zubrod found activity in only 4/39 patients at 0.2 mg/kg/week, after a loading course [67], but a response rate of 42% was seen by Hurley at 0.4 mg/kg/week [68]. Melphalan was found to have 30% activity when used by Sears at a dose of 0.2–0.3 mg/kg given for 4–6 days every 3–6 weeks [69]. The Eastern Cooperative Oncology Group gave melphalan at 6 mg/m^2 PO daily for 5 days every 6 weeks with a 20% response rate in 91 treated patients [70]. These alkylating agents may be substituted for cyclophosphamide in the event of cystitis with that drug. They also are used in some combination programs. Evidence that alkylating agents enter experimental tumors by different transport mechanisms supports the possible differences among these drugs in individual cases.

Antimetabolites

Extensive work has been published on the use of the antimetabolite 5-fluorouracil (5-FU). Early work with 5-FU involved daily administration of 15 mg/kg (600 mg/m^2) $\times$ 5 days followed by 7.5 mg/kg (300 mg/m^2) every third day until slight toxicity appeared or until 11 half-doses were given. Treatment given after the appearance of mild toxicity, such as stomatitis, often produced prolonged life-threatening toxicity [71]. Subsequent courses followed at monthly intervals. A less toxic schedule with 12 mg/kg/day (480 mg/m^2) with a maximum total dose at 800 mg $\times$ 5 days followed by 6 mg/kg/day (240 mg/m^2) on alternate days until slight toxicity or 11 half-doses gave equal results with less toxicity [72]. To reduce toxicity further, colon and breast cancer have been treated with 15 mg/kg/week without a loading dose [73]. Four schedules of 5-FU dosage were tested in a prospective randomized study by Ansfield. The rank order of response rates showed

33% for the loading schedule, 24% for a weekly dose of 15–20 mg/kg without loading, 20% for a fixed dose of 500 mg weekly after a loading course of 4 days of 500 mg/day, and 19% for an oral schedule [74]. Toxicity was comparable to effectiveness. In another randomized trial of 51 patients who received 15–20 mg/kg/week, significant differences were not seen in response or survival whether patients were treated orally or intravenously [75]. The overall response rate for 5-FU is 20–30%. When compared directly to cyclophosphamide, the response rate is about equal [47,76].

Methotrexate is the other widely used antimetabolite. When given daily for 5–10 days it has had its most consistently high response rate—about 40% [62]. This type of schedule has not been used extensively in combinations. Several attempts have been made to increase the effectiveness of methotrexate. High-dose methotrexate (2.5–7.5 gm/m^2) followed by folinic acid rescue has been studied in 27 women refractory to doxorubicin-containing regimens [77]. There was a 29% response rate, one-third of whom had had prior methotrexate exposure. Toxicity, particularly renal impairment and stomatitis, was not formidable. Significantly, hematologic toxicity was mild, an advantage that may be exploited in combination therapy. The major drawbacks are the cost of the large quantity of the drug and the usual inpatient status. Modulation of moderate-dose methotrexate toxicity by the protein synthesis inhibitor L-asparaginase has also been studied [78,79]. Giving 120–300 mg/m^2 of methotrexate, Yap [79] found a 28% response rate in patients who had received prior methotrexate and a 31% response rate with no prior methotrexate. The median duration of response was 8 months.

Vinca Alkaloids

The *Vinca* alkaloids are a group of plant derivatives with efficacy against breast cancer. The activity of vincristine is on the order of 20% and appears to be dose-dependent [80,81] with little benefit below 0.0125 mg/kg or 1 mg total dose. The limiting toxicity is neurologic, with paresthesias, ileus, deep bone pain, and motor disturbances all possible. Areflexia is nearly universal but appears to have no adverse clinical effect. Seizures and other central nervous system phenomena, as distinct from peripheral nervous system effects, occur only at excessively high doses. Vinblastine has similar effectiveness, but less neurotoxicity [62]. The major disadvantage of vinblastine in combination is its myelosuppression, which accentuates the marrow effects of other cytotoxic compounds. Five-day infusions of vinblastine have been reported by Yap to increase the efficacy of vinblastine to 40% and to produce some responses in patients refractory to conventional dose schedules [82,83]. This was not confirmed in a trial by Tannock in which none of the 17 patients responded [84]. Infusion with vincristine at a dose of 0.25 mg/m^2/day for 5 days every 3 weeks resulted in no responses in 18 patients [85]. Vindesine is a recently synthesized *Vinca* derivative with activity in experimental systems similar to vincristine but with much less neurotoxicity. In phase II trials, the response rate in patients refractory to conventional chemotherapy has been 25–30% with a suggestion of partial lack of cross resistance with other *Vinca* alkaloids [86–89].

Anthracyclines

The most effective single agent available today is doxorubicin (Adriamycin). Single-agent data are available from several trials with clear and accepted criteria of response. The use of concurrent controls and in some studies of previously untreated women allows a more precise analysis of the activity of this drug. Adriamycin can be expected to produce 35–50% responses in previously untreated cases and 20–35% where prior chemotherapy has been given [90]. Table I lists several of these studies and the doses used. The standard dose is 60–75 mg/m^2 every 3 weeks. In previously treated patients Creech achieved a 27% response rate with 20 mg/m^2 on days 1 and 8 each month [96]. This same dose and schedule of adriamycin was inferior to 60 mg/m^2 given every 21 days in previously untreated patients [97]. The SWOG was unable to demonstrate a dose-response relationship in good-risk patients when the doses ranged from 45 to 75 mg/m^2 every 3 weeks [155]. In contrast, Jones et al. [100] have reported preliminary results of a study of adriamycin, administered over 3 successive days every 4 weeks, in which the total dose was escalated in increments of 15 mg/m^2 per course,

TABLE I. Doxorubicin in Metastatic Breast Cancer

Author	Prior chemotherapy	Dose (mg/m^2, every n weeks)		No. patients	Response frequency (%)	Median response duration (weeks)
Hoogstraten [91]	No	60	3	79	39	16
Nemoto [95]	No	75	3	32	38	30
Ahmann [99]	No	60	3–4	20	50	32
Creech [96]	Yes	20	[a]	60	27	28
Knight [93]	Yes	70	3–5	36	44	20
Legha [98]	Yes	60	3[b]	27	48	28
Ingle [94]	Yes	60	4	19	21	35
Gottlieb [92]	Yes	60–75	3	40	38	28

[a]dl, eight every 28 days.
[b]48–96 h infusion.

from 75 to 135 mg/m^2 unless a white blood cell nadir under $1{,}000/mm^3$ was reached. Of 20 women reported, 85% responded, of whom 30% reached complete response. The duration of remission has not yet been determined. The limiting toxicity in this study is subclinical decline of cardiac ejection fraction measured by gated pool isotopic scanning. Intravenous infusions of adriamycin have been given in order to reduce the cardiotoxicity; results at 60 mg/m^2 over 96 h showed a 48% response rate in 27 patients [98].

Other Agents

The anthracenes, a new class of synthetic compounds structurally similar to the anthracyclines without an amino sugar moiety, have broad antitumor activity. Dihydroxyanthacenedione (Mitoxantrone, DHAD) was studied in 29 patients with breast cancer, most of whom had received prior chemotherapy [101]. Responses occurred in 28% including two patients unresponsive or refractory to doxorubicin. Toxicity after Mitoxantrone appeared less than after the anthracycline doxorubicin, including absent alopecia. In 92 heavily pretreated patients (median of seven drugs), the Southwest Oncology Group found minimal evidence of activity: only three partial responses [102]. In patients without prior chemotherapy, DHAD produced 19/59 responses (32%) with only a single case of questionable cardiotoxicity [103]. Bisantrene, another anthracene compound, showed a 40% response rate in a small group of ten previously treated evaluable patients [104]. In a larger group of previously treated patients 9/40 women had partial responses, without cardiotoxicity [105]. In this study 2/23 patients refractory to adriamycin responded.

Several compounds are listed in Table II that have been tested in clinical trials. Because of the large number of drugs known to provide effective palliation, sometimes for several years, it will be increasingly difficult ethically to test new drugs in women who have not received prior chemotherapy. Phase II trials will, therefore, usually be performed first in women with prior exposure to chemotherapy. The possibility is real that some active and possibly less toxic drugs will be mistakenly considered inactive in this setting. For example, hexamethylmelamine was used as primary chemotherapy by the Central Drug Evaluation Group in the 1960s. A 30% response rate was found at a dose of 8 mg/kg/day for 90 days [114]. When later used in previously treated women, admittedly on a different schedule, there was virtually no activity [115–117]. Despite these limitations, testing of new chemotherapeutic agents and other treatments must remain a high priority in women who can no longer benefit from conventional treatment.

TABLE II. Single Chemotherapeutic Agents in Metastatic Breast Cancer

Drug	Prior chemotherapy	Dose IV mg/m^2	Freq. (q n weeks)	No. patients	Response frequency (%)
Mitomycin C [106]	Yes	[a]	—	42	36
Mitomycin C [107]	Yes	10	4	46	18
Ansacrine[b] [108]	Yes	120	3	40	2.5
Ansacrine[b] [109]	Yes	30 daily × 3	3	26	16
Etoposide[c] [110]	Yes	100–125 every other day × 3	4	19	0
Etoposide[c] [111]	Yes	45–75 daily × 5	3	119	7
Methyl-G[d] [112]	Yes	500	1	29	7
Cisplatin [113]	Yes	100	3,4	14	0
		20 daily continuous infusion × 5	4	12	0
Cisplatin [118]	Yes	60	3	18	0
		120	3	19	20
CCNU[e]		100–130 PO	6	29	14
Hexamethylmelamine [114]	Minimal (No alkylating agents)[f]		—	31	32
Hexamethylmelamine [115]	Yes	320 daily × 21	6	15	0
Hexamethylmelamine [116]	Yes	300 daily × 14	3	15	0
Hexamethylmelamine [117]	Yes	240–320 daily × 21	6	89	2

[a] 0.05 mg/kg daily × 6, then every other day until toxicity or 50 mg (not repeated).
[b] AMSA.
[c] VP-16.
[d] Methylglyoxal bis-guanylhydrazone.
[e] Lomustine.
[f] 8 mg/kg daily × 90.

COMBINATION THERAPY

The strategy of combining multiple active drugs in order to achieve a greater effect has been successful in curing some neoplasms once considered uniformly fatal. Similar attempts have been made to treat metastatic breast cancer more effectively, but the results have been subcurative thus far.

Theoretic considerations involving combination chemotherapy include biochemical, cytokinetic, and pharmacologic advantages to the simultaneous or sequential use of multiple drugs [119]. The most important advantage of combination treatment is the delay in development of drug resistance when agents with different mechanisms of action are employed. If one in a million tumor cells is resistant to a drug, then the chance of any specific cell being resistant is 10^{-6}, and the chance of its being resistant simultaneously to two agents is 10^{-12}. In vitro and in vivo work support these propositions [119].

The combinations have included, to the extent possible, active single agents with different mechanisms of action and nonadditive host activity. Generally, in the most widely used combinations, there has been little selection of drugs based upon well-understood biochemical mechanisms of action.

The work at Mount Sinai by Greenspan is recognized as inaugurating the era of combination chemotherapy in breast cancer. Using the alkylating agent Thio-TEPA and the antimetabolite methotrexate, with testosterone and prednisone, he reported responses in 60% of 40 women [120]. With refractory disease, treatment with 5FU and cyclophosphamide was successfully used in 59/73 cases (81%).

Cooper introduced a five-drug regimen based on the combined effect of individually active drugs. His scheme sought to provide cumulative tumor toxicity with toxic side effects that were not so additive for the marrow, gut, or other organs such as to diminish tolerated drug doses below effective levels. The drugs chosen, each with 20–30% activity, were cyclophosphamide, methotrexate, 5-fluorouracil, vincristine, and prednisone (CMFVP) [122]. Cooper's initial data were exceptionally interesting, since he reported a 90% response rate, a result that has not been equaled. All the patients were treated by a single capable oncologist, however, and Cooper's exact design has never been duplicated (Table III).

An attempt was made to reproduce Cooper's protocol in a study of 110 women, mainly postmenopausal [52]. Initially, the doses were used just as Cooper described, but they were reduced in subsequent patients because of hematologic toxicity early in the study. The overall response rate of 64% was not further analyzed in terms of those receiving the initial dose versus the later reduced doses. Davis tested a similar five-drug program given on a weekly basis and his results were also credible with 69% responses in untreated patients and 52% in those who had received prior single-agent chemotherapy [123].

The optimal scheduling of this type of program has been studied. The Southeastern Cancer Study Group compared CMFVP given on a weekly schedule with the same drugs given intermittently [124]. The weekly regimen had more responses (46% vs. 27%), but the response duration and overall survival were similar. Because of less toxicity in the intermittent arm of the trial, this treatment was selected as the control arm in further studies

TABLE III. Cooper Type Regimens

Regimen	Dose	Cycle repeated every n weeks	No. patients	Response frequency (%)	Response duration (weeks)
CMFVP [122]					
C	2 mg/kg PO daily				
M	0.7 mg/kg IV weekly × 8, then q 2 weeks		60	90	—
F	12 mg/kg IV weekly × 8, then q 2 weeks				
V	0.035 mg/kg IV weekly × 5, on week 8, then q 4 weeks				
P	0.75 mg/kg PO daily tapered to 0 in 8 weeks				
CMFVP vs. FVP [121]					
C	2 mg/kg PO daily				
M	0.75 mg/kg IV weekly × 8[a]				
F	12 mg/kg IV weekly × 8[a]		123	51	26
V	0.035 mg/kg IV weekly × 8[a]				
P	0.75 mg/kg PO daily × 3 weeks, then tapered to 0 over 1 week				
Versus					
F	12 mg/kg IV weekly × 8[a]				
V	0.035 mg/kg IV weekly × 8[a]		129	37	14
P	0.75 mg/kg PO daily × 3 weeks, then tapered to 0 over 1 week				
CFP ± V [126]					
C	4 mg/kg IV dl-5				
F	8 mg/kg IV dl-5				
V	1.4 mg/kg IV, dl,5	4	41	46	39
P	30 mg PO daily, tapered to 10 mg PO daily				
Versus					
C	4 mg/kg IV dl-5				
F	8 mg/kg IV dl-5	4	49	59	35
P	30 mg PO daily, tapered to 10 mg PO daily				
CMFVP [123]					
C	2 mg/kg (100 mg max) PO daily				
M	0.5 mg/kg (25 mg max) IV weekly		74	42	19
F	10 mg/kg (500 mg max) IV weekly		(16)[b]	(69)[b]	(21)[b]
V	1 mg IV weekly				
P	45 mg PO daily tapered to 15 mg				

(continued)

TABLE III. Cooper Type Regimens *(Continued)*

Regimen	Dose	Cycle repeated every n weeks	No. patients	Response frequency (%)	Response duration (weeks)
CMFP [128]					
C	100 mg/m^2 PO dl-14				
M	60 mg/m^2 IV dl,8	4	40	68	32
F	700 mg/m^2 IV dl,8				
P	40 mg/m^2 PO dl-14				
CMFVP [125]					
C	80 mg/m^2 PO dl-42				
M	40 mg/m^2 IV weekly × 6				
F	500 mg/m^2 IV weekly × 6	12	21	66	46
V	1.4 mg/m^2 (2 mg max) IV weekly × 6				
P	40 mg/m^2 PO daily and tapered over 6 weeks to 0				
CMFVP [52]					
C	100 mg PO daily				
M	25 mg IV weeks 1–12, then q 3 weeks				
F	500 mg IV weeks 1–12, then q 3 weeks		97	64	36
V	1 mg IV weeks 1–6, then q 6 weeks				
P	0.75 mg/kg PO daily, then tapered over 1 month to 0				

Abbreviations: C—cyclophosphamide; M—methotrexate; F—5-fluorouracil; V—vincristine; P—prednisone.

[a]Followed by maintenance therapy at greater intervals.

[b]With no prior chemotherapy.

by that group. It might alternatively have been concluded that the weekly treatment, by exhibiting a greater response rate, was capable of achieving a higher percentage of tumor cell kill. High cell kill is the necessary prerequisite for complete response and eventual curative strategies. Clues must be taken from the regimens found to be most active, even if at this stage of development survival benefit is not achieved. The hypothesis of increased cell kill by more intensive regimens is the basis for the report by Perloff et al. of the increased response duration of CMFVP given as 6-week courses with rest periods of 6 weeks compared to prior work with 2-week courses of therapy [125]. The response rate to the 6-week regimen of 59% was associated with a response duration of nearly double the 28 weeks found with the 2-week program.

Of the drugs in the CMFVP programs, vincristine has been the most challenged in terms of toxicity-benefit ratio. Ahmann compared CFP with CFPV and found no significant differences in the response rates [126]. The response rate without vincristine was 59% and with vincristine 46%. The utility of prednisone was demonstrated by Tormey in comparing CMF to CMFP. [127]. The group receiving all four drugs had 63% responses compared to 57% without prednisone. Duration of response was almost twice as long in the CMFP arm, however (8.4 months). In an uncontrolled study at the National Cancer Institute, Canellos reported a 68% response rate in 40 consecutive patients treated with CMFP [128].

A low-dose variant of CMF, using about 50% of the conventional drug doses, was tested in an uncontrolled trial by Creech involving 46 patients [129]. A response rate of 46%, low compared to CMFVP or CMFP, with a duration of response of about 9 months was reported.

There have been many variations of the type CMFVP program tested. The highest responses have been seen in those regimens giving the drugs at higher doses and greater dose delivery rates. This has not yet resulted in a satisfactory improvement in survival. It is reasonable to expect that 50–70% of patients will respond to a CMFVP-type treatment if they have not received prior chemotherapy. The duration of response is generally under 1 year.

Doxorubicin-Containing Regimens

The initial enthusiasm for the high response rates to doxorubicin as a single agent was largely due to the expectation that the drug would have major impact when used with other active agents. Response rates and response durations appear slightly higher in doxorubicin-containing regimens than in other programs but not to the extent initially hoped.

The combinations of doxorubicin and cyclophosphamide are usually given intravenously on an intermittent schedule, every 3–4 weeks. Jones treated 55 consecutive women and reported an 80% response rate with a median duration of response of 10 months [130]. When the Southwest Oncology Group used the same dose and schedule in a controlled trial, however, they achieved only a 44% response rate [131] with a median duration of response of 29 weeks. Differences in response criteria may account for the differences in response rate, since the SWOG had stricter criteria for response in bone disease. When the dose of doxorubicin was decreased by 50% [132] or the cyclophosphamide reduced [133], response rates were even lower.

When compared in a randomized trial of previously untreated patients, the combination of vincristine and doxorubicin (AV) was as effective as

CMF given on a day 1, day 8 schedule [134]. The response rate was 53% and the duration of response 8 months. There was a doubling of the rate of complete responses to 16% when partially responding or stable patients were switched to CMF after eight cycles of AV. More liberal criteria of response were used in a study of AV plus prednisolone, where there were 67% responders among 48 women, some of whom had had prior chemotherapy [135].

Doxorubicin, vincristine, and cyclophosphamide have been combined in several VAC regimens, with a wide range of response rates reported. In the pilot study, Rainey demonstrated a 72% response rate with a notable 22-month median duration of response [136]. When used with a slightly higher dose of vincristine and a single day of intravenous cyclophosphamide, VAC was no better than CMFP [137]. More significant than the 56% response rate was the decrease in duration of response to 12 months.

There is a similar variability in results reported with combinations including doxorubicin and 5FU. In an uncontrolled trial by the M.D. Anderson group, there was a 73% reponse rate in 44 women treated [138]. The combinations of AF, CAF, and CAFM were almost equivalent in response rates for the four-drug treatment which was 35 weeks [138a]. The median survival of 64 weeks for all patients in the study was similar in the three treatment arms. A high response rate of 82% was obtained by Bull using CAF in a 2-weeks-on, 2-weeks-off format [48]. The low response rate of 25% reported by Nemoto [133] might be accounted for by random variation with a small number of patients or by the considerable dosage reductions employed compared to the original report.

Randomized controlled comparisons have been made between regimens with and without doxorubicin (Table IV). At the National Cancer Institute, Bull compared the utility of doxorubicin versus methotrexate in combination giving CAF or CMF on day 1, day 8 schedules [48]. With the sample sizes employed, the response rate of 82% to CAF was not significantly better than the 62% rate with CMF. The duration of response was about 9 months in each arm. When stable disease was considered too, the CAF combination provided a longer time of disease control and offered a longer survival (median 27.2 months vs. 17 months), although this also failed to reach statistical significance.

In a study with a high rate of unevaluable patients, the Southeastern Cancer Study Group found CAF to be superior to their intermittent low-dose CMFVP [139]. Although the low response rate for intermittent low-dose CMFVP contrasts with most other reports, it had a survival curve equal to weekly CMFVP in a prior study by that same group [124].

TABLE IV. Comparisons of Doxorubicin- and Non-Doxorubicin–Containing Regimens

Regimen/ Reference	Dose (mg/m^2 IV)			Frequency (q n weeks)	No. Patients	Response frequency (%)	Response duration (weeks)	Comments
C [48]	100	PO	d1-14	4	40	62	34	Difference in response rate not significant with this sample size.
M	40		d1,8					
F	600		dl,8					
Versus								
C	100	PO	d1-14	4	38	82	36	
A	30		d1,8					
F	500		d1,8					
C [140]	100	PO	d1-14	4	96	34	28	
M	40		d1,8					
F	500		d1,8					
Versus								Both doxorubicin-containing regimens produced significantly more responses than CMF
C	100	PO	d1-14	4	80	54	54	
A	25		d1,8					
F	500		d1,8					
Versus								
C	100	PO	d1-14	4	77	57	40	
A	25		d1,8					
F	500		d1,8					
V	1		d1,8					
P	40	PO	d1-14					

(continued)

TABLE IV. Comparisons of Doxorubicin- and Non-Doxorubicin–Containing Regimens *(Continued)*

Regimen/ Reference	Dose (mg/m^2 IV)			Frequency (q n weeks)	No. Patients	Response frequency (%)	Response duration (weeks)	Comments
F [139]	500		d1	3	59	64	32	
A	50		d1					
C	500		d1					
Versus								Low doses used in the CMFVP regimen
C	400		d1	4	54	37	22	
M	30		d1,8					
F	400		d1,8					
V	1	(total)	d1,8					
P	20	mg PO qid	d1-7					
V [137]	1.4		d1,8	3	25	56	48	
A	40		d1					
C	500		d1					
Versus								
C	100	PO	d1-15, 30–45	[a]	26	65	48	
M	20		Weekly × 20					
F	500		Weekly × 20					
P	20	PO	Then tapered					

Abbreviations: A–adriamycin (doxorubicin) (and see Table III).
[a]Followed by maintenance treatment 3 weeks out of 6.

The Cancer and Acute Leukemia Group B has compared CMF with CAF and CAFVP and found that the doxorubicin-containing regimens had higher response rates (34% for CMF; 54% for CAF, 57% for CAFVP) as well as longer response durations [140].

The combination of vinblastine, doxorubicin, thiotepa, and fluoxymesterone (VATH) has been used in patients refractory to CMF, CAF, CMFVP, or CAFVP. The regimen was originally given over 5 days and repeated monthly. Among 19 patients there were ten responders (52%) with a median duration of response of 11.5 months [141]. A one-day VATH regimen was designed to make the program more logistically acceptable [142]. The overall response rate was 45% among 29 patients with a median duration of response of 11 months, thus preserving the effectiveness of the original program. As second-line treatment following other multidrug chemotherapy, these results are impressive.

The addition of doxorubicin to the other effective drugs does not appear to have resulted in the desired additional cell killing to provide truly long-term remission or cure to a substantial number of women with metastatic breast cancer. It has increased the options available to the practitioner, and its use probably results in a greater proportion of women surviving over 2 years from the onset of treatment. There are no persuasive data that demonstrate whether it is preferable to use doxorubicin first, second, or interspersed between other courses using the criteria of total survival or total months of disease control. Indeed, even the optimal dose of doxorubicin is not established.

Direct comparison of single-agent and multiagent chemotherapy has been performed in only a few trials. Interpretation of these studies is dependent on the end point of interest. Rubens compared CMF plus vinblastine with oral cyclophosphamide given daily [143]. Although the criteria for response are not precisely specified and appear more liberal than commonly used, 55% responses were seen in the cyclophosphamide group and 62% in the combination chemotherapy group. By using the four-drug regimen to treat women who had relapsed from cyclophosphamide, the authors were able to achieve survival results identical to those found when the four drugs were used as initial therapy. However, the median survival of 6 months for all patients is low and suggests that these drug regimens were suboptimal. The Eastern Cooperative Oncology Group achieved a 53% response rate with CMF compared to 20% with L-phenylalanine mustard [144]. This was associated with a higher one-year survival in the group treated with combination chemotherapy.

The most active single agent, doxorubicin, has been compared with combinations in two studies. Ahmann found response rates of 50% for doxorubicin and 46% for CFP (with or without vincristine), but the duration of response was significantly shorter in the doxorubicin alone arm (31 weeks vs. 39 weeks) [99]. Survival was also shorter, although not significantly, with single-agent treatment first. The Southwest Oncology Group compared CMFVP to doxorubicin [91] and found a 59% response rate for the combination given weekly, 40% for the intermittent combination treatment, and 39% for doxorubicin alone. The doxorubicin arm had the shortest duration of response—4 months.

The use of sequential drugs, each used until disease progression occurs, was studied by the Southeastern Cancer Study Group [124]. Patients receiving the combination CMFVP at relatively low doses had twice the response rate (36% vs. 18%) and survival time as those receiving the drugs sequentially. By 2 years, however, almost all of the patients treated either way had died. Baker found no survival differences between patients treated with sequential or combination 5FU, cyclophosphamide, and vincristine, but the combination was less toxic [145]. The Western Oncology Group found that although response rates were higher overall with combination chemotherapy, only the subsets of patients with liver, lung, or central nervous system involvement benefited in terms of survival from the use of the combination [146].

In attempts to overcome the apparent plateau of response rate and the low number of long-term survivors, several new strategies have been employed. It has been theorized that, just as combination chemotherapy delayed the emergence of resistant cell lines, the use of alternating non-cross-resistant combinations might prolong response duration. It was hoped also that because of activity against different subsets of the cell population, the use of alternating therapies would result in higher response rates. Abeloff treated 34 women with four courses of doxorubicin-cyclophosphamide (AC) followed by the alternation of three courses of methotrexate-5FU with single courses of AC [147]. The result was a 56% response rate with responses lasting a median of only 8 months. The Eastern Cooperative Oncology Group randomly allocated patients to receive CMF, CMFP, or CMF alternating with AV [148]. The respective response rates were 55%, 70%, and 58% (not significantly different). The median response duration of 12.4 months in the group receiving alternating therapy was, however, greater than the 6 to 7 months seen in the other groups, although they were, perthaps by chance, unusually short. The combination of CAF was alternated with a putatively cycle-active regimen of vincristine, methotrexate, folinic acid, and cytosine arabinoside [149]. The initial response to the CAF was 84%, but the median duration of remission was only 50 weeks.

At M.D. Anderson, three cycles of vincristine, adriamycin, cyclophosphamide-BCG were followed by three courses of 5FU-methotrexate and another three courses of VAC-BCG [150]. Maintenance was then given with CMF-BCG. The 67% response rate lasting 14 months was not superior to the 76% rate seen in an historical control group who received FAC-BCG alone.

The use of moderate or high doses of methotrexate with folinic acid rescue results in little marrow toxicity and has been used in combination to allow higher doses of other cytotoxic drugs than could be given with conventional methotrexate doses. An intensive regimen using cyclophosphamide, 5FU, and high-dose methotrexate alternating with doxorubicin was particularly effective in prolonging response duration in a pilot study [151]. Use of this "super-CMF"–doxorubicin sequence allowed 27% complete responses, 51% partial responses, and a median response duration of 24.5 months. Toxicity was similar to conventional CMF therapy.

A firmer understanding of the biochemical consequences of the use of cytotoxic drugs should allow a more rational application of combination chemotherapy. Work done with the proper sequencing of methotrexate and 5FU demonstrates potential clinical advantages that may follow such investigation. The observation has been made that methotrexate increased the levels of phosphoribosylpyrophosphate (PRPP) in L1210 leukemia cells, possibly by a decrease in de novo purine biosynthesis [152]. If 5FU was given after this effect had occurred, a greater toxic effect on the tumor cell line was seen which was associated with an increased concentration of intracellular 5FU ribonucleotides and enhanced incorporation of 5FU into RNA. Using a dose of methotrexate of 200 mg/m^2 followed in 1 h by 5FU 600 mg/m^2 Gewirtz et al. demonstrated responses in 9/17 evaluable women, many of whom had received prior chemotherapy including 5FU or methotrexate [153]. Similar results were reported independently in a group of women refractory to CMF and doxorubicin [154], but Perrault found only 8% response in 25 women, most refractory to CMF [156]. The optimal dose and sequencing are still to be worked out; this line of research demonstrates the potential for more active combinations as our understanding of mechanisms of drug action improves.

COMBINATION OF HORMONAL THERAPY AND CHEMOTHERAPY

Since both hormonal and chemotherapeutic approaches to the treatment of metastatic breast cancer are effective in overlapping patient subgroups, strategies for their optimal use, sequentially and in combinations, are under investigation. In a controlled trial of low-dose AC (doxorubicin and cyclophosphamide) with or without calusterone, the response rate was 65% when the hormone was added and 53% without it [132]. There was a 21.5-months median duration of response with combined treatment and only 11.5 months with chemotherapy alone. A similar survival advantage was seen for the hormone plus chemotherapy. A trial of CMFVP with one-half of the patients receiving other simultaneous endocrine treatment was reported by Brunner [157]. In premenopausal women, 74% of those treated with CMFVP plus oophorectomy responded, with a median survival time of 19.9 months compared to a 43% response for chemotherapy alone with a median survival of 13.2 months. The group of postmenopausal patients treated with combined hormonal and chemotherapy had more responses (63% vs. 54%) and lived longer (26.7 vs. 19.2 months median) than those treated without hormonal therapy. The addition of fluoxymesterone (Halotestin) to CMF, CMFP, or AV resulted in a slight prolongation of time to treatment failure from 6.7 to 9.5 months [29]. This may have been due to the marrow-stimulating effect of the androgen allowing a higher percentage of scheduled chemotherapy to be delivered, or due to a direct antitumor effect of the androgen. The overall survival of patients of CMFH was 23.3 months compared to 19.8 for CMF, a difference not statistically significant. The Cancer and Acute Leukemia Group B has not found the addition of tamoxifen to CAF to be beneficial in postmenopausal women [158] even with positive receptors. The North Central Cancer Treatment Group achieved a 66% response to CFP and only a 60% response to CPF-tamoxifen [159]. Cocconi, however, did find that the combination CMF-tamoxifen was more effective at achieving initial response than CMF alone (74% vs. 51%). The sequential use of CMF followed, at the time of progression, by CMF-T resulted in a slightly longer time to treatment failure and survival, neither reaching statistical significance.

Several investigators have addressed the question of whether there is any harm in delaying chemotherapy until the patient either fails to respond to or relapses from endocrine therapy. The CALGB studied oophorectomy plus CMFVP versus oophorectomy followed later by CMFVP after lack of response or disease progression was established in 92 premenopausal women [161]. While the patients receiving immediate combined treatment had more responses with a longer remission duration of 17 months, overall survival was the same at 36 months. CFP given at the time of oophorectomy in premenopausal women, although producing longer progression-free intervals (53 weeks with CFP + oophorectomy vs. 17 weeks with oophorectomy alone), was later found to evoke no survival difference [162,163]. Glick treated 89 estrogen receptor–positive or receptor–unknown patients with tamoxifen and then randomized one-half of those responding or with stable disease to receive low-dose CMF together with the tamoxifen [164]. The tamoxifen alone group had a median time to treatment failure of 12.5 months, compared to 17 months (N.S.) with low-dose CMFT, but survival in the two groups was no different.

It is likely that because patients in the past have been unselected for receptor status, benefit in the receptor–positive subgroup is obscured by inefficacy of hormonal therapy in the receptor–negative patients. Limitation of a trial to receptor–positive patients (> 3 fmol per mg of protein), 88% of whom were postmenopausal, resulted in equal effectiveness of tamoxifen (T) followed at relapse by CMF or initial therapy with CMFT [165]. In this randomized trial 15/24 women responded to tamoxifen alone compared to 17/26 with combined treatment. The median survivals of the two groups were similar at 17 months. Thus, unless immediate life-threatening disease is present, such as lymphangitic pulmonary or hepatic metastases, receptor-positive patients may benefit by a trial of hormonal therapy first. There may be a period of benefit without the toxicity of chemotherapy which can be employed later. Such an approach is appropriate for a patient unwilling to participate in a research program aimed at increasing the fundamental information which will be necessary for cure by initial therapy.

Treatment strategies have also been designed based on the concept that low doses of estrogen therapy may increase cell division rates and increase the effectiveness of subsequent chemotherapy. Allegra has used tamoxifen followed by estrogen challenge to synchronize cells, stimulating them to synthesize DNA, thus increasing the growth fraction and theoretically enhancing the response to subsequent sequential methotrexate-5FU [166]. Response rates to this innovative program are encouraging with 15 complete responses and seven partial responses among the first 32 evaluable patients, predominantly with skin and soft-tissue metastases, and without significant toxicity. Whether the results will obtain for patients with the ordinary frequency of visceral and skeletal metastases, or will be better than those obtained without estrogen stimulation, is not yet known.

Lippmann used a program of cyclophosphamide and doxorubicin on day 1 with methotrexate and 5FU given on day 8 in each 21-day cycle [167]. One-half of the 93 patients were randomly assigned to receive tamoxifen on days 2–6 and Premarin on day 7. Objective response rates were 62% for CAMF and 60% for CAMFTP. Time to progression (13 vs. 17 months) and survival (17 vs. 23 months) slightly favored the CAMFTP arm.

COMBINATIONS OF IMMUNOTHERAPY AND CHEMOTHERAPY

In attempts to enhance host immunity against metastatic breast cancer, investigators have combined putative immunostimulators with conventional chemotherapy. Scarification with Bacillus-Calmette-Guerin (BCG) was added to FAC and the results compared to a recent historical group [168]. Response rate was not improved, but duration of remission and survival were longer with the addition of immunotherapy in this noncomparative trial. The methanol extraction residue of BCG (BCG-MER) has been tested by two cooperative groups in randomized trials and been found devoid of benefit. The Piedmont Oncology Association studied 239 women, of whom 179 were evaluable, and found that the response rate to CAFVP was 56% and CAFVP (BCG-MER) 54% [169]. Median response duration was 16.2 months with chemotherapy alone and 14.0 months with immunotherapy. Similarly, immunotherapy provided no survival advantage. The Cancer and Leukemia Group B compared each of the three regimens CMF, CAF, and CAFVP with or without BCG-MER [140]. The response rates were CMF 34%, CMF-MER 44%; CAF 54%, CAF-MER 41%, and CAFVP 57%, CAFVP-MER 32%. There was neither increased duration of response nor survival advantage with MER. The efficacy of BCG and BCG-MER remain unproved.

Levamisole is an oral synthetic compound used as a nonspecific stimulant of cell-mediated immunity. The addition of levamisole to FAC was reported to be as effective as BCG in prolonging remissions and improving survival compared to historical controls, and it was less toxic [170]. In this nonrandomized study, the response rates for FAC-levamisole and FAC-BCG-levamisole were both 72%, identical to an historical FAC treatment group. The duration of response to the historical FAC was 9 months, FAC-levamisole 13 months, and FAC-levamisole-BCG 14 months. In sequential randomized trials in Helsinki, Klefstrom found levamisole to improve both response rate and survival when added to CMF-vinblastine, or vincristine-adriamycin-cyclophosphamide (VAC) given at low-dose schedules [171]. VAC-levamisole gave 63% responses with a greater than 120-weeks survival (projected) compared to 47% with a 90-weeks median survival for VAC alone. These are provocative results in appropriately controlled studies and should encourage other comparative trials.

ADJUVANT THERAPY

The use of chemotherapy to prevent the development of clinically overt recurrent disease following treatment of primary breast cancer represents a major advance in cancer management. The use of such adjuvant chemotherapy is grounded in the knowledge that systemic dissemination has already occurred before (or during) the operation. The inadequacy of local treatment of breast cancer is obvious. Even when the mastectomy leaves no evident tumor behind, 24% of the women with negative axillary nodes will relapse by 10 years [172]. For 1–3 positive nodes and greater than 3, the relapse rates by 10 years are 65% and 86% respectively. Surgical sampling of the axilla is mandatory since clinical exam is incorrect over one-fourth of the time [173], and alternative visualization techniques have not yet been devised. Positive nodal status has been the usual entry requirement into adjuvant studies, since this is associated with a 76% chance of relapse by 10 years [172]. It would be advantageous to predict which of the node-negative women is likely to be in the one-fourth who will relapse by 10 years. Among factors said to be predictive of relapse are elevated preoperative CEA [174], blood vessel invasion [175], primitive nuclear structure [176], lobular carcinoma [181], and the size of primary [173]. The presence of an estrogen receptor may indicate a less aggressive tumor and a longer time to relapse [177–179], but this is disputed [180]. Gallagher found no significance to intralymphatic invasion [181].

In 1964, the Scandinavian Adjuvant Chemotherapy Group began treating one-half the patients undergoing surgery for breast cancer with a single 6-day course of cylophosphamide [182]. All the patients received adjuvant radiotherapy to the chest following chemotherapy save one group, which had their chemotherapy delayed several weeks until after the radiotherapy was finished. The group receiving the chemotherapy immediately postoperatively had an advantage of an 11% lower relapse rate and a 13.2% lower death rate than controls, which has persisted for the 14 years reported. This benefit was seen in pre- and postmenopausal women as well as those with positive or negative nodes. Only the group whose chemotherapy was delayed by radiotherapy did not benefit from adjuvant treatment. This has been taken to support the concept that the systemic treatment should be given very shortly after treatment of the primary. Another alkylating agent, L-phenyalanine mustard (L-PAM), was tested by the National Surgical Adjuvant Breast Program in women with positive homolateral axillary lymph nodes [183]. In randomized comparisons involving 1,030 patients, women who received 2 years of L-PAM had a relapse rate of 45% compared to 50% of placebo-treated patients at 5 years, a statistically significant difference [183]. When subgroup analysis was done, the benefit occurred only in premenopausal women. A trial involving L-PAM plus 5FU and L-PAM, 5FU and methotrexate showed these regimens to be superior to L-

PAM alone in that they provided significant increases in disease-free survival for postmenopausal as well as premenopausal women [183].

In the most widely known of the adjuvant breast trials, the Milan group gave CMF for 1 year and compared this to no treatment. Although the initial publication claimed benefit in all subgroups [184], further follow-up revealed improvement in relapse-free and overall survival only in premenopausal women (Table V) [185]. The explanation proposed by Bonadonna is that the older women received less of the planned chemotherapy, often for inadequate reasons [186]. Those postmenopausal women who received over 85% of the optimal dosage outlined in the protocol had a significant benefit from the chemotherapy. In a subsequent study treatment with the CMF regimen for 6 months was as effective as 12 months when assessed at a median follow-up of 56 months [187]. The relapse-free survival in the 6-months group was 66% and in the 12-months group 60%. The Southeastern Cancer Study Group randomly treated 267 patients with 1–3 involved nodes, with either 6 or 12 months of CMF [187a]. With 24 months follow-up 16% and 20% of the patients have relapsed in the 6- and 12-months groups respectively.

Cooper reported long term follow-up of 100 women with four or more positive axillary nodes treated with his original CMFVP regimen [188]. Using several historical control groups, the results of his work indicate benefit in both pre- and postmenopausal groups. A deleterious effect of postoperative radiotherapy was striking [189]. Following this lead, the Cancer and Leukemia Group B compared modified CMFVP to modified CMF [190] in women with stage II breast cancer. Only those with over three positive nodes have been reported, a group at high risk for relapse. Overall, the CMFVP provided significantly better relapse-free survival with the advantage most marked when ten or more nodes were positive. Immunotherapy with MER-BCG was not beneficial [61]. The Southwest Oncology Group compared CMFVP to L-PAM and found the combination to be superior in all subgroups with a median follow-up of 5 years [190a,191].

The combination of doxorubicin and cyclophosphamide was used for 6 months in 159 women with positive axillary nodes [192]; it proved superior to historical controls. The addition of radiotherapy seemed to benefit the group with 1–3 positive nodes, but was deleterious with four or more positive nodes [192]. These drugs also appear effective in node-negative women with 94% relapse-free survival at a median follow-up of 44 months [193]. Because only 24% of these women will relapse by 10 years without therapy, a controlled trial is needed before these results are applied broadly. No decline in cardiac ejection fraction was noted in 39 women treated with

TABLE V. Randomized Adjuvant Chemotherapy Trials in Breast Cancer

	Scand[a] (14 years) [182]		NSABP (5 years) [183]		Milan (5 years) [185]		CALGB (4[b] years) [203]		SWOG (5 years) [191]		Milan (5 years) [187]	
	Placebo	Cyclo	Placebo	L-PAM	Control	CMF	CMF	CMFVP	L-PAM	CMFVP	CMF-12	CMF-6
DFS												
Overall	—	—	50	55	45	60	45	60	54	70	59	66
Premenopausal 1–3	51	57	52	75	43	66	—	—	51	68	72	80
Premenopausal ⩾4			30	40			52	65			38	46
Postmenopausal 1–3	40	52	—	—	50	56	—	—	56	71	72	66
Postmenopausal ⩾4			35	35			36	53			34	55
Survival												
Overall	—	—	60	60	66	78	—	—	58	73	73	77
Premenopausal 1–3	—	—	74	85	—	—	—	—	—	—	72	77
Premenopausal ⩾4	—	—	43	49	—	—	—	—	—	—		
Postmenopausal 1–3	—	—	—	—	—	—	—	—	—	—	74	76
Postmenopausal ⩾4	—	—	50	34	—	—	—	—	—	—		

[a]Includes node-negative patients.
[b]Only patients with four or more positive nodes.

300 mg/m^2 of doxorubicin as part of an adjuvant FAC regimen [194]. A brief report of 226 node-positive women treated with AVCF reports superiority of relapse-free survival to CMF ($P < 0.015$) in a randomized trial [195].

The addition of immunotherapy with BCG to FAC was studied in a randomized trial by the M.D. Anderson group in 238 patients [196]. With a median follow-up of 32 months, stage II and III patients respectively had 13% and 30% recurrences with FAC, and 22% and 35% with FAC-BCG. In their first reported controlled trial of BCG, therefore, immunotherapy provided no benefit.

Hormonal manipulation alone has been less impressive in the adjuvant setting. Prophylactic oophorectomy increased the disease-free interval following surgery for primary breast cancer only from 8 to 12 months and had no effect on survival [197]. Preliminary results from Denmark with a small number of patients in each subgroup show an advantage to DES or tamoxifen in terms of relapse-free survival when receptors for estrogen are high [198]. The addition of tamoxifen to L-PAM and 5FU by the NSABP added significantly to preventing relapses during the observation period in postmenopausal women only (15% vs. 29% at 2 years [199]. Higher receptor levels were associated with greater benefit from the addition of tamoxifen [199]. A beneficial effect with the addition of tamoxifen was also reported in a study involving 318 women comparing low-dose CMF plus tamoxifen to low-dose CMF [200]. Whether the tamoxifen effect will be recognizable if major chemotherapy is given is not yet known.

The long-term adverse results of adjuvant chemotherapy are not yet established. There appears to be no increased risk of second malignant neoplasms so far [185,201], although acute myelocytic leukemia would appear to be an expected outcome in a small percentage of patients treated with alkylating agents. Salvage treatment with chemotherapy following relapse after adjuvant chemotherapy is possible with both hormonal and cytotoxic treatments [202]. If several years of tumor-free survival can be obtained at the cost of a short period of chemotherapy, the adjuvant therapy will surely be of value. Demonstration of improved long-term survival with a true plateau on the relapse curve will be evidence that many women with subclinical metastatic cancer are being cured. Such a plateau is not yet seen in the 14-year data for cyclophosphamide by Nissen-Meyer, nor for the 12-year CMFVP data of Cooper.

SUMMARY

Carcinoma of the breast will prove fatal to over 37,000 women in the United States in 1983 [1], despite attempts at early diagnosis.

Hormonal manipulation, known to provide effective palliation for many years, can now be effectively aimed at receptor-positive women, who have a 50–70% chance of responding. Newer agents, such as tamoxifen and aminoglutethimide, offer the benefits of older treatments with less morbidity. Investigations of drugs acting at the level of the central nervous system are ongoing.

Single-agent chemotherapy is clearly effective in causing tumor regression, but effective combination chemotherapy provides more responses and a longer duration of response. The most effective combination regimens at present contain doxorubicin. Pharmacologic studies at the cellular level can be expected to provide more effctive combinations.

The most effective way to combine hormonal and chemotherapeutic treatments is not known. In receptor-positive women without life-threatening disease, beginning with hormonal treatment may be effective in providing palliation at low toxic cost without jeopardizing overall survival. New efforts to cure clinically manifest metastatic breast cancer may eschew palliation as a prime goal. Techniques of synchronizing and of stimulating breast cancer to increase its susceptibility to cytoxic drugs are under investigation.

Immunotherapy is not established as a beneficial modality in the treatment of breast cancer, although levamisole has led to suggestive benefit in small controlled trials.

The use of chemotherapy, and possibly of some hormonal treatments in appropriate patients, as an adjuvant to surgery prolongs disease-free survival. This approach, using established chemotherapeutic and hormonal agents when the metastatic disease is subclinical, is consonant with abundant evidence from experimental systems and other human cancers that are curable. Expectation of curing human breast cancer will likely require aggressive action at the time when the total body tumor burden is at a minimum.

REFERENCES

1. Silverberg E: Cancer statistics, 1983, Ca-A. Cancer J Clin 33:9–25.
2. Haagensen C, Bodian C, Haagensen D: Reproductive factors in breast carcinoma. In: "Breast Carcinoma: Risk and Detection." Philadelphia: WB Saunders, 1981, pp 30–51.
3. Osborne C, Yochmowitz M, Knight W, McGuire W: The value of estrogen and progesterone receptors in the treatment of breast cancer. Cancer 40 (Suppl):2884–2888, 1980.
4. Lippman M, Allegra J: Quantitative estrogen receptor analyses: The response to endocrine and cytotoxic chemotherapy in human breast cancer and the disease-free interval. Cancer 46 (Suppl):2829–2834, 1980.

5. Dao T, Nemoto T: Steroid receptors and response to endocrine ablations in women with metastatic cancer of the breast. Cancer 46 (Suppl):2779–2782, 1980.
6. Manni A, Arafah B, Pearson O: Estrogen and progesterone receptors in the prediction of response of breast cancer to endocrine therapy. Cancer 46 (Suppl):2838–2841, 1980.
7. Johnson P, Bonomi P, Anderson K, Walter J, Rossof A, Economou S: Megestrol acetate (MA) in advanced breast cancer: Response rate related to estrogen receptor (ER) and progesterone receptor (PR) levels. Proc ASCO 1:89, 1982.
8. Rubens R, Hayward J: Estrogen receptors and response to endocrine therapy and cytotoxic chemotherapy in advanced breast cancer. Cancer 46 (Suppl):2922–2924, 1980.
9. Young P, Ehrlich C, Einhorn L: Relationship between steroid receptors and response to endocrine therapy and cytotoxic chemotherapy in metastatic breast cancer. Cancer 46 (Suppl):2961–2963, 1980.
10. Paridaens R, Sylvester R, Ferrazzi E, Legros N, Leclercq G, Henson J: Clinical significance of the quantitative assessment of estrogen receptors in advanced breast cancer. Cancer 46 (Suppl):2889–2895, 1980.
11. McFarlane J, Fleiszer D, Fazekas A: Studies on estrogen receptors and regression in human breast cancer. Cancer 45:2998–3003, 1980.
12. Skinner L, Barnes D, Ribeiro G: The clinical value of multiple steroid receptor assays in breast cancer management. Cancer 46:2939–2945, 1980.
13. Leake R, Laing L, Calman K, Macbeth F, Crawford D, Smith D: Oestrogen-receptor status and endocrine therapy of breast cancer: Response rates and status stability. Br J Cancer 43:59–66, 1981.
14. Degenshein G, Bloom N, Tobin E: The value of progesterone receptor assays in the management of advanced breast cancer. Cancer 46 (Suppl):2789–2793, 1980.
15. Bloom N, Tobin E, Schreibman B, Degenshein G: The role of progesterone receptors in the management of advanced breast cancer. Cancer 45:2992–2997, 1980.
16. Sarrif A, Durant J: Evidence that estrogen-receptor–negative, progesterone-receptor–positive breast and ovarian carcinomas contain estrogen receptor. Cancer 48:1215–1220, 1981.
17. Johnson P, Bonomi P, Bacon L, Walter J, Anderson K, Economou S: Quantitative progesterone receptor level as a predictor of response to megestrol acetate or tamoxifen in advanced breast cancer. Proc ASCO 2:108, 1983.
18. Paridaens R, Leclercq G, Legros N, Sylvester R, Henson J, Toma S: Estrogen receptor variation in neoplastic tissue during the course of disease in patients with recurrent breast cancer. Proc AACR 23:151, 1982.
19. Gross G, Clark G, McGuire W: Multiple progesterone (PR) assays in human breast cancer. Proc ASCO 2:110, 1983.
20. Kennedy B, Fortuny I: Therapeutic castration in the treatment of advanced breast cancer. Cancer 17:1197–1203, 1964.
21. Harris H, Spratt J: Bilateral adrenalectomy in metastatic mammary cancer: An analysis of sixty-four cases. Cancer 23:145–151, 1969.
22. Fracchia A, Randall H, Farrow J: The results of adrenalectomy in advanced breast cancer in 500 consecutive patients. Surg Gynecol Obstet 125:747–756, 1967.
23. Manni A, Pearson O, Brodkey J, Marshall J: Transphenoidal hypophysectomy in breast cancer: Evidence for an individual role of pituitary and gonadal hormones in supporting tumor growth. Cancer 44:2330–2337, 1979.
24. Council on Drugs, Subcommittee on Breast and Genital Cancer, Committee on Research, AMA: Androgens and estrogens in the treatment of disseminated mammary

carcinoma: Retrospective study of nine hundred forty-four patients. JAMA 171:1271–1283, 1960.
25. Kennedy B: Hormone therapy for advanced breast cancer. Cancer 18:1551–1557, 1965.
25a. Cooperative Breast Cancer Group: Results of studies of the Cooperative Breast Cancer Group, 1961–63. Cancer Chemother Rep 41 (Suppl):1–20, 1964.
26. Carter A, Sedransk N, Kelley R, Ansfeld F, Ravdin R, Talley R, Potter N: Diethylstilbestrol: Recommended dosages for different categories of breast cancer patients: Report of the Cooperative Breast Cancer Group. JAMA 237:2079–2085, 1977.
27. Ingle J, Ahmann D, Green S, Edmonson J, Bisel H, Krols L, Nichols W, Creagan E, Hahn R, Rubin J, Frytak S: Randomized clinical trial of diethylstilbestrol vs tamoxifen in postmenopausal women with advanced breast cancer. N Engl J Med 304:16–21, 1981.
28. Westerberg H: Tamoxifen and fluoxymesterone in advanced breast cancer. A controlled clinical trial. Cancer Treat Rep 64:117–121, 1980.
29. Tormey D, Gelman R, Band P, Sears M, Bauer M, Arseneau J, Falkson G: A prospective evaluation of chemohormonal therapy remission maintenance in advanced breast cancer. Breast Cancer Res Treat 1:111–119, 1981.
30. Manni A, Pearson O: Antiestrogen-induced remission in premenopausal women with stage IV breast cancer: Effects on ovarian function. Cancer Treat Rep 64:779–785, 1980.
31. Pritchard K, Thompson D, Myers R, Sutherland D, Mobbs B, Meakin J: Tamoxifen therapy in premenopausal patients with metastatic breast cancer. Cancer Treat Rep 64:787–796, 1980.
32. Hoogstraten B, Fletcher W, Gad-el-Mawla N, Maloney T, Altman S, Vaughn C, Foulkes M: Tamoxifen and oophorectomy in the treatment of recurrent breast cancer: A Southwest Oncology Group Study. Cancer Res 42:4788–4791, 1982.
33. Beex L, Pieters G, Koenders A, Benraad T, Kloppenborg P: Tamoxifen versus ethinyl estradiol in the treatment of postmenopausal women with advanced breast cancer. Cancer Treat Rep 65:179–185, 1981.
34. Legha S, Carter S: Antiestrogens in the treatment of breast cancer. Cancer Treat Rev 3:205–216, 1976.
35. Manni A, Arafah B: Tamoxifen-induced remission in breast cancer by escalating the dose to 40 mg daily after progression on 20 mg daily: A case report and review of the literature. Cancer 48:873–875, 1981.
36. Fabian C, Sternson L, El-Serafi M, Cain L, Hearne E: Clinical pharmacology of tamoxifen in patients with breast cancer: Correlation with clinical data. Cancer 48:876–882, 1981.
36a. Santen R, Worgul T, Lipton A, Harvey H, Boucher A, Samojlik E, Wells S: Aminoglutethimide as treatment of postmenopausal women with advanced breast carcinoma. Ann Intern Med 96:94–101, 1982.
37. Asbury R, Bakemeier R, Folsch E, McCune C, Savlov E, Bennett J: Treatment of metastatic breast cancer with aminoglutethimide. Cancer 47:1954–1958, 1981.
38. Santen R, Worgul T, Samojlik E, Interrante A, Boucher A, Lipton A, Harvey H, White D, Smart E, Cox C, Wells S: A randomized trial comparing surgical adrenalectomy with aminoglutethimide plus hydrocortisone in women with advanced breast cancer. N Engl J Med 305:545–551, 1981.
39. Lipton A, Harvey H, Santen R, Boucher A, White D, Bernath A, Dixon R, Richards G, Shafik A: A randomized trial of aminoglutethimide versus Tamoxifen in metastatic breast cancer. Cancer 50:2265–2268, 1982.

40. Nagel G, Wander H, Blossey HC: Phase II study of aminoglutethimide and medroxyprogesterone acetate in the treatment of patients with advanced breast cancer. Cancer Res 42 (Suppl):3442–3444, 1982.
41. Alexiera-Figusch J, van Gilse H, Hop W, Phoa C, Wijst S, Treurniet R: Progestin therapy in advanced breast cancer: Megestrol acetate—An evaluation of 160 treated cases. Cancer 46:2369–2372, 1980.
42. Pannuti F, Martoni A, Lenaz G, Piana E, Nanni P: A possible new approach to the treatment of metastatic breast cancer: Massive doses of medroxyprogesterone acetate. Cancer Treat Rep 62:499–504, 1978.
43. Izuo M, Iino Y, Endo K: Oral high dose medroxyprogesterone acetate (MAP) in treatment of advanced breast cancer. Breast Cancer Res Treat 1:125–130, 1981.
43a. Wander H, Blossey C, Koberling J, Nagel G: High dose medroxyprogesterone acetate in metastatic breast cancer: Correlations between tumor response and endocrine parameters. Klinische Wochenschrift, 1983 (in press).
43b. Pellegrini A, Massidda B, Mascia V, Ionta M, Lippi M, Muggiano A, Carboni E, della Cuna G, Bernardo G, Strada M, Pavesi L: Ethinyl estradiol and medroxyprogesterone treatments in advanced breast cancer: A pilot study. Cancer Treat Rep 65:135–136, 1981.
44. Klijn J, De Jong F: Treatment with a luteinizing hormone–releasing-hormone analogue (Buserelin) in premenopausal patients with metastatic breast cancer. Lancet 1:1213–1216, 1982.
44a. Harvey H, Lipton A, Santen R, Escher G, Hardy M, Glade L, Segaloff A, Landan R, Schreier H, Max D: Phase II study of a gonadotropin-releasing hormone analogue (Leuprolide) in postmenopausal advanced breast cancer patients. Proc ASCO 22:444, 1981.
45. Paladine W, Ayres V, Price L, Drapkin R, Sokol G, Kriz E, Scheinbaum M: Danazol, an inhibitor of LH and FSH in the treatment of recurrent or metastatic breast carcinoma. Proc ASCO 22:447, 1981.
46. Nagel G, Holtkamp W, Wander H, Blossey C: Hyperprolactinemia and bromocryptine in metastatic breast cancer. Proc AACR 22:139, 1982.
47. Nemoto T, Dao T: 5-Fluorouracil and cyclophosphamide in disseminated breast cancer. NY State J Med 71:554–558, 1971.
48. Bull J, Tormey D, Li S, Carbone P, Falkson G, Blom J, Perlin E, Simon R: A randomized comparative trial of adriamycin versus methotrexate in combination drug therapy. Cancer 41:1649–1657, 1978.
49. Swenerton K, Legha S, Smith T, Hortobagyi G, Gehan E, Yap H, Gutterman J, Blumenschein G: Prognostic factors in metastatic breast cancer treated with combination chemotherapy. Cancer Res 39:1552–1562, 1979.
50. Nash C, Jones S, Moon T, Davis S, Salmon S: Prediction of outcome in metastatic breast cancer treated with adriamycin combination chemotherapy. Cancer 46:2380–2388, 1980.
51. Tormey D: Single agent chemotherapy and comparison with combination therapy in advanced breast cancer (pp 790–791 in Young R (moderator): Perspectives in the treatment of breast cancer: 1976). Ann Int Med 86:784–798, 1977.
52. Manni A, Trujillo J, Pearson O: Sequential use of endocrine therapy and chemotherapy for metastatic breast cancer: Effects on survival. Cancer Treat Rep 64:111–116, 1980.

53. Legha S, Buzdar A, Smith T, Swenerton K, Hortobagyi G, Blumenschein G: Response to hormonal therapy as a prognostic factor for metastatic breast cancer treated with combination chemotherapy. Cancer 46:438–445, 1980.
54. Steiner R, Stewart J, Rubens R: Does response to endocrine therapy predict response to chemotherapy in advanced breast cancer? Proc AACR 23:143, 1982.
55. Lippman M, Allegra J, Thompson E, Simon R, Barlock A, Green L, Huff K, Do H, Aitken S, Warren R: The relation between estrogen receptors and response rate to cytotoxic chemotherapy in metastatic breast cancer. N Engl J Med 298:1223–1228, 1978.
56. Kiang D, Frenning D, Gay J, Goldman A, Kennedy B: Estrogen receptor status and response to chemotherapy in advanced breast cancer. Cancer 46 (Suppl):2814–2817, 1980.
57. Mortimer J, Reimer R, Greenstreet R, Groppe C, Bukowski R: Influence of estrogen receptor status on response to combination chemotherapy for recurrent breast cancer. Cancer Treat Rep 65:763–766, 1981.
58. Chang J, Wergowske G: Correlation of estrogen receptors and response to chemotherapy of cyclophosphamide, methotrexate and 5-fluorouracil (CMF) in advanced breast cancer. Cancer 48:2503–2506, 1981.
59. Jonat W, Maass H, Stolzenbach G, Trams G: Estrogen receptor status and response to polychemotherapy in advanced breast cancer. Cancer 46 (Suppl):2809–2813, 1980.
60. Hilf R, Feldstein M, Savlov E, Gibson S, Seneca B: The lack of relationship between estrogen receptor status and response to chemotherapy. Cancer 46 (Suppl):2797–2800, 1980.
61. Holland JF: Breaking the cure barrier. J Clin Oncol 1:75–89, 1983.
62. Carter S: Single and combination nonhormonal chemotherapy in breast cancer. Cancer 30:1543–1555, 1972.
63. Coggins P, Eisman S, Elkins W, Ravdin R: Cyclophosphamide therapy in carcinoma of the breast and ovary—A comparative study of intermittent massive vs continuous maintenance dosage regimens. Cancer Chemother Rep 15:3–8, 1961.
64. Stoll B: Evaluation of cyclophosphamide dosage schedules in breast cancer. Br J Cancer 24:478–483, 1970.
65. Skipper H, Schabel F, Wilcox W: Experimental evaluation of potential anticancer agents. XIII. On the criteria and kinetics associated with "curability" of experimental leukemia. Cancer Chemother Rep 35:1–52, 1964.
66. Moore G, Bross D, Ausman R, Nadler S, Jones R, Slack N, Rimm H: Effects of chlorambucil (NSC-3088) in 374 patients with advanced cancer: Eastern Clinical Drug Evaluation Programs. Cancer Chemother Rep 52:661–666, 1968.
67. Zubrod C: Appraisal of methods for the study of chemotherapy in man: Comparative therapeutic trial of nitrogen mustard and triethylene thiophosphoramide. J Chron Dis 11:7–33, 1966.
68. Hurley J: A method of selecting patients for cancer chemotherapy. Arch Surg 83:611–619, 1961.
69. Sears M, Haut A, Eckles N: Melphalan (NSC-8806) in advanced breast cancer. Cancer Chemother Rep 50:271–279, 1966.
70. Canellos G, Pocock S, Taylor S, Sears M, Klaasen D, Band P: Combination chemotherapy for metastatic breast carcinoma: Prospective comparison of multiple drug therapy with L-phenylalanine mustard. Cancer 38:1882–1886, 1976.
71. Curreri A, Ansfield F, McIver F, Waisman H, Heidelberger C: Clinical studies with 5-fluorourcil. Cancer Res 18:478–484, 1958.

72. Ansfield F: A less toxic fluorouracil dosage schedule. JAMA 190:686–688, 1964.
73. Jacobs E, Reeves W, Wood D: Treatment of cancer with weekly intravenous 5-fluorouracil. Cancer 27:1302–1305, 1971.
74. Ansfield F, Klotz J, Nealon T, Ramirez G, Minton J, Hill G, Wilson W, Davis H, Cornell G: A phase III Study comparing the clinical utility of four regimens of 5-fluorouracil: A preliminary report. Cancer 39:34–40, 1977.
75. Chlebowski R, Pugh R, Weiner J, Bateman J: Treatment of advanced breast cancer with 5-fluorouracil: A randomized comparison of two routes of delivery. Cancer 48:1711–1714, 1981.
76. Talley R, Vaitkevicius V, Leighton G: Comparison of cyclophosphamide and 5-fluorouracil in the treatment of patients with metastatic breast cancer. Clin Pharm Ther 6:740–748, 1965.
77. Yap H, Blumenschein G, Yap B, Hortobagyi G, Tashima C, Waring A, Benjamin R, Bodey G: High-dose methotrexate for advanced breast cancer. Cancer Treat Rep 63:757–761, 1979.
78. Capizzi R: Improvement in the therapeutic index of methotrexate (NSC-740) by L-asparaginase (NSC-109229). Cancer Chemother Rep 6:37–41, 1975.
79. Yap H, Benjamin R, Blumenschein G, Hortobagyi G, Tashima C, Buzdar A, Bodey G: Phase II study with sequential L-asparaginase and methotrexate in advanced refractory breast cancer. Cancer Treat Rep 63:77–83, 1979.
80. Holland JF, Scharlan C, Gailani S, Krant M, Olson K, Horton J, Schnider B, Lynch J, Owens A, Carbone P, Colsky J, Grob D, Miller S, Hall T: Vincristine treatment of advanced cancer: A cooperative study of 392 cases. Cancer Res 33:1258–1264, 1973.
81. Grinberg R, Nemoto T, Dao T: Vincristine (NSC-67574): Dosage and response in advanced breast cancer. Cancer Chemother Rep 45:57–61, 1965.
82. Yap H, Blumenschein G, Keating M, Hortobagyi G, Tashima C, Loo T: Vinblastine given as a continuous 5-day infusion in the treatment of refractory advanced breast cancer. Cancer Treat Rep 64:279–283, 1980.
83. Fraschini G, Yap H, Barnes B, Buzdar A, Hortobagyi G, Blumenschein G: Continuous 5-day infusion of vinblastine for refractory metastatic breast cancer. Proc ASCO 1:78, 1982.
84. Tannock I, Erlichman C, Perrault D, Quirt I, King M: Failure of 5-day vinblastine infusion in the treatment of patients with advanced refractory breast cancer. Cancer Treat Rep 66:1783–1784, 1982.
85. White D, Hopkins J, Jackson D, Muss H, Richards F, Cooper M, Stuart J, Spurr C: Vincristine by continuous infusion in refractory breast cancer: A phase II study. Proc ASCO 1:83, 1982.
86. Walker B, Raich P, Fontana J, Subramanian V, Rogers J, Knost J, Denning B: Phase II study of Vindesine in patients with advanced breast cancer. Cancer Treat Rep 66:1729–1732, 1982.
87. Smith I, Hedley D, Powles T, McElwain T: Vindesine: A phase II study in the treatment of breast carcinoma, malignant melanoma, and other tumors. Cancer Treat Rep 62:1427–1433, 1978.
88. Cobleigh M, Williams S, Einhorn L: Phase II study of Vindesine in patients with metastatic breast cancer. Cancer Treat Rep 65:659–663, 1981.
89. Yap H, Blumenschein G, Bodey G, Hortobagyi G, Buzdar A, DiStefano A: Vindesine in the treatment of refractory breast cancer: Improvement in therapeutic index with continuous 5-day infusion. Cancer Treat Rep 65:775–779, 1981.

90. Tormey D: Adriamycin (NSC-123127) in breast cancer: An overview of studies. Cancer Chemother Rep 6:319–327, 1975.
91. Hoogstraten B, George S, Samal B, Rivkin S, Costanzi J, Bonnet J, Thigpen T, Braine H: Combination chemotherapy and adriamycin in patients with advanced breast cancer. A Southwest Oncology Group study. Cancer 38:13–20, 1976.
92. Gottlieb J, Rivkin S, Spigel S, Hoogstraten B, O'Bryan R, Delaney F, Singhakowinta A: Superiority of adriamycin over oral nitrosoureas in patients with advanced breast cancer: A Southwest Cancer Chemotherapy Group study. Cancer 33:519–526, 1974.
93. Knight E, Horton J, Cunningham T, Rhie F, Lagakos S, Rosenbaum C, Taylor S, Tennant J: Adriamycin: Comparison of a 5-week schedule with a 3-week schedule in the treatment of breast cancer. Cancer Treat Rep 63:121–122, 1979.
94. Ingle J, Ahmann D, O'Fallon J, Bisel H, Rubin J, Krols L, Giuliano E: Randomized phase II trial of Rubidazone and adriamycin in women with advanced breast cancer. Cancer Treat Rep 63:1701–1705, 1979.
95. Nemoto T, Rosner D, Diaz R, Dao T, Sponzo R, Cunningham T, Horton J, Simon R: Combination chemotherapy for metastatic breast cancer: Comparison of multiple drug therapy with 5-fluorouracil, Cytotoxan and prednisone with adriamycin or adrenalectomy. Cancer 41:2073–2077, 1978.
96. Creech R, Catalano R, Shah M: An effective low-dose adriamycin regimen as secondary chemotherapy for metastatic breast cancer patients. Cancer 46:433–437, 1980.
97. Creech R, Catalano R, Hopson R: A comparison of standard dose adriamycin (SDA) and low dose adriamycin (LDA) as primary chemotherapy for metastatic breast cancer. Proc AACR 21:142, 1980.
98. Legha S, Benjamin R, Mackay B, Yap H, Wallace S, Ewer M, Blumenschein G, Freireich E: Adriamycin therapy by continuous intravenous infusion in patients with metastatic breast cancer. Cancer 49:1762–1766, 1982.
99. Ahmann D, Bisel H, Eagan R, Edmonson T, Hahn R: Controlled evaluation of adriamycin (NSC-123127) in patients with disseminated breast cancer. Cancer Chemother 58:877–882, 1979.
100. Jones R, Norton L, Bhardwaj S, Mass T, Holland J: Single agent adriamycin for metastatic breast cancer. A steep dose-response relationship. Proc ASCO 2:107, 1983.
101. Stuart-Harris R, Smith I: Mitoxantrone: A phase II study in the treatment of patients with advanced breast carcinoma and other solid tumors. Cancer Chemother Pharm 8:179–182, 1982.
102. Knight W, Von Hoff D, Tranum B, O'Bryan R: A phase II trial of dihydroxyanthracenedione (DHAD, Mitoxantrone) in breast cancer. A Southwest Oncology Group (SWOG) study. Proc ASCO 1:87, 1982.
103. Stuart-Harris R, Smith I, Cornbleet M, Smyth J, Rubens R: Mitoxantrone, an active well tolerated new drug in advancing breast cancer: A phase II study in patients receiving no previous chemotherapy. Proc ASCO 19:100, 1982.
104. Osborne C, Von Hoff D, Sandback J: Activity of bisantrene in a phase II study in advanced breast cancer. Proc ASCO 18:87, 1982.
105. Yap H, Yap B, Blumenschein G, Barnes B, Schell F, Bodey G: Bisantrene, an active new drug in the treatment of metastatic breast cancer. Cancer Res 43:1402–1404, 1983.
106. Moore G, Bross D, Ausman R, Nadler S, Jones R, Slack N, Rimm A: Effects of mitomycin C (NSC-26980) in 346 patients with advanced cancer. Eastern Clinical Oncology Evaluation Program. Cancer Chemother Rep 52:675–683, 1968.

107. Creech R, Catalano R, Shah M, Dayal H: A randomized trial of adriamycin vs. mitomycin at low doses in CMF refractory metastatic breast cancer patients. Proc ASCO 1:88, 1982.
108. Currie V, Howard J, Wittes R: A phase II evaluation of m-AMSA, 4'-(9-acridinylamino) methane-sulfon-m-anisidide, in patients with breast cancer. Cancer Clin Trials 4:249–251, 1981.
109. Legha S, Blumenschein G, Buzdar A, Hortobagyi G, Bodey G: Phase II study of 4'-(9-acridinylamino) methane-sulfon-m-anisidide (AMSA) in metastatic breast cancer. Cancer Treat Rep 63:1961–1964, 1979.
110. Ahmann D, Bisel H, Bacon R, Edmonson J, Hahn R, O'Connell M, Frytak S: Phase II evaluation of VP-16-213 (NSC-141540) and cytembena (NSC-104801) in patients with advanced breast cancer. Cancer Treat Rep 60:633–635, 1976.
111. Vaughn L, Panettiere F, Thigpen T, Bottomley R, Hoogstraten B, Samal B: Phase II evaluation of VP-16-213 in patients with advanced breast cancer: A Southwest Oncology Group study. Cancer Treat Rep 65:443–445, 1981.
112. Yap H, Blumenschein G, Schnell F, Bodey G: Phase II evaluation of methyl-GAG in patients with refractory metastatic breast cancer. Cancer Treat Rep 65:465–467, 1981.
113. Yap H, Salem P, Hortobagyi G, Bodey G, Buzdar A, Tashima C, Blumenschein G: Phase II study of cis-dichlorodiammineplatinum (II) in advanced breast cancer. Cancer Treat Rep 62:405–408, 1978.
114. Shingleton W, Sedransk N, Johnson R: Systemic chemotherapy of mammary carcinoma. Ann Surg 173:913–919, 1971.
115. Denefrio J, Vogel C: Phase II Study of hexamethylmelamine in women with advanced breast cancer refractory to standard cytotoxic therapy. Cancer Treat Rep 62:173–175, 1978.
116. Legha S, Buzdar A, Hortobagyi G, Di Stefano A, Wiseman C, Yap H, Blumenschein G, Bodey G: Phase II study of hexamethylmelamine alone and in combination with mitomycin C and vincristine in advanced breast carcinoma. Cancer Treat Rep 63:2053–2056, 1979.
117. Fabian C, Rasmussen S, Stephens R, Haut A, Smith F, Balcerzak S, Tranum B: Phase II evaluation of hexamethylmelamine in advanced breast cancer: A Southwest Oncology Group study. Cancer Treat Rep 63:1359–1361, 1977.
118. Forestiere A, Hakes T, Wittes J, Wittes R: Cisplatin in the treatment of metastatic breast carcinoma. A prospective randomized trial of two dosage schedules. Am J Clin Oncol 5:243–247, 1982.
119. Blum R, Frei E, Holland JF: Principles of dose schedule and combination chemotherapy. In Holland JF, Frei E (eds): "Cancer Medicine." Philadelphia: Lea and Febiger, 1982, pp 730–752.
120. Greenspan E: Combination cytotoxic chemotherapy in advanced disseminated breast carninoma. J Mt Sinai Hosp 33:1–27, 1966.
121. Leone L, Falkson G, Glidewell I, Holland JF: CALGB unpublished data.
122. Cooper R: Combination chemotherapy in hormone resistant breast cancer. Proc AACR 10:15, 1969.
123. Davis H, Ramirez G, Ellerby R, Ansfield F: Five-drug therapy in advanced breast cancer. Factors influencing toxicity and response. Cancer 34:239–245, 1974.
124. Smalley R, Murphy S, Huguley C, Bartolucci A: Combination versus sequential five-drug chemotherapy in metastatic carcinoma of the breast. Cancer Res 36:3911–3916, 1976.

125. Perloff M, Norton L, Bushkin E, Holland J: Intensive six-week courses of combination chemotherapy in stage IV breast carcinoma. Proc ASCO 1:73, 1982.
126. Ahmann D, Bisel H, Hahn R, Eagan T, Edmonson J, Steinfeld J, Tormey D, Taylor W: An analysis of a multiple drug program in the treatment of patients with advanced breast cancer utilizing 5-fluorouracil, cyclophosphamide and prednisone with or without vincristine. Cancer 36:1925–1935, 1975.
127. Tormey D, Gelman R, Band P, Sears M, Rosenthal S, De Wys W, Perlia C, Rice M: Comparison of induction chemotherapies for metastatic breast cancer: An Eastern Cooperative Oncology Group trial. Cancer 50:1235–1244, 1982.
128. Canellos G, De Vita V, Gold G, Chabner B, Schein P, Young R: Combination chemotherapy for advanced breast cancer: Response and effect on survival. Ann Intern Med 84:389–392, 1976.
129. Creech R, Catalano R, Mastrangelo M, Engstrom P: An effective low-dose intermittent cyclophosphamide, methotrexate and 5-fluorouracil treatment regimen for metastatic breast cancer. Cancer 35:1101–1107, 1975.
130. Jones S, Dupre B, Salmon S: Combination chemotherapy with adriamycin and cyclophosphamide for advanced breast cancer. Cancer 36:90–97, 1975.
131. Tranum B, McDonald B, Thigpen T, Vaughn C, Wilson H, Maloney T, Costanzi J, Bickers J, el Mawli N, Palmer R, Hoogstraten B, Heilburn L, Rasmussen S: Adriamycin combination in advanced breast cancer. A Southwest Oncology Group study. Cancer 49:835–839, 1982.
132. Lloyd R, Jones S, Salmon S: Comparative trial of low-dose adriamycin plus cyclophosphamide with or without additive hormonal therapy in advanced breast cancer. Cancer 43:60–65, 1979.
133. Nemoto T, Horton J, Simon R, Dao T, Rosner D, Cunningham T, Sponzo R, Snyderman M: Comparison of four-combination chemotherapy programs in metastatic breast cancer: Comparison of multiple drug therapy with Cytoxan, 5FU, and prednisone versus Cytoxan and adriamycin versus Cytoxan, 5FU and adriamycin, versus Cytoxan, 5FU and prednisone alternating with Cytoxan and adriamycin. Cancer 49:1988–1993, 1982.
134. Brambilla C, De Lena M, Rossi A, Valagussa P, Bonadonna G: Response and survival in advanced breast cancer after two non-cross-resistant combinations. Br Med J 1:801–804, 1976.
135. Russell J, Baker J, Dady P, Ford H, Gazet J, McKinna J, Nash A, Powles T: Combination chemotherapy of metastatic breast cancer with vincristine, adriamycin and prednisolone. Cancer 41:396–399, 1978.
136. Rainey J, Jones S, Salmon C: Combination chemotherapy for advanced breast cancer utilizing vincristine, adriamycin, and cyclophosphamide (VAC). Cancer 43:66–71, 1979.
137. Carmo-Pereira J, Costa F, Henriques E: Chemotherapy of advanced breast cancer: A randomized trial of vincristine, adriamycin, and cyclophosphamide (VAC) versus cyclophosphamide, methotrexate, 5-fluorouracil, and prednisone (CMFP). Cancer 48:1517–1521, 1981.
138. Blumenschein G, Cardenas J, Freireich E, Gottlieb J: FAC chemotherapy for breast cancer. Proc Am Assoc Clin Oncol 10:193, 1974.
138a. Tranum B, Hoogstraten B, Kennedy A, Vaughan C, Samal B, Thigpen T, Rivkin S, Smith F, Palmer R, Costanzi J, Tucker W, Wilson H, Moloney T: Adriamycin in combination for the treatment of breast cancer: A Southwest Oncology Group study. Cancer 41:2078–2083, 1978.

139. Smalley R, Carpenter J, Bartolucci A, Vogel C, Krauss S: A comparison of cyclophosphamide, adriamycin, 5-fluorouracil (CAF) and cyclophosphamide, methotrexate, 5-fluorouracil, vincristine, prednisone (CMFVP) in patients with metastatic breast cancer: A Southeastern Cancer Study Group Project. Cancer 40:625–632, 1977.
140. Aisner J, Weinberg V, Perloff M, Weiss R, Raich P, Perry M, Wiernik P: Chemoimmunotherapy for advanced breast cancer: A randomized comparison of 6 combinations (CMF, CAF vs CAFVP) each with or without MER immunotherapy. A CALGB study. Proc ASCO 22:443, 1981.
141. Perloff M, Hart R, Holland J: Vinblastine, adriamycin, thiotepa, and halotestin (VATH): Therapy for advanced breast cancer refractory to prior therapy. Cancer 32:2534–2537, 1978.
142. Hart R, Perloff M, Holland J: One-day VATH (vinblastine, adriamycin, thiotepa, and halotestin) therapy for advanced breast cancer refractory to chemotherapy. Cancer 48:1522–1527, 1981.
143. Rubens R, Knight R, Hayward J: Chemotherapy of advanced breast cancer: A controlled randomized trial of cyclophosphamide versus a four-drug combination. Br J Cancer 32:730–736, 1975.
144. Canellos G, Pocock S, Taylor S, Sears M, Klaasen D, Bard P: Combination chemotherapy for metastatic breast carcinoma: Prospective comparison of multiple drug therapy with L-phenylalanine mustard. Cancer 38:1882–1886, 1976.
145. Baker L, Vaughn C, Al-Sarraf M, Reed M, Vaitkevicius V: Evaluation of combination vs sequential cytotoxic chemotherapy in the treatment of advanced breast cancer. Cancer 33:513–518, 1974.
146. Chlebowski R, Irwin L, Pugh R, Sadoff L, Hestorff R, Wiener J, Bateman J: Survival of patients with metastatic breast cancer treated with either combination or sequential chemotherapy. Cancer Res 39:4503–4506, 1979.
147. Abeloff M, Ettinger D: Treatment of metastatic breast cancer with adriamycin-cyclophosphamide induction followed by alternating combination therapy. Cancer Treat Rep 61:1685–1689, 1977.
148. Tormey D, Gelman R, Falkson G: Prospective evaluation of rotating chemotherapy in advanced breast cancer. An Eastern Cooperative Oncology Group trial. Am J Clin Oncol (CCT) 6:1–18, 1983.
149. Vogel C, Love N, East D, Moore M, Smalley R: Phase II study of alternating cytoreductive and cycle-active combination chemotherapy for metastatic breast cancer. Cancer Treat Rep 63:2077–2079, 1979.
150. Blumenschein G, Hartobagyi G, Richman S, Gutterman J, Tashima C, Buzdar A, Burgess M, Livingston R, Hersh E: Alternating non-cross-resistant combination chemotherapy and active nonspecific immunotherapy with BCG or MER-BCG for advanced breast cancer. Cancer 45:742–749, 1980.
151. Henderson L, Gelman R, Canellos G, Frei E: Prolonged disease-free survival in advanced breast cancer treated with "super-CMF" adriamycin: An alternating regimen employing high-dose methotrexate with citrovorum factor rescue. Cancer Treat Rep 65 (Suppl):67–75, 1981.
152. Cadman E, Heimes R, Davis L: Enhanced 5-fluorouracil nucleotide formation after methotrexate administration: Explanation for drug synergism. Science 205:1135–1137, 1979.
153. Gewirtz A, Cadman E: Preliminary report on the efficacy of sequential methotrexate and 5-fluorouracil in advanced breast cancer. Cancer 47:2552–2555, 1981.
154. Herrmann R, Westerhausen M, Bruntsch U, Jungi F, Manegold C, Fritze D: Sequential methotrexate (MTX) and 5-fluorouracil (FU) is effective in extensively pretreated breast cancer. Proc ASCO 1:86, 1982.

155. O'Bryan R, Baker L, Gottlieb E, Rivkin S, Balcerzak S, Grumet G, Salmon S, Moon T, Hoogstraten B: Dose response evaluation of adriamycin in human neoplasia. Cancer 39:1940–1948, 1977.
156. Perrault D, Erlichman C, Hasselback R, Tannock I, Boyd N: Sequenced methotrexate (MTX) and 5-fluorouracil (5FU) in refractory metastatic breast cancer: A phase II study. Proc ASCO 2:100, 1983.
157. Brunner K, Sonntag R, Alberto P, Senn H, Martz G, Obrecht P, Maurice P: Combined chemo- and hormonal therapy in advanced breast cancer. Cancer 39:2923–2933, 1977.
158. Kardinal C: Personal communication, 1983.
159. Krook J, Ingle J, Green S, Bowman W, Duluth M: Randomized trial of cyclophosphamide, 5-fluorouracil, prednisone (CFP) plus or minus tamoxifen (T) in postmenopausal women with advanced breast cancer. Proc. ASCO 2:106, 1983.
160. Cocconi G, De Lisi V, Boni C, Mori P: CMF vs CMF plus tamoxifen (T) in postmenopausal metastatic breast cancer. A prospective randomized study. Proc. ASCO 18:75, 1982.
161. Falkson G, Falkson H, Glidewell O, Weinberg V, Leone L, Holland JF: Improved remission rates and remission duration in young women with metastatic breast cancer following combined oophorectomy and chemotherapy. A study by the Cancer and Leukemia Group B. Cancer 43:2215–2222, 1979.
162. Ahmann D, O'Connell M, Hahn R, Bisel H, Lee R, Edmonson J: An evaluation of early or delayed adjuvant chemotherapy in premenopausal patients with advanced breast cancer undergoing oophorectomy. N Engl J Med 397:356–360, 1977.
163. Ahmann, D, Green S, Bisel H, Ingle J: An evaluation of early or delayed adjuvant chemotherapy in premenopausal breast cancer undergoing oophorectomy. A later analysis. Am J Clin Oncol (CCT) 5:355–358, 1982.
164. Glick J, Creech R, Torri S, Holroyde C, Brodovsky H, Catalano R, Varano M: Tamoxifen plus sequential CMF chemotherapy versus tamoxifen alone in postmenopausal patients with advanced breast cancer: A randomized trial. Cancer 45:735–741, 1980.
165. Bezwoda W, Derman D, Moor N, Lange M, Levin J: Treatment of metastatic breast cancer in estrogen receptor positive patients. A randomized trial comparing tamoxifen alone versus tamoxifen plus CMF. Cancer 50:2747–2750, 1982.
166. Allegra J, Woodcock T, Richman S, Patel J, Wittliff J: A phase II evaluation of tamoxifen, Premarin, methotrexate (MTX) and 5-fluorouracil (5FU) in stage IV breast cancer. Proc ASCO 22:441, 1981.
167. Lippman M, Cassidy J, Wesley M, Young R: A randomized attempt to increase the efficacy of cytotoxic chemotherapy in metastatic breast cancer by hormonal synchronization. Proc ASCO 1:79, 1982.
168. Hortobagyi G, Gutterman J, Blumenschein G, Tashima C, Burgess M, Einhorn L, Buzdar A, Richman P, Hersh F: Combination chemoimmunotherapy of metastatic breast cancer with 5-fluorouracil, adriamycin, cyclophosphamide and BCG. Cancer 44:1955–1962, 1979.
169. Muss H, Richards F, Cooper R, White D, Jackson D, Howard V, Shore A, Rhyne A, Spurr C: Chemotherapy vs. chemoimmunotherapy with methanol extraction residue of *Bacillus* Calmette-Guerin (MER) in advanced breast cancer: A randomized trial by the Piedmont Oncology Association. Cancer: 47:2295–2301, 1981.
170. Hortobagyi G, Gutterman J, Blumenschein G, Yap H, Buzdar A, Tashima C, Burgess M, Hersh E: Combined chemoimmunotherapy for advanced breast cancer. A comparison of BCG and levamisole. Cancer 43:1112–1122, 1979.
171. Klefstrom P: Combination of levamisole immunotherapy and polychemotherapy in advanced breast cancer. Cancer Treat Rep 64:65–72, 1980.

172. Fisher B, Slack N: Number of lymph nodes examined and the prognosis in breast cancer. Surg Gynecol Obstet 131:79, 1970.
173. Stenkvist B, Bengtsson E, Dahlquist B, Eklund G, Eriksson O, Jarkrans T, Nordin B: Predicting breast cancer recurrence. Cancer 50:2884–2893, 1982.
174. Hager J, Furmanski P, Heppner G, Roi L, Brennan M, Rich M, Breast Cancer Prognostic Study Assoc: Correlation between elevated preoperative CEA levels and early recurrence in breast cancer patients. Proc AACR 23:144, 1982.
175. Weigand R, Isenberg W, Russo J, Rich M, Breast Cancer Prognostic Study Assoc: Blood vessel invasion as a prognostic indicator in human breast cancers. Proc AACR 21:155, 1980.
176. Black M, Speer F: Survival in breast cancer cases in relation to the structure of the primary tumor and regional lymph nodes. Surg Gynecol Obstet 100:543, 1955.
177. Kinne D, Ashikari R, Butler A, Menendez-Botet C, Rosen P, Schwartz M: Estrogen receptor protein in breast cancer as a predictor of recurrence. Cancer 47:2364–2367, 1981.
178. Blamey R, Bishop H, Blake J, Doyle P, Elston C, Haybittle J, Nicholson R, Griffiths K: Relationship between primary breast tumor receptor status and patient survival. Cancer 46:2765–2769, 1980.
179. Leake R, Laing L, McArdle C, Smith D: Soluble and nuclear oestrogen receptor status in human breast cancer in relation to prognosis. Br J Cancer 43:67–71, 1981.
180. Hilf R, Feldstein M, Gibson S, Savlov E: The relative importance of estrogen receptor analysis as a prognostic factor for recurrence or response to chemotherapy in women with breast cancer. Cancer 45:1993–2000, 1980.
181. Gallagher H: Current controversies in breast cancer. Presented at M.D. Anderson, Nov. 3–5, 1982.
182. Nissen-Meyer R, Kjellgren K, Mansson B: Adjuvant chemotherapy in breast cancer. In Mathe G, Bonadonna G, Salmon S (eds): "Recent Results in Cancer Research: Adjuvant Therapies of Cancer." New York: Springer-Verlag, 1982, pp 142–148.
183. Fisher B, Redmond C, Fisher E: The contribution at recent NSABP clinical trials of primary breast cancer therapy to an understanding of tumor biology—An overview of findings. Cancer 46:1009–1025, 1980.
184. Bonadonna G, Brusamolino E, Valagussa P, Rossi A, Brugnatelli L, Brambilla C, De Lena M, Tancini G, Bajetta E, Musumeci R, Veronesi U: Combination chemotherapy as an adjuvant treatment in operable breast cancer. N Engl J Med 294:405–410, 1976.
185. Rossi A, Bonadonna G, Valagussa P, Veronesi U: Multimodal treatment in operable breast cancer: Five-year results of the CMF programme. B Med J 282:1427–1431, 1981.
186. Bonadonna G, Valagussi P: Dose-response effect of adjuvant chemotherapy in breast cancer. N Engl J Med 304:10–15, 1981.
187. Tancini G, Bonadonna G, Valagussa P, Marchini S, Voronesi U: Adjuvant CMF in breast cancer: Comparative 5-year results of 12 versus 6 cycles. J Clin Oncol 1:2–10, 1982.
187a. Velez-Garcia E, Moore M, Marcial V, Bartolucci A, Ketcham A, Smalley R: Adjuvant chemotherapy and radiotherapy in stage II breast cancer. Proc ASCO 18:80, 1982.
188. Cooper, R, Holland J, Glidewell O: Adjuvant chemotherapy of breast cancer. Cancer 44:793–798, 1979.
189. Holland J, Glidewell O, Cooper R: Adverse effect of radiotherapy on adjuvant chemotherapy for carcinoma of the breast. Surg Gynecol Obstet 150:817–821, 1980.
190. Tormey D, Holland J, Weinberg V, Weiss R, Falkson G, Glidewell O, Leone L, Perloff M: 5-Drug vs. 3-drug ± MER postoperative chemotherapy for mammary carcinoma.

In Salmon S, Jones S (eds): "Adjuvant Therapy of Cancer III." New York: Grune and Stratton, 1981, pp 377–384.

190a. Glucksberg H, Rivkin S, Rasmussen S, Tranum B, Gad-el-Mawla N, Costanzi J, Hoogstraten B, Athens J, Maloney T, McCracken J, Vaughn C: Combination chemotherapy (CMFVP) versus L-phenylalanine mustard (L-PAM) for operable breast cancer with positive axillary nodes. A Southwest Oncology Group study. Cancer 50:423–434, 1982.

191. Rivkin S, Glucksberg H, Foulkes M: Adjuvant chemotherapy for operable breast cancer with positive axillary nodes. Proc ASCO 2:100, 1983.

192. Allen H, Brooks R, Jones S, Chase E, Heuskinkveld R, Giordano G, Ketchel S, Jackson R, Davis S, Moon T, Salmon S: Adjuvant treatment for stage II (node-positive) breast cancer with adriamycin, cyclophosphamide (AC) ± radiotherapy (XRT). In Salmon S, Jones S (eds): "Adjuvant Therapy of Cancer III." New York: Grune and Stratton, 1981, pp 453–462.

193. Brooks R, Jones S, Salmon S, Chase E, Davis S, Moon T, Giordano G, Ketchel S: Doxorubicin and cyclophosphamide adjuvant therapy of node negative breast cancer. Proc ASCO 1:85, 1982.

194. Ali M, Cheng R, Buzdar A, Ewer M, Haynie T: Non-invasive cardiac studies before and after adriamycin containing chemotherapy (FAC) for stages II and III breast cancer. Proc ASCO 1:77, 1982.

195. Misset J, Delgado M, Plagne R, Belpomme D, Guerrin J, Fumoleau P, Metz R, Mathe G: Three year results of a randomized trial comparing CMF to adriamycin (ADM), vincristine (VCR), cyclophosphamide (CPM) and 5-fluorouracil (5-FU) (ACVF) as adjuvant therapy for operated N+ breast cancer. Proc ASCO 1:84, 1982.

196. Buzdar A, Blumenschein G, Smith T, Powell K, Hortobagyi G, Yap H, Hersh E: Adjuvant chemotherapy for breast cancer with fluorouracil, adriamycin, cyclophosphamide (FAC) with or without BCG and with or without postoperative radiation (XRT). A prospective randomized study. Proc AACR 23:142, 1982.

197. Ravdin R, Lewison E, Slack N, Dao T, Gardner B, State D, Fisher B: Results of a clinical trial concerning the worth of prophylactic oophorectomy for breast carcinoma. Surg Gynecol Obstet 131:1055–1064, 1970.

198. Palshof T, Mouridsen H, Daehnfeldt S: Adjuvant endocrine therapy of primary operable breast cancer. Report on the Copenhagen Breast Cancer Trials. Eur J Cancer Suppl 1:183–187, 1980.

199. Fisher B, Redmond C, Brown A, Wolmark N, et al.: Treatment of primary breast cancer with chemotherapy and tamoxifen. N Engl J Med 305:1–6, 1981.

200. Hubay C, Pearson O, Marshall J, Rhodes R, De Banne S, Rosenblatt J, Mangone E, Hermann R, Jones J, Glynn W, Eckert C, McGuire W: Adjuvant chemotherapy antiestrogen therapy and immunotherapy for stage II breast cancer: 45-month follow-up of a prospective, randomized clinical trial. Cancer 46:2805–2808, 1980.

201. Kardinal C, Donegan W: Second cancers after prolonged adjuvant thiotepa for operable carcinoma of the breast. Cancer 45:2042–2046, 1980.

202. Wendt A, Jones S, Salmon S: Salvage treatment of patients relapsing after breast cancer adjuvant chemotherapy. Cancer Treat Rep 64:269–273, 1980.

Use of Human Tumor Stem Cell Assay in Gynecologic Cancer Chemotherapy

Earl A. Surwit, David S. Alberts, and Sydney E. Salmon

Division of Gynecologic Oncology, Department of Obstetrics and Gynecology (E.A.S.); Section of Hematology and Oncology (D.S.A., S.E.S.); and Cancer Center (E.A.S., D.S.A., S.E.S.); College of Medicine, University of Arizona, Tucson, Arizona 85724.

The concept of using a clonogenic assay for the study of tumor stem cells was first delineated by Bruce et al. [1,2] and was followed by a series of studies by investigators at the Ontario Cancer Institute [3,4]. They demonstrated that tumor stem cells responsible for population renewal and the colonization of a metastatic neoplasm could be assayed in vivo and in vitro with colony-forming assays. Measurement of in vitro colony-forming ability after exposure to drugs showed that differential sensitivity was present between various mouse myeloma cell lines, and results of a quantitative in vitro colony assay were predictive of in vitro results [3]. Thus, these clonogenic assays appeared a reliable measure of cytotoxicity [5].

Since a clinically relevant assay for in vitro drug sensitivity evaluation had not been developed, it seemed rational to develop an assay for human myeloma stem cells analogous to the technique of Park et al. [4] for murine myeloma. In 1975 Salmon and Hamburger at the University of Arizona used cells from BALB/c mice that had been primed with mineral oil to condition medium to induce clonal proliferation of human myeloma cells [6]. They discovered that adherent spleen cells from such animals did, in fact, condition medium that would then support the growth of human myeloma colonies in soft agar. Morphologic assessment of the adherent spleen cell population indicated that it was composed predominantly of macrophages.

In control experiments wherein biopsies from various other human cancers were tested, the Arizona group discovered that the culture system

Chemotherapy of Gynecologic Cancer, pages 301–320

facilitated colony growth by a wide variety of human cancers [7]. Some of these (e.g., ovarian cancer, myeloma, bladder cancer, lung cancer, and neuroblastoma) have now been studied in greater depth (without the use of conditioned medium) in clonogenic assays. Overall, approximately 70% of all tumors plated in the clonogenic assay exhibit colony formation, but in over 50% of cases the cloning efficiency has been too low (e.g., < 0.01%) to permit detailed drug sensitivity testing. In general, samples from malignant ascites or widespread metastatic disease have had the highest cloning efficiencies. The low clonogenicity that has been observed in some solid tumors containing heavy stroma (e.g., breast) may, in part, result from difficulties experienced in attempting to mechanically disaggregate these solid tumors.

MOUSE-SPLEEN–CONDITIONED MEDIUM DISCONTINUED

During the course of subsequent studies, Salmon and Hamburger found that the mouse-spleen–conditioned medium was not required for the growth of solid cancers, perhaps because the presence of endogenous macrophages and/or other host cells within the tumor may provide conditioning factors directly. In fact, in ovarian cancer studies [8], removal of phagocytic macrophages from ascites has reproducibly reduced the cloning efficiency for the tumor colony-forming units (TCFUs). This led to a hypothesis that the macrophage might be a "two-edged sword" regulating and promoting the growth of both immune cells and clonogenic tumor cells via soluble factors [9–11]. It also appears likely that a variety of hormones (e.g., insulin) and growth factors (e.g., epidermal growth factor) modulate clonogenicity of tumor stem cells.

With our current technology, less than 0.1% of tumor cells are usually clonogenic. Although the cloning efficiency will likely be improved somewhat with better techniques for cell disaggregation, adjustment in medium components, addition of appropriate growth factors and hormones or change in incubation conditions, a low cloning efficiency (e.g., less than 0.1%) may be an inherent feature of spontaneous human tumors that have not been subjected to serial in vitro passages or animal transplantation.

PROVING THAT THE HUMAN TUMORS "BREED" TRUE IN VITRO

In the study of human tumors it is very important to look for a series of features that would permit the identification of the colonies growing as being of neoplastic origin. In all instances, morphology of the colonies on dried slides, standard histologic sections, or electron microscopy has been consistent with the cell types present in the original tumor. In many tumors it has been possible to identify additional markers (e.g., protein, hormone secretion, or cytogenetic) to further confirm the neoplastic origin of the colonies. As described and detailed by Trent [12], the development of techniques to analyze cytogenetics in tumor colonies has substantially amplified and broadened the applications of karyology to human solid tumors.

Investigations of drug sensitivity were begun shortly after the first successes at growing TCFUs from biopsies. When we have studied drugs active in cancer chemotherapy, we have limited ourselves to assessment of pharmacologically achievable concentrations. Of interest, prior studies of solid tumors with the use of dye exclusion or thymidine incorporation into whole tumor cell populations have generally employed substantially higher dosages of cytotoxic agents than are clinically achievable. We believe that our success in predicting clinical drug sensitivity or resistance has resulted from using an assay of just the clonogenic tumor cells, clinically relevant drug concentrations, and a precise method of quantitating in vitro sensitivity and resistance [13–17].

STUDIES OF OVARIAN CANCER UTILIZING THE HUMAN TUMOR CLONOGENIC ASSAY

Using the human tumor clonogenic assay (HTCA) [18], we have studied the in vitro sensitivity rates of anticancer drugs used in the treatment of patients with previously untreated and relapsing ovarian cancer. Our pharmacologic and clinical trial results have been reported elsewhere [19–21] and are reviewed here because of their relevance to future developments in gynecologic oncology. The data from these studies have identified patterns of cross resistance and sensitivity between these agents [19] and have allowed the prospective selection of active agents (i.e., sensitive in vitro) for the treatment of relapsing disease [19–21]. In addition, we have used the HTCA to evaluate the activity of two drug combinations for in vitro testing against epithelial ovarian cancers.

Use of HTCA in Screening of New Drugs for Anticancer Drug Activity

Until the present, experimental mouse tumor systems have constituted the primary approach for screening new drugs for anticancer activity. However, this approach depends heavily on the use of a few signal mouse tumors and may well have missed compounds that were inactive in the L1210 or P388 leukemia prescreen. We have used the HTCA to carry out in vitro screening studies of new compounds and in vitro phase II trials of new agents that have been entered into phase I and clinical trials.

Clinical Protocol Designed on Basis of In Vitro Data

Another potential use of the HTCA is to design new multiagent chemotherapy regimens for patients with relapsing ovarian cancer. Drugs can be selected on the basis of overall in vitro drug sensitivity patterns observed in previously treated patients.

MATERIALS AND METHODS

Patients

Drug sensitivity tests were successfully carried out on tumor specimens from 165 women with surgically and histologically proven epithelial ovarian adenocarcinoma. Sixty-five patients had had no prior chemotherapy, and 100 had received previous anticancer drug treatment. No patient had received chemotherapy within 3 weeks of drug assay. These studies were concluded in 1980.

In Vitro Clonogenic Assay

Tumor samples for culture were obtained from both solid tissues and malignant pleural and peritoneal effusions. Techniques for preparing single-cell suspensions, for drug incubations, and for plating the cells in the "tumor stem cell" agar cultures were as reported [22, 23] except that conditioned medium was not used since sufficient ovarian tumor colony growth (e.g., 30–200 colonies per 35-mm Petri dish) was usually obtained within 7–10 days. For the drug assay, cells were exposed to varying concentrations of drugs in tissue culture tubes for 1 h at 37°C before they were washed and plated [23]. Standard agents for in vitro drug testing included melphalan, adriamycin, cis-platinum, methotrexate, vinblastine, bleomycin, and mAMSA, which were all tested at low doses up to an upper limit of pharmacologically achievable concentrations [13]. Freshly plated cultures were examined by inverted light microscopy to ascertain that aggregates were not present. Plates were cultured under standard assay conditions. Clusters (15–30 cells) were apparent within 3 days, and colonies (30-cell aggregates $> 60\ \mu m$ in diameter) were usually present in sufficient numbers and size to be counted by inverted microscopy with the Bausch and Lomb FASII image analyzer 7–10 days after plating.

Representative plates were prepared for morphological analysis with a dried slide technique using Papanicolaou staining. Evidence for neoplastic origin of the TCFUs was observed with morphologic and cytogenetic analysis [12].

Data Analysis

Data from all in vitro experiments were stored in a laboratory computer used for statistical analysis and graphic output. Interpretation of in vitro sensitivity to standard drugs was based on the area under linear survival concentration curves (i.e., sensitivity index) obtained in a group of 96 patients who had been studied earlier [23]. Tumor stem cell assay and drug sensitivity measurements on biopsy samples from these patients showed that, overall, TCFUs from about 50–60% of ovarian tumor samples undergo in vitro clonogenic growth in the culture system and provide sufficient colony growth to permit assessment of drug-induced lethality [22, 23]. There were 1,224 dose-response curves to known anticancer drugs performed on tumor specimens from the 165 ovarian tumors which formed > 30 tumor colonies per plate in the assays. Ovarian cancers were considered sensitive to a drug in vitro if the sensitivity index for specific anticancer drugs was less than the following relative area units: 5.3 for melphalan, 9.5 for adriamycin, 11.4 for cis-platinum, 6.5 for methotrexate, 7.5 for 5-fluorouracil, and 3.8 for bleomycin.

On the basis of the studies of Moon et al. [23], we now use the following criteria for evaluating anticancer drug activity in the HTCA: 1) 100–51% TCFUs survival represents a resistant zone; 2) 50–30% TCFUs survival represents an intermediate sensitivity zone; and 3) $< 30\%$ TCFUs survival represents a sensitive zone. The drug concentration selected to identify the resistant or sensitive zone represents 10% or less of the peak plasma concentration or total in vivo plasma concentration time product following a standard clinical dose of the drug. Throughout our studies, we have considered a tumor to be sensitive in vitro to a specific agent if a low concentration of that drug is associated with 50% or less survival of TCFUs.

Studies of the Additive Effects of Two Drug Combinations

The HTCA was used to assess the additive effects of adriamycin–cis-platinum, cis-platinum–vinblastine, and vinblastine-bleomycin on the inhibition of TCFU growth from these patients with epithelial ovarian cancer. Each drug in the combination was tested for a 1-h incubation at two or three different drug concentrations (low, intermediate, and high). The two drugs were also combined simultaneously for 1-h incubations at one or two of the concentrations used for single agents. Quantitation of in vitro drug effects was carried out according to the methods of Valeriote and Lin [24] and Momparler [25]. The surviving fraction of TCFUs resulting from each drug individually (SF_A or SF_B) and the surviving fraction of the drug combination (SF_{A+B}) are determined experimentally. If the (SF_{A+B}) is equal to $(SF_A) \cdot (SF_B)$, the combined drug effects are additive. If the SF_{A+B} is less than $(SF_A) \cdot (SF_B)$, the combined effect is defined as greater than additive or synergistic. If the SF_{A+B} is greater than $(SF_A) \cdot (SF_B)$ [23], the combination interaction is defined as less than additive or inhibiting.

Prospective Clinical Trial

Of the 100 patients with previously treated epithelial ovarian cancer, 32 have undergone 44 clinical trials with single agents that were tested in vitro [19]. All 32 of these patients had clinically measurable disease which had recurred following chemotherapy. All correlations between in vitro and in vivo drug sensitivity were made prospectively, whereas correlations of drug resistance were made both prospectively and retrospectively. The clinical data for these 32 patients had been published previously [19–21]. Standard criteria were used to evaluate objective response. Partial remissions were defined as at least 50% reduction in the size of all measurable tumor masses for longer than one month.

RESULTS

Patterns of Anticancer Drug Cross Sensitivity and Resistance

In the previously untreated patients, there was evidence of in vitro cross resistance between melphalan and adriamycin and between melphalan and bleomycin. Of the 28 previously untreated patients who were tested in vitro for adriamycin sensitivity, 20 were resistant and eight sensitive in vitro to melphalan. Of the 20 melphalan-resistant patients, only three (15%) were sensitive to adriamycin, whereas all eight melphalan-sensitive patients were also sensitive to adriamycin (100%) ($P < 0.001$ for difference in adriamycin sensitivity rates). Similar data apply to bleomycin-melphalan in vitro cross resistance. Of 13 melphalan-resistant patients, only two (15%) were sensitive to bleomycin, whereas four of five (80%) melphalan-sensitive patients were also sensitive to bleomycin ($P < 0.01$).

In relapsing ovarian cancer patients, vinblastine was as active as cis-platinum in the inhibition of TCFUs when resistance was seen in vitro to other drugs ($P > 0.20$; Tables I, II). The range of sensitivity rates to vinblastine was 19–36% (mean 26%) for these patients. Vinblastine and cis-platinum did not appear cross-resistant with 25% of the tumors being sensitive to the former agent in the setting of in vitro resistance to the latter. On the other hand, vinblastine did appear cross-resistant ($P = 0.44$) with the related *Vinca* alkaloid Vindesine. None of ten ovarian cancers resistant to vinblastine were sensitive in vitro to Vindesine.

TABLE I. Frequency of Sensitivity of Vinblastine by TCFUs "Resistant" to Standard Agents[a]

Resistant drug	Total No. tested	Number sensitive to vinblastine
Adriamycin	36	10 (28%)
Bleomycin	36	13 (36%)
Cis-platinum	36	9 (25%)
mAMSA	15	5 (33%)
Melphalan	30	9 (30%)
Methotrexate	16	3 (19%)
Vindesine	10	0 (0%)

[a]Data on TCFUs from 86 patients in relapse are included in this analysis. Reproduced from "Cancer Chemotherapy and Pharmacology" [Alberts DS et al., 6:279–285, 1981] with permission of the publisher.

TABLE II. Frequency of Sensitivity to Cis-Platinum by TCFUs "Resistant" to Standard Agents[a]

Resistant drug	Total No. tested	Number sensitive to cis-platinum
Adriamycin	40	7 (18%)
Bleomycin	38	11 (29%)
mAMSA	11	3 (27%)
Melphalan	37	6 (16%)
Methotrexate	18	3 (17%)
Vinblastine	34	7 (21%)

[a]Data on TCFUs from 86 patients in relapse are included in this analysis. Reproduced from "Cancer Chemotherapy and Pharmacology" [Alberts DS et al., 6:279–285, 1981] with permission of the publisher.

DRUG COMBINATION STUDIES

The results of the drug combination studies are shown in Table III [26, 27]. There were 88 in vitro combination drug trials using cancers from 23 patients. Adriamycin plus cis-platinum at concentrations of 0.1 μg/ml was suggestive of being additive in the inhibition of TCFU growth in 13 of 15 trials and less than additive in two trials.

In addition, both the vinblastine-bleomycin and the vinblastine–cis-platinum combinations were at least additive in the majority of patients in this trial.

Design of a Clinical Protocol Based on In Vitro Data

On the basis of the in vitro chemosensitivity described above, we have designed a multiagent regimen for the treatment of patients relapsing after

TABLE III. Quantitation of the Additive Effects of Two-Drug Combination Versus Single-Agent Therapy on the Inhibition of Human TCFUs[a]

No. studies	Drug 1	Drug 2	SF_{1+2}[b] vs. $SF_1 \cdot SF_2$[c] experimental vs. calculated effect of two-drug RX		
			Inhibitory	Additive	Synergistic
15	Adriamycin	Cis-platinum	2	13	0
9	Bleomycin	Vinblastine	2	6	1
9	Cis-platinum	Vinblastine	3	6	0

[a]Statistical analyses compare the inhibition of each patient's TCFUs by one- and two-drug therapy using the methods of Drewinko et al. [48].
[b]SF_{1+2} represents the "surviving fraction" of TCFU resulting from the experimental addition of drug 1 and drug 2.
[c]$SF_1 \cdot SF_2$ represents the calculated effect of multiplying the "surviving fraction" of TCFUs resulting from drug 1 and drug 2 separately.
Reproduced from "Cloning of Human Tumor Stem Cells" [Salmon SE (ed), Alan R. Liss, New York, 1980, pp 3–13] with permission of the publisher.

primary or secondary anticancer drug treatment. Three of the four drugs were included because of their high degree of activity in vitro.

Although the activity of bleomycin in the assay was low (16%) in previously treated patients, it was included in our drug combination because of its potential additive effects with vinblastine and cis-platinum, which has been noted in both testicular tumors and germ cell tumors of the ovary [28], and its lack of myelotoxicity. The additive effects of bleomycin-vinblastine have also been documented in studies using the HTCA, as noted earlier. Although at the time this regimen was designed hexamethylmelamine had not been tested in the HTCA, it was included in the regimen because of its known activity in relapsing ovarian cancer patients [29].

Day 1	Vinblastine 5 mg/m^2 IV
	Bleomycin 15 mg/m^2 IV
	Cis-platinum 50 mg/m^2 IV in 1 liter normal saline with 40 g Manitol at 1 mg/min
Days 1–14	Hexamethylmelamine 150 mg/m^2 PO

Courses of therapy were repeated at 4-week intervals for up to 1 year. Patients with epithelial-type carcinomas of the ovary who previously failed to respond to or had relapsed from single agent alkylating agent or adriamycin plus alkylating agent therapy were eligible for this study. To be eligible, all patients had to have measurable disease demonstrated by physical examination or radiologic techniques (i.e., CT scanning) or undergo "third-look" laparotomy.

Laboratory criteria to initiate each course of therapy were WBC ⩾ 3,000/mm^3, platelets ⩾ 100,000/mm^3, and serum creatinine ⩽ 1.5 mg/dl. Drug treatment was discontinued if there was progression of disease following two courses of therapy, while those patients achieving response continued to receive therapy for up to 12 courses. Those patients who were considered in complete clinical remission were eligible for "third-look" laparotomy within 8–12 courses of therapy.

Patients were considered to have clinical complete response if there was complete disappearance of all measurable disease for at least 1 month. Patients were considered to have a partial response if they had ⩾ 50% reduction in measurable tumor mass or complete disappearance of cytologically proven malignant effusions for more than 1 month.

Thirty-five patients were evaluable for response. See Tables IV and V for staging data and prior chemotherapy exposures. Nine patients experienced a partial response and eight had a complete clinical response for an overall response rate of 49%. The median duration of response was 10 months for partial responders and 13.5 months for complete responders. Three of the

TABLE IV. Initial Staging Characteristics

Stage	No. patients
I	2
II	3
III	24
IV	7

TABLE V. Previous Chemotherapy

Treatment	No. patients
Melphalan	7
Adriamycin, cyclophosphamide ± BCG	22
Adriamycin, cyclophosphamide, cis-platinum	2
Adriamycin, cyclophosphamide, melphalan, cis-platinum	1
Cyclophosphamide, cis-platinum	1
Adriamycin, 5-FU, methotrexate, cyclophosphamide, melphalan	1
Hexamethylmelamine, cyclophosphamide, methotrexate, 5-fluorouracil	2

complete responders remain free of disease at 10+, 17+, and 22+ months after the start of therapy (Table VI). Survival data are shown in Table VII. The median survival for responders was 14+ months as compared to 5.8 months for nonresponders.

The partial and complete responders in this study were evenly divided (8/16 vs. 9/19) between patients who had responded to their primary chemotherapy and relapsed and those who were initially nonresponders, respectively. It is of interest that of the four patients having had previous cis-platinum therapy, all had a partial response—two continuing on cis-platinum and two who received vinblastine, bleomycin, and hexamethylmelamine without cis-platinum.

Third-look laparotomy was performed in five patients in clinical complete remission. There was no pathologic evidence of disease in two of these patients, who remain free of disease for 10+ and 13+ months.

Complications of therapy are listed in Table VIII. The major dose-limiting toxicity was peripheral neuropathy with four of the 36 patients requiring cessation of cis-platinum or hexamethylmelamine because of severe foot numbness and/or ataxia. Nausea and vomiting were well controlled utilizing various antiemetic regimens including Decadron, droperidol, and metaclopramide.

In Vitro–In Vivo Tumor Sensitivity Correlations

The relation between results of in vitro drug sensitivity assays and outcome of prospective treatment using single anticancer agents in 32 patients

TABLE VI. H-C-V-B–Evaluable Patients

Response	No. patients	Duration
Partial	9/35 (26%)	7.3 m[a]
Complete	8/35 (23%)	13.5 m[b]
PR + CR	17/35 (49%)	10.2 m

[a]Two patients sustained at 9+, 12+ months.
[b]Three patients sustained at 13+, 10+, 22+ months.

TABLE VII. H-C-V-B Survival Duration

	Medial survival (months)
Partial responders	12.3+
Complete responders	16 +
PR + CR	14 +
Nonresponders	5.8

TABLE VIII. H-C-V-B Toxicity

	No.	percent
Neurotoxicity	4	11%
Myelosuppression	2	6%
Nephrotoxicity	1	3%
Severe nausea and vomiting	3	9%

TABLE IX. Correlation of In Vitro Sensitivity and Clinical Response in 32 Patients With Ovarian Cancer

No. patients	No. clinical trials	Sensitive in vitro, sensitive in vivo	Sensitive in vitro, resistant in vivo	Resistant in vitro, sensitive in vivo	Resistant in vitro, resistant in vivo
32	44	8 (true positives)	3 (false positives)	0 (false negatives)	33 (true negatives)

Total No. trials, 44.
Predictive accuracy for sensitivity = × 100 = 73% (P 0.0001).
Predictive accuracy for resistance = × 100 = 100% (P 0.0001).
Reproduced from "Cancer Chemotherapy and Pharmacology" [Alberts DS et al., 6:279–285, 1981] with permission of the publisher.

is summarized in Table IX. In 11 of the 32 patients, in vitro testing predicted sensitivity to single agents; eight of these treated prospectively with the most active agent had partial remissions lasting a median of 3.3 months. Three patients whose tumors were sensitive in vitro to specific anticancer drugs failed to respond clinically to these drugs used as single agents (false-positive assays). Thus, the predictive accuracy of the in vitro assay for objective response was 73% (i.e., 8/11). Responses were predicted for such occasionally used single agents as 13-cis-retinoic acid, Vindesine, bleomycin, and vinblastine, and the more commonly used adriamycin, melphalan, and cisplatin.

Among the 32 patients, there were 33 instances of lack of clinical response successfully predicted by in vitro drug resistance (true negatives). Since there were no instances of in vitro resistance associated with in vivo sensitivity to the same drug, the accuracy of the assay for predicting lack of clinical response was 100%. The statistical test of association between all the in vitro and in vivo study results was highly significant ($P < 0.0001$).

Use of In Vitro Assay for New Drug Screening

To maximize the sensitivity to identify potential new anticancer drugs, we have established a protocol to test new agents against fresh or cryopreserved TCFUs from human tumors by continuous contact of the drug with cells in the agar. If a drug concentration of 10 μg/ml is used in the initial test (and the drug is stable in vitro), the concentration time product achieved will be in the range of 3,400 μg/h/ml when the cultures are incubated for 14 days prior to counting. TCFUs that proliferate from a single cell suspension and form tumor colonies of 30 cells or more in the presence of such drug exposure are clearly resistant to the agent tested. Virtually all the standard cytotoxic drugs (which do not require bioactivation) that we have tested are readily detected with this type of screening assay when tested against tumors from previously untreated patients with neoplasms of the types for which the given agent is used clinically. For example, doxorubicin often reduces survival of TCFUs (from tumors of types known to be frequently sensitive to anthracyclines) to less than 1% of control at 10 μg/ml by continuous contact. This test appears quite sensitive, and therefore should miss relatively few active agents if a variety of previously untreated tumors are used in the testing. If TCFU survival is reduced to less than 30% of control, the unknown agent is retested at lower concentrations, and also by 1-h exposure against a broadened panel of tumors of the same type in which sensitivity was observed as well as other tumor types.

Following the lead of Epstein et al. [30], our laboratory initiated studies of human leukocyte interferon and, more recently, other more highly purified interferons prepared by purification procedures and/or recombinant DNA techniques. The preliminary results of continuous exposures of Interferon A (La Roche) in ovarian cancers reveals a sensitivity rate of 21% with an additional 14% of patients having intermediate sensitivity [31]. Interferon is clearly as active as some cytotoxic agents against TCFUs from certain patients with ovarian cancer. Although the mechanism responsible for the in vitro activity remains unknown, the assay has the potential to select new interferon preparations for clinical trial in relation to in vitro oncolytic activity. Previously, such selections have been made primarily on the basis of the antiviral activity of interferons.

Another promising application of the in vitro assay for screening is in testing agents that have already been selected for clinical trial. In concept, a phase II in vitro trial could markedly reduce the scale of initial clinical trials wherein new agents are given to patients to determine whether they would have antitumor effects [10]. At present, much of the expense and toxicity of such agents unfortunately involves patients who achieve no benefit from the agent administered. Patients could receive such agents only if they appear active in initial screening against a particular tumor type in the assay.

On the basis of preliminary data, it would appear that 4′-deoxydoxorubicin [32], Vinzolidine [33], would be potentially active drugs in the treatment of ovarian cancer.

DISCUSSION

In Vitro Drug Sensitivity Data

The analysis of drug sensitivity and resistance patterns in previously untreated and relapsing ovarian cancer patients provides evidence that the development of resistance to even one drug may be associated with the acquisition of resistance to several classes of compounds (Tables I, II). Furthermore, acquisition of resistance to various classes of anticancer agents may occur despite apparently different mechanisms of drug action. Clearly the development of resistance to cis-platinum conveyed tumor resistance to adriamycin. However, both these agents exert cytotoxicity by interacting with DNA. Resistance to these apparently diverse drugs could be due to enhanced DNA repair mechanisms in resistant TCFUs, although other mechanisms might also apply. Clinical reports have also shown that adriamycin is ineffective as a second-line therapy for ovarian cancer patients previously exposed to alkylating agents [28,34,35]. These in vitro and in vivo findings suggest adriamycin resistance in patients who have received alkylating agent or adriamycin therapy [36]. Similar studies of cross-sensitivity and resistance patterns in more patients may be useful to identify those drugs that may be most effective in both previously untreated and relapsing ovarian cancer patients.

In addition to revealing important cross-resistance relationships between different classes of anticancer agents, these in vitro studies have identified vinblastine and bleomycin as potentially useful agents in the therapy of ovarian cancer patients. Vinblastine had similar in vitro activity to cis-platinum and was not cross-resistant with it. Finally, preliminary data on TCFUs from ten ovarian cancer patients showed that Vindesine and vinblastine were completely cross-resistant with one another. At least for ovarian cancer, it is unlikely that Vindesine will prove more useful than vinblastine [37].

In Vitro Drug Combinations

In these studies, the HTCA has been used to assess the additive effects of adriamycin–cis-platinum, cis-platinum–vinblastine, and vinblastine-bleomycin on the inhibition of TCFU growth from epithelial ovarian cancers. The results correlate with the findings of broad phase II clinical trials of adriamycin plus cis-platinum in the treatment of solid cancers, which suggested at least additive effects for this two-drug combination. In addition, the additive effects seen in vitro with Velban–cis-platinum and Velban-bleomycin correlate with the known high activity of these drugs in combination in testicular tumors [28].

On the basis of these preliminary data, we conclude that the HTCA can be used to assess the potential additive effects of two-drug combination chemotherapy for specific tumors and can help identify those chemotherapy regimens that might be additive or potentiating in the clinic.

The evaluation of in vitro combination studies should either use cancers from previously untreated patients or take into account the prior therapy record. Prior therapy, even with a single agent, can cause cross resistance to a large number of anticancer drugs and may invalidate or weaken the interpretation of the results of such studies. In our preliminary in vitro work in this area, we have avoided using drugs and drug combinations to which the patients had been previously exposed, but these preliminary studies were not limited to samples from patients who had not received prior chemotherapy. The data derived from such studies may be of value in defining new approaches to combination chemotherapy of ovarian cancer. Finally, to validate this in vitro method of analyzing two-drug combination efficacy, it will be necessary to carry out correlative clinical trials.

In Vitro–In Vivo Clinical Correlations

All clinical correlate trials were carried out in ovarian cancer patients who had relapsed following treatment with an alkylating agent or multiple drug regimens, containing adriamycin, cyclophosphamide, or cis-platinum. Clinical response rates to empirical second-line single-agent therapy in such patients are very low, averaging 0–25% in large series of patients [28,34,35]. In view of these data, the HTCA's 73% predictive accuracy for objective tumor response was considered quite good. It is important to point out that some patients included in this trial were entered using a prospective correlative design [38] rather than randomization. With this design, clinical trials of a single agent are carried out independently and generally simultaneously with laboratory testing. However, when assay results permitted selection of an agent to which the patient's TCFUs were sensitive, this agent was then prospectively selected in a decision-aiding mode [10] in relation to the clinical trial. Unfortunately, only 11 of the 24 in vitro assays [25] detected tumor sensitivity to a single drug, which could then be used in a decision-aiding clinical trial. As might be anticipated as the number of drugs tested in vitro increases, the percentage of patients sensitive in vitro to at least one drug also increases.

The extremely high true negative rate (100%) accuracy of the in vitro assay in predicting clinical drug resistance in patients with advanced ovarian cancer clearly indicates that this assay can exclude anticancer drugs that will not be clinically useful for tumor response but which could cause toxicity. Unfortunately, the partial remissions in our patients were relatively short in duration (median of 3.3 months), reflecting the poor results attainable with currently available agents for second-line therapy even when drug sensitivity is predicted.

When applied in a research center, use of the HTCA for the prediction of response to anticancer agents appears to have at least a comparable accuracy rate to the estrogen receptor assay for the prediction of response to hormonal manipulation in breast cancer [39]. However, additional studies are needed before the assay can be considered to be optimized for routine clinical and research applications. Some of these study areas include 1) the use of pharmacokinetic principles to design clinically relevant drug dosing for the in vitro assay system [13–17, 40], and 2) the evaluation of individual agents for possible schedule-dependent antitumor activity [13, 14].

Clinical Protocol Designed on the Basis of In Vitro Data

We have used chemotherapy data obtained from studies of ovarian cancers in the HTCA to help design a multiagent regimen for patients who had failed primary chemotherapy. The rationale for selecting agents for this regimen on the basis of HTCA data was based in part on the assay's 60–70% accuracy in the prediction of clinical response to single-agent chemotherapy, noted previously [9]. The success of this regiment in producing high response rates and durable complete remissions suggests that chemosensitivity data obtained from the HTCA can be useful in designing combination drug regimens for the treatment of ovarian and other solid cancers.

Variable success rates have been reported with multiagent chemotherapy in patients with ovarian cancer who have relapsed after Alkeran alone [41–43]. However, the majority of patients (80%) in our study had previously received multiagent chemotherapy. In patients previously treated with adriamycin and Cytoxan, Lopez et al. [44] reported only two of 13 patients having a partial response with the combination of hexamethylmelamine and cis-platinum, and Vogl [45] noted a median survival of only 3 months with hexamethylmelamine and cis-platinum in patients having previously received adriamycin and cyclophosphamide. In contrast, nearly one-quarter of the patients in the present study had a complete clinical response lasting a median of 13.5 months and had a median duration of survival in excess of 16 months, suggesting superiority for this new four-drug regimen.

Vinblastine appears to be a major contributor to the improved activity of the cis-platinum–hexamethylmelamine drug regimen. Vinblastine was the most active drug evaluated in the HTCA in ovarian cancer for patients who had failed primary chemotherapy. It should be noted that only limited cross resistance existed in the HTCA studies between vinblastine and either adriamycin or alkylating agents. It is difficult to know how important bleomycin was in the success of this drug combination. However, owing to its lack of bone marrow suppression and its potential synergism with vinblastine and cis-platinum, it continues as part of the regimen. We conclude that this four-drug regimen is effective in the treatment of relapsing ovarian cancer patients and should be considered for study as a front-line drug combination for previously untreated patients.

Further Development of Assay System: Practical Considerations

Although progress in understanding of growth regulation and tumor biology is being made in many research laboratories at the present time, the tumor stem cell assay has only just begun to become clinically useful. In view of the many clinical correlations to disease status and treatment response that have already been made with this system, it is reasonable to project that this assay system could become a standard diagnostic procedure in the future. However, much work lies ahead before this assay can be removed from the research setting. Practical considerations usually weigh heavily on the transition of a research procedure into a routine clinical tool. Although the semisolid culture systems support growth of a wide variety of tumors in vitro, it is apparent that the cluster-colony growth currently observed is still suboptimal for most tumor types. Clearly, there is much promise in studying growth factors for various tumor types. For example, epidermal growth factor (EGF) has been reported to enhance the growth of a variety of neoplastic cell lines [46]. Sarcoma growth factor, nerve growth factor, T-cell growth factor, and somatomedin are other specific factors that also warrant detailed study in the clonogenic assay with various tumor types, as do specific prostaglandins and cyclic nucleotides. Detailed studies of the macrophage-elaborated tumor growth factor from BALB/c mouse spleen cells and the factor or factors elaborated by human macrophages in malignant effusions are clearly of high priority. The utilization of macrophage underlayer for cervix cancer also holds promise for future work with this tumor type [47].

CONCLUSIONS

In summarizing the overall experience using the HTCA for gynecologic cancers, it appears that clinical correlations with the system seem extremely encouraging for ovarian cancer. The assay now appears to be very accurate for predicting what drug will not work against an individual patient's tumor. Application of this finding to clinical oncology should reduce morbidity and eliminate costs associated with drug administration to patients who could be confidently predicted not to respond to those agents clinically. Additionally, the assay is very promising for predicting what drug will work against an individual patient's tumor. Although the current major applicability of this system in gynecologic cancer is in protocol development and drug screening, it is showing increasing applicability for prospective clinical trials.

ACKNOWLEDGMENTS

Supported by grants CA 17094, CA 21839, and CA 23074 from the National Institutes of Health, Bethesda, Maryland.

REFERENCES

1. Bruce WR, Lin H: An empirical cellular approach to improvement of cancer therapy. Cancer Res 29:2308–2310, 1969.
2. Bruce WR, Valeriote FA: Comparison of the sensitivity of normal hematopoietic and transplanted lymphoma colony-forming cells to chemotherapeutic agents administered in vivo. J Natl Cancer Inst 37:233–245, 1966.
3. Ogawa M, Bergsagel DE, McCulloch EA: Chemotherapy of mouse myeloma: Quantitative cell culture predictive of response in vivo. Blood 41:7–15, 1973.
4. Park CH, Bergsagel DE, McCulloch EA: Mouse myeloma tumor stem cells: A primary cell culture assay. J Natl Cancer Inst 46:411–422, 1971.
5. Roper PR, Drewinko B: Comparison of in vitro methods to determine drug-induced lethality. Cancer Res 36:2182–2188, 1976.
6. Potter M, Boyce CR: Induction of plasma-cell neoplasms in strain BALB/c mice with mineral oil and mineral oil adjuvants. Nature 193:1086–1087, 1962.
7. Salmon SE, Alberts DS, Meyskens FL Jr, Soehnlen B, Young L, Chen HSG, Moon TE: Clinical correlations of in vitro drug sensitivity. In Salmon SE (ed): "Cloning of Human Tumor Stem Cells." New York: Alan R. Liss, 1980, pp 223–245.
8. Hamburger AW, Salmon SE, Kim MB, Trent JM, Soehnlen BJ, Alberts DS, Schmidt HJ: Direct cloning of human ovarian carcinoma cells in agar. Cancer Res 38:3438–3444, 1978.
9. Salmon SE: Background and overview. In Salmon SE (ed): "Cloning of Human Tumor Stem Cells." New York: Alan R. Liss, 1980, pp 3–13.

10. Salmon SE: Applications of the human tumor stem cell assay to new drug evaluation and screening. In Salmon SE (ed): "Cloning of Human Tumor Stem Cells." New York: Alan R. Liss, 1980, pp 291–312.
11. Salmon SE: Perspectives on future directions. In Salmon SE (ed): "Cloning of Human Tumor Stem Cells." New York: Alan R. Liss, 1980, pp 315–317.
12. Trent JM: Cytogenetic analysis of human tumor cells cloned in agar. In Salmon SE (ed): "Cloning of Human Tumor Stem Cells." New York: Alan R. Liss, 1980, pp 165–167.
13. Alberts DS, Chen HSG, Salmon SE: In vitro drug assay: Pharmacologic considerations. In Salmon SE (ed): "Cloning of Human Tumor Stem Cells." New York: Alan R. Liss, 1980, pp 197–207.
14. Alberts DS, Griffith K, Goodman G, Herman T, Murray E: Phase I clinical trial of methoxantrone: A new antracenedione anticancer drug. Cancer Chemother Pharmacol 5:11–15, 1980.
15. Moon TE: Quantitative and statistical analysis of the association between in vitro and in vivo studies. In Salmon SE (ed): "Cloning of Human Tumor Stem Cells." New York: Alan R. Liss, 1980, pp 209–221.
16. Moon TE, Salmon SE, White CD, Chen G, Meyskens FL Jr, Durie BGM, Alberts DS: Quantitative association between the in vitro human tumor stem cell assay and clinical response to cancer chemotherapy. Cancer Chemother Pharmacol 6:211–218, 1981.
17. Moon TE, Salmon SE, Alberts DS, Chen G, Durie B, Meyskens FL Jr: Quantitative analysis of the human tumor stem cell assay (HTSCA) and the degree of association with clinical response. Proc Am Soc Clin Oncol 22:C–61, 1981.
18. Hamburger AW, Salmon SE: Primary bioassay of human tumor stem cells. Science 197:461–463, 1977.
19. Alberts DS, Chen HSG, Salmon SE, Surwit EA, Young L, Moon TE, Meyskens FL Jr, Co-investigators from the Arizona-New Mexico Cloning Group: Chemotherapy of ovarian cancer directed by the human tumor stem cell assay. Cancer Chemother Pharmacol 6:279–285, 1981.
20. Alberts DS, Salmon SE, Chen HSG, Surwit EA, Soehnlen B, Young L, Moon TE: In vitro clonogenic assay for predicting response of ovarian cancer to chemotherapy. Lancet 2:340–342, 1980.
21. Surwit EA, Alberts DS, Salmon SE: Studies of ovarian cancer utilizing the human tumor stem cell assay: A review. In Fischer G (ed): "Cancer of the Ovary: Cancer Campaign," Vol 7. New York: Verlag & Stuttgart, 1982.
22. Hamburger AW, Salmon SE, Kim MB, Trent JM, Soehnlen BJ, Alberts DS, Schmidt HJ: Direct cloning of human ovarian carcinoma cells in agar. Cancer Res 38:3438–3444, 1978.
23. Moon TE, Salmon SE, White CS, Chen HSG, Meyskens FL Jr, Durie BGM, Alberts DS: Quantitative association between the in vitro human stem cell assay and clinical response to cancer chemotherapy. Cancer Chemother Pharmacol 6:211–218, 1981.
24. Valeriote F, Lin H: Synergistic interaction of anticancer agents: A cellular perspective. Cancer Chemother Rep 59:895–900, 1975.
25. Momparler R: In vitro systems for evaluation of combination chemotherapy. Pharmacol Ther 8:21–35, 1980.
26. Alberts DS, Salmon SE, Chen HSG, Moon TE, Young L, Surwit EA: Pharmacologic studies of anticancer drugs using the human tumor stem cell assay. Cancer Chemother Pharmacol 6:253–264, 1981.

27. Alberts DS, Salmon SE, Surwit EA, et al: Combination chemotherapy in vitro with the human tumor stem cell assay (HTSCA). Proc Am Assoc Cancer Res 22:607, 1981.
28. Einhorn KH, Donohue JJ: Cis-diammine-dichloroplatinum, vinblastine, and bleomycin. Combination chemotherapy in disseminated testicular cancer. Ann Intern Med 87:293, 1977.
29. Wampler GL, Mellett SJ, Kupermine M, Regelson W: Hexamethylmelamine in the treatment of advanced ovarian cancer. Cancer Chemother Rep 56:505, 1972.
30. Epstein LB, Shen JT, Abele JS, Reese CC: Further experience in testing the sensitivity of human ovarian carcinoma cells to interferon in an in vitro semi-solid and ascitic forms of the tumor. In Salmon SE (ed): "Cloning of Human Tumor Stem Cells." New York: Alan R. Liss, 1980, pp 277–290.
31. Salmon SE, Durie BGM, Young L, Liu R, Trown PW, Stebbins N: Effects of cloned human leukocyte interferon in the human tumor stem cell assay. J Clin Oncol 1:217–225, 1983.
32. Salmon SE, Young L, Liu R: Antitumor activity of 4′ deoxydoxorubicin in the human tumor clonogenic assays with comparisons to doxorubicin. Submitted for publication, 1983.
33. Takasugi B, Salmon SE, Young L, Liu R: In vitro phase II trial of Vinzolidine with comparison to vinblastine. Proc ASCO, San Diego, 1983.
34. Hubbard SM, Barkes P, Young RC: Adriamycin therapy for advanced ovarian carcinoma recurrent after chemotherapy. Cancer Treat Rep 62:1375–1377, 1978.
35. Bolis G, D'Incalci M, Gramellini F, Magniota C: Adriamycin in ovarian cancer patients resistant to cyclophosphamide. Eur J Cancer 14:1401–1402, 1978.
36. Ozols RF, Willison JKV, Grotzinger KR, Young RC: Cloning of human ovarian cancer cells in soft agar from malignant effusions and peritoneal washings. Cancer Res 40:2743–2747, 1980.
37. Miller TP, Jones SE, Chester A: Phase II trial of Vindesine in the treatment of lymphomas, breast cancer, and other solid tumors. Cancer Treat Rep 64:1001–1003, 1980.
38. Salmon SE: Clinical correlation of drug sensitivity. In Salmon SE (ed): "Cloning of Human Tumor Stem Cells." New York: Alan R. Liss, 1980, pp 223–245.
39. McGuire W: Hormone receptors: Their role in predicting prognosis and response to endocrine therapy. Semin Oncol 5:428–433, 1978.
40. Salmon SE, Hamburger AW, Soehnlen BJ, Durie BGM, Alberts DS, Moon TE: Quantitation of differential sensitivity of human tumor stem cells to anticancer drugs. N Engl J Med 298:1321–1327, 1978.
41. Vogl SE, Greenwald E, Kaplan BH, Moukhtar M, Wollner D: Ovarian cancer. Effective treatments after alkylating agent failure. JAMA 241:1908, 1979.
42. Kane R, Harvey H, Andrews T, Bernath A, Curry S, Dixon R, Gottleib R, Kukrika M, Lipton A, Mortel R, Ricci J, White D: Phase II trial of cyclophosphamide, hexamethylmelamine, adriamycin, and cis-dichloroplatinum (II) combination chemotherapy in advanced ovarian cancer. Cancer Treat Rep 63:307, 1979.
43. Vogl SE, Pagano M, Davis TE, Einhorn N, Tunca JC, Kaplan BH, Arseneau JC: Hexamethylmelamine and cisplatin in advanced ovarian cancer after failure of alkylating-agent therapy. Cancer Treat Rep 66:1285, 1982.
44. Lopez JA, Krikorian JG, Dias SF, Spiers ASD, Finkel HE, Barnard DE: Cis-platinum–hexamethylmelamine therapy of advanced ovarian cancer. Gynecol Oncol 11:64, 1981.
45. Vogl SE, Pagano M, Kaplan BH, Einhorn N, Arseneau J, Moukhtar M, Greenwald E: Combination chemotherapy of advanced ovarian cancer with hexamethylmelamine, cis-platinum, and doxorubicin after failure of prior therapy. Obstet Gynecol 56:635, 1980.

46. Hamburger AW, White SP: Interaction between macrophages and human tumor clonogenic cells. Stem Cells 1:209–223, 1981.
47. Welander CE, Natale RB, Lewis JL Jr, Old LJ: In vitro growth stimulation of human ovarian cancer cells by xenographic peritoneal macrophages. In press.
48. Drewinko B, Loo TL, Brown B, Gottleib JA, Freireich EJ: Combination chemotherapy in vitro with adriamycin. Observations of additive, antagonistic, and synergistic effects when used in two-drug combinations on cultured human lymphoma cells. Cancer Biochem Biophys 1:187–195, 1976.

Intraperitoneal Chemotherapy in Gynecologic Malignancies

Leslie A. Walton

Division of Gynecologic Oncology, Department of Obstetrics and Gynecology, University of North Carolina School of Medicine, Chapel Hill, North Carolina 27514

Active research into upgrading or expanding drug delivery methods is presently underway. The basic goal of this research is to improve efficacy and reduce toxicity. The intraperitoneal administration of chemotherapeutic drugs is one such delivery method undergoing clinical trials. This therapeutic method is undergoing a resurgence because of refinement in technique, the availability of potent new drugs, and advancement in the understanding of the physiology and pharmacodynamics of the peritoneal cavity. Intraperitoneal (IP) chemotherapy has been used in a variety of cancers, including cancers of the gastrointestinal tract and lymphomas. However, ovarian carcinoma has been the most prevalent disease entity in the historical and contemporary use of this method of therapy. Some reasons for the selection of this disease category will be forthcoming.

THE RATIONALE FOR IP THERAPY IN OVARIAN CARCINOMA

Ovarian carcinoma is disseminated in 60–70% of patients at the time of initial diagnosis. The exfoliating ovarian cancer cell has immediate access to all peritoneal surface membranes and later to the lymphatic and vascular systems. However, the classic surface spreading ability of this disease entity is a dominant route of spread. Death in patients with ovarian carcinoma usually results from gastrointestinal complications due to localized disease.

While surgery and chemotherapy have resulted in regression of clinically apparent disease, approximately 20–35% of patients have macroscopic or

Chemotherapy of Gynecologic Cancer, pages 321–330

microscopic disease, again confined to the peritoneal cavity. This group of patients is difficult to treat, and historical and present-day trials advocate the delivery of the chemotherapeutic agent to the peritoneal cavity.

THE PERITONEAL CAVITY AS A VEHICLE FOR IP THERAPY

The peritoneal cavity covers a square area as large as that covered by the skin. Intraperitoneally injected substances follow one of two major absorption routes depending on the peritoneal absorption surface. Absorption via the visceral peritoneum, mesentery, and omentum lead to drainage into the portal venous system while parietal peritoneum and lymphatic absorption terminate in the systemic circulation (Fig. 1). Since the square surface of the first is larger, the portal system is the recipient of the larger volume of IP material. Drugs undergoing detoxification by the liver will have reduced plasma concentration and decreased systemic toxicity.

IP-administered drugs cross the peritoneal membrane either via the intercellular pores or via transcellular migration. The first method of passage is influenced by molecular size while lipid solubility affects cellular transport. Thus, the larger the molecule the higher the IP retention and the more soluble the molecule, the higher the peritoneal exit capacity.

In addition to molecule size and lipid solubility, the following factors would influence IP drug absorption: 1) volume of drug administered; 2)

Fig. 1. Peritoneal absorption.

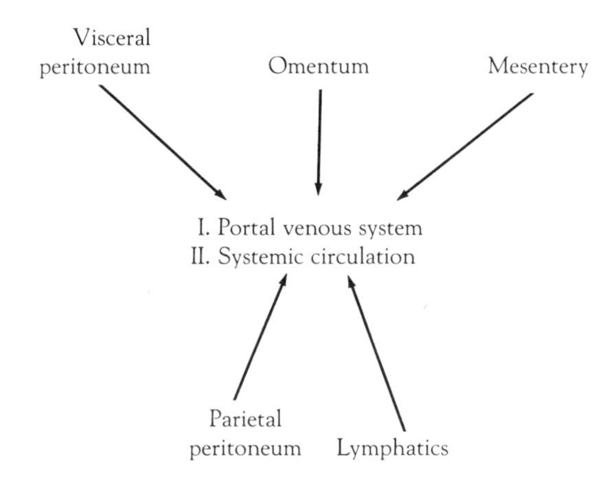

position of the patient; 3) hydrostatic pressure; 4) multiple adhesive areas; and 5) drugs competing for same sites of organ excretion.

Large molecules with low lipid solubility remain in the peritoneal cavity for a long time (Table I). Adequate drug volumes have to be administered. Animal studies have established cytotoxic doses. These doses have to be added to large volumes of administered fluid in the range of 1.5 to 3 liters so that the numerous peritoneal recesses will be distended and all peritoneal surfaces bathed with the medication. Thus, this method of therapy has been dubbed the "belly bath." The presence of adhesions will reduce the free circulation of the cytotoxic agent. The Trendelenberg position in the presence of adequate drug and fluid volume enhances the bathing of peritoneal recesses, especially the subdiaphragmatic and perihepatic spaces. With inspiration, the pressure in these two latter recesses falls and fluid can be aspirated out of the pelvis and pericolic gutters so that circulation and distribution are fostered.

Finally, drugs competing for renal or hepatic clearance mechanisms should not be concomitantly administered with IP drugs. Systemic toxicity due to higher serum levels would result.

A HISTORICAL LOOK AT IP THERAPY

In the early and mid 1950s, the concept of intracavitary injection of chemotherapy began to emerge with the use in mice of drugs such as hemisulfur mustard (close structural relationship to nitrogen mustard) [1]. In 1959, using this drug intraperitoneally in a series of 11 patients with ovarian carcinoma, Green obtained a 55% palliation of ascites and improvement in general well-being [2]. A reduction in systemic toxicity was also observed. Green postulated that the drug was effective because of its effect

TABLE I. IP Drug Absorption in Rats

Drug	Percent retained IP at 1 h	Molecular weight	Lipid solubility
5FU	72	130	Low
Platinum	75	300	Low
Methotrexate	85	472	Low
Adriamycin	89	544	Low
Actinomycin D	79	1,255	Intermediate
Bleomycin	87	1,400	Low
(Cyclophosphamide)	63	261	Intermediate
(Hexamethylmelamine)	8	210	High

on the peritoneal surface and its activity on superficially located tumor cells. He observed that the size of palpable masses was not appreciably diminished.

Hodgkinson in 1966 used a daily intraperitoneal injection of methotrexate in a liter of normal saline followed by citrovorum factor rescue for 14 days in 15 patients with ovarian carcinoma [3]. He reported that two of three patients initially treated had long survival periods. Kottmeier in 1968 commented on his experience with intraperitoneal thiotepa in a series of patients who received postoperative irradiation and intravenous chemotherapy [4]. He did not ascribe any success to intraperitoneal therapy.

Thereafter, IP therapy was sporadic, not standardized, used as an adjunct to surgery and radiation therapy, and a hodgepodge of patients were treated. Usually, the drugs were administered single-shot. Thus, this method of therapy waned for a while.

Using laboratory animals and carefully selected patients, investigators at the National Institutes of Health in the late 1970s sparked a resurgence in intraperitoneal therapy. Chabner et al. [5] and Dedrick et al. [6] documented the pharmacodynamics of intraperitoneal drug administration, and suggested that patients with small volume of disease were more likely to obtain remission after therapy. Jones et al. [7] used methotrexate IP in selected patients with ovarian carcinoma as a "belly bath" technique. Ozols et al. [8], using a murine ovarian carcinoma model, elaborated on adriamycin penetration into tumors when the drug was administered intraperitoneally.

SUMMARY OF THE RATIONALE FOR IP DRUG THERAPY

Drugs used for IP therapy must have a demonstrated efficacy in ovarian carcinoma. The effectiveness of these drugs will depend on their ability to diffuse from the surface to the center of the tumor mass and the blood perfusion of the mass. In addition, specific reasons for the efficacy of tumor kill via IP administation are as follows: 1) Stem cell cytotoxicity studies have shown that both initial conventional drug dose resistance and resistance after therapy can be overcome by higher doses which can only be achieved with IP levels; 2) topical cytotoxicity has been shown to be a mechanism of cell kill for drugs such as adriamycin; and 3) immunoreactive macrophages in the peritoneal cavity ingest the chemotherapeutic drug and migrate to tumor masses where they reside for 2–3 days with release of the drug molecule.

Furthermore, with IP drug administration 1) there is a reduction in specific organ toxicity due to reduced serum levels, and 2) cumulative toxicity doses (using intravenous levels as a guide) will be reached after multiple treatments.

IP DRUGS STUDIED

Three drugs have received wide attention in the treatment of ovarian carcinoma—adriamycin, 5FU, and cis-platinum.

When adriamycin was given IP, it rapidly localized in free-floating cells, it penetrated up to six cell layers of small tumors, and it localized in the outermost layer of solid masses. At 4 h, the IP level was about 474 times higher than the intravenous level.

5FU was also studied. The 4-h IP level is approximately 298 times higher than the equivalent dose given intravenously. The patients with effusions who have responded to 5FU in clinical trials were those patients with large numbers of free-floating cells.

Cis-platinum was also studied. While its concentration in the peritoneal fluid was 3–6 times higher IP than serum, no drug was detected in the central portion of a 2 × 3 cm intraperitoneal nodule. Thus, this drug's diffusion capacity is somewhat impaired [9]. Systemic toxicity seems to be the same whether the drug is given via the intravenous or intraperitoneal route.

METHOD OF IP DRUG ADMINISTRATION

A Tenckhoff catheter is inserted into the peritoneal cavity under local anesthesia or at the time of exploratory celiotomy. The drug in a peritoneal dialysate is allowed to "dwell" in the peritoneal cavity for varying time intervals and then removed. The average "dwell" time is about 4 h. Large volumes in the range of 1.5–3 liters are necessary to distend the peritoneal cavity and fill the numerous peritoneal recesses. The number of exchanges per treatment and the number of treatment cycles vary with the drug. Hospitalization for each treatment cycle varies from 24 to 72 h. Patients can be treated every 2 weeks. The treatment period can last for up to 6 months. Assays of dialysate and the serum can be measured. The distribution of the dialysate can be monitored via CT scanning, ultrasound, contrast media administration.

Toxicity of IP Chemotherapy

Systemic drug absorption produces some of the known side effects of chemotherapy, such as nausea, vomiting, and hematopoietic depression. Thrombocytopenia and leukopenia were observed in some patients. However, abdominal pain and peritonitis are complications peculiar to this method of therapy. The abdominal pain is due to distention of the peritoneal cavity and peritoneal membrane irritation occasionally resulting in aseptic peritonitis. The administration of steroids relieves the pain of aseptic peritonitis. Bacterial peritonitis also occurs and is related to catheter disconnection-connection and responds readily to antibiotic therapy.

Contraindications for IP Therapy

Intraperitoneal chemotherapy should not be offered to patients with a history of whole abdominal irradiation or peritonitis or known intra-abdominal adhesions. Similarly, patients with congestive heart failure or arrhythmias or patients with compromised respiratory, renal, or hepatic function should not be offered this method of therapy. Obviously, patients with palpable abdominal masses and patients with disease beyond the abdomen are excluded. In addition, if marrow function is compromised, initiation of therapy should be deferred until satisfactory baseline values are present.

CLINICAL TRIALS OF IP CHEMOTHERAPY

Data on the results of IP therapy are accumulating at the present time. Because of the treatment of small series of patients, the presence of advanced disease, lack of standardization of technique, and the use of IP therapy after failure with prior agents, the role of IP therapy is not firmly established. However, ongoing standardized clinical trials are in progress at centers across the United States. The emerging role for IP therapy seems to be in situations where there is microscopic, macroscopic, or disease not exceeding 1–2 cm in volume. The following tables will look at historical (Table II) and contemporary trials (Table III). The historical trials used single-shot, small doses in most instances whereas contemporary trials used the belly-bath technique.

Table II looks at the clinical response in 121 patients in whom intraperitoneal chemotherapy was combined with postoperative irradiation or adjunctive oral or intravenous chemotherapy. No clear conclusions could be drawn. The patients with no residual or small residual disease would be expected to have an enhanced survival with any form of adjunctive therapy, and so the contribution of intraperitoneal chemotherapy is questioned except in Green's series.

On the other hand, 19 patients reported on in the contemporary trials (Table III) were treated solely with intraperitoneal chemotherapy after failure of prior therapy. The patients with small residual disease have shown responses to this type of therapy. There was concomitant relief of ascites.

TABLE II. Intraperitoneal Chemotherapy—Historical Summary: Irradiation and Chemotherapy Constituted Adjunctive Therapy After Surgical Exploration

Year	Author	Drug	How given	No. patients	Disease status (ovarian carcinoma)	Relief of ascites	Diminution of masses	Previous (P)/concomitant (C)/ additional (A) therapy
1959	Green [2]	5FU	Single shot	11	Bulky	6/11	0/11	P, A in 2 failure
1966	Hodgkinson [3]	Methotrexate	Infusion	15 (reported follow-up on 3)	Bulky	Not applicable	2/3	A
1968	Kottmeier [4]	Thiotepa	Single shot and infusion	49	No residual	Not applicable	Not applicable[a]	A, radiation
		Thiotepa (IV, IP)	Multiple shots IP	32	Small residual	Not applicable	No response[a]	A, radiation
1973	Walton (unpublished)	Thiotepa, Nitrogen mustard	Single shot	10[b]	No residual	Not applicable	Not applicable	A, 9/10 radiation
				4	Small residual	Not applicable	2/4	A

[a]Author said survival (in years) not improved by IP therapy.
[b]Ten of ten survived 2–5 years.

TABLE III. Intraperitoneal Chemotherapy—Contemporary Trials

Year	Author	Drug	How given	No. patients	Disease status (ovarian carcinoma)	Clinical outcome		
						Relief of ascites	Diminution of masses	Previous (P)/concomitant (C)/ additional (A) therapy
1978	Jones et al. [7]	Methotrexate	IP exchanges	3	Small residual	Not applicable	2/3	P
1980	Speyer et al. [10]	5FU	IP exchanges	6	Bulky—4 Small residual—2	Not applicable	2/6	P
1982	Ozols et al. [11]	Adriamycin	IP exchanges	10	Bulky—8 Small residual—2	2/10	3/10	P

SUMMARY

The delivery of chemotherapy to the host via the intraperitoneal route has evoked interest, especially in disease conditions where the bulk of disease remains intra-abdominal—e.g., ovarian carcinoma. Suitable drugs for usage are those with large molecular weights and low lipid solubility. Higher doses of drugs could be delivered by the IP route. The real and potential toxicity is reduced. The delivery of the drugs involves techniques similar to peritoneal dialysis, and the use of the Tenckhoff catheter has permitted repeated treatments over a period of many months.

Historical and contemporary trials have documented success with IP therapy when there is small volume of disease. IP's therapy role in alleviating recurrent ascites has not been intensively pursued because large tumor masses are usually present when ascites is evident. However, IP therapy should play a role in decreasing the number of repeated taps required in the management of refractory ascites of ovarian carcinoma.

Many clinical trials of IP therapy are ongoing. When larger series have accumulated, the exact role of this method of therapy in the therapeutic armamentarium of cancer, especially ovarian cancer, will be clarified.

REFERENCES

1. Seligman AM, Rutenburg AM, Persky L, Friedman OM: Effect of 2 chloro 2^1 hydroxy-diethyl sulfide (hemisulfur mustard) on carcinomatosis with ascites. Cancer 5:354–363, 1952.
2. Green TH: Hemisulfur mustard in the palliation of patients with metastatic ovarian carcinoma. Obstet Gynecol 383–393, 1959.
3. Rutledge F, Burns BC: Chemotherapy for advanced ovarian cancer. Am J Obstet Gynecol 96:761–772, 1966, (Comments by Hodgkinson).
4. Kottmeier HL: Treatment of ovarian cancer with thio tepa. Clin Obstet Gynecol 11:428–438, 1968.
5. Chabner BA, Stoller RG, Jacobs S, Young RC: Methotrexate disposition in humans: Case studies in ovarian cancer and following high-dose infusion. Drug Metab Rev 8:107–117, 1978.
6. Dedrick RL, Myers CE, Bungay PM, DeVita VT Jr: Pharmacokinetic rationale for peritoneal drug administration in the treatment of ovarian cancer. Cancer Treat Rep 62:1–11, 1978.
7. Jones RB, Myers CE, Guarino AM, Dedrick RL, Hubbard SM, DeVita VT: High volume intraperitoneal chemotherapy ("belly bath") for ovarian cancer. Cancer Chemother Pharmacol 161–166, 1978.
8. Ozols RF, Locker GY, Doroshow JH, Grotzinger KR, Myers CE, Young RC: Pharmacokinetics of adriamycin and tissue penetration in murine ovarian cancer. Cancer Res 39:3209–3214, 1979.

9. Lagasse LD, Pretorius RG, Petrilli ES, Ford LC, Hoeschele J, Kean C: The metabolism of cis-dichloro-diammineplatinum (11): Distribution, clearance, and toxicity. Am Obstet Gynecol 139:791–798, 1981.
10. Speyer JL, Collins JM, Dedrick RL, Brennan MF, Buckpitt AR, Lander H, DeVita VT, Myers CE: Phase I and pharmacologic studies of 5-fluorouracil administered intraperitoneally. Cancer Res 40:567–572, 1980.
11. Ozols RF, Young RC, Speyer CF: Phase I and pharmacological studies of adriamycin administered intraperitoneally to patients with ovarian cancer. Cancer Res 42:4265–4269, 1982.

Monoclonal Antibodies and Their Potential Role in Gynecologic Cancer Chemotherapy

Robert M. Galbraith and Gregory W. Warr

Departments of Basic and Clinical Immunology and Microbiology, Medicine, and Biochemistry, Medical University of South Carolina, Charleston, South Carolina 29425

The increasing use of sensitive immunological methods for the detection, analysis, and measurement of a wide variety of biologically important molecules has repeatedly prompted the suggestion that such techniques might be useful in the detection and treatment of cancer. This is not a new concept, since similar approaches were originally postulated almost 100 years ago [see Pressman, 1980]. However, before such routine methods as radioimmunoassay and ELISA can become useful tools in the clinical management of cancer, it is necessary to have access to large supplies of reproducible antibodies, which are preferably highly specific for the tumor in question. This one factor has often seemed, even to the more enthusiastic pioneers in the field, to present a daunting, and possibly insurmountable, obstacle. The introduction by Köhler and Milstein [1976] of hybridoma methods which can be used for the large-scale preparation of highly specific monoclonal antibodies has therefore been greeted with much interest. Although very few relevant studies have yet been performed, some important lessons have already surfaced, and the time appears ripe for a brief discussion of the potential usefulness of monoclonal antibodies in gynecological cancer chemotherapy.

CONVENTIONAL VERSUS MONOCLONAL ANTIBODIES

Conventional heteroantisera prepared by deliberate immunization of laboratory animals with more or less pure antigen preparations have been

Chemotherapy of Gynecologic Cancer, pages 331–340

employed successfully for many years, but, with newer knowledge and increasing requirements for clearer discrimination between antigens, the shortcomings of these reagents have become progressively more apparent. It is now clear that the normal immune system can produce antibodies with specificities for up to a million or more different antigens. This fact, coupled with the realization that each typical macromolecular protein antigen actually possesses a multiplicity of antigenic determinants (epitopes), means that an animal immunized with a single, purified antigen can produce hundreds of antibodies of differing specificities that recognize the protein from virtually any imaginable direction. The consequent heterogeneity of antibodies in such conventional antisera tends to cause unwanted cross reactivities, the definition of the latter being to the immunologist what the definition of a weed is to a gardener—a personal judgment based on specific needs, circumstances, and prejudice. The usual cause of such unwanted cross reactions is that the original antigen was contaminated. However, even when antigens are available in sufficiently pure form—an unusual circumstance for tumor antigens—genuine but inexplicable cross reactions may occur between unrelated molecules. Cross reactions are also frequent between members of related molecular families, a good example being the multiple immunoglobulin classes themselves. This heterogeneous reactivity of conventional antisera can obscure the otherwise clear-cut differences between unique antigens.

Theoretically, unwanted cross reactions can be removed by adsorption with materials selected for content of *unwanted* antigens. However, although this strategy undoubtedly works in some situations, its successful application in many other cases requires a greater degree of knowledge of antigenic structures than we currently possess. Viewed in this light, the major advance realized by Köhler and Milstein [1976] with the introduction of hybridization for formation of monoclonal antibodies is the possibility of generating large amounts of single antibody species with single binding-site specificities for a theoretically limitless number of different antigens.

PRINCIPLES OF MONOCLONAL ANTIBODY PRODUCTION

Antibodies are produced by cells of the B (bone marrow–derived) lymphocyte lineage, and according to the generally accepted dogma one cell and its progeny can secrete antibody of only one specificity. Therefore, by selecting one appropriate lymphocyte and clonally expanding it, "monoclonal" antibody with a preselected specificity can be produced. The attractiveness of this concept is that it avoids the necessity of immunizing with a pure antigen, and in principle offers the possibility of avoiding unwanted cross reactions. Interestingly enough, monoclonal antibodies, in some cases, still show totally unexpected cross reactivities [Pillemer and Weissman, 1981], but as long as this possibility is borne in mind and excluded by appropriate controls, monoclonal antibodies will, by and large, perform the tasks we ask of them.

The selection and expansion of a single lymphocyte clone is very difficult to achieve by straightforward tissue culture of B-lymphocytes, and the technique adopted by Köhler and Milstein [1976] and elegantly described in a general review by Milstein [1980] involves the immortalization of antibody-producing cells by fusion with lymphoid tumor lines that have been adapted to long-term tissue culture. Monoclonal antibodies are primarily produced in mouse and rat systems, although studies in other species including human [Kozbor and Rodor, 1983] are now being performed.

Cell fusion is accomplished by mixing normal spleen or lymph node lymphocytes and tumor cells in the presence of agents promoting such fusion. Although Sendai virus was originally used, polyethylene glycols in the molecular weight range of 1,000–6,000 are generally the current reagents of choice. Suppose, then, that we successfully fuse the lymphocytes from a mouse immunized with antigen X, with in vitro grown lymphoid tumor cells. We have, in our test tube, normal mouse lymphocytes, unfused tumor cells, tumor cells fused with each other, mouse lymphocytes fused with each other, and the desired normal lymphocytes fused with tumor cells. Unfortunately, the latter category of cells comprise only a small fraction (< 1%) of the total. The next steps are therefore to select out the fused tumor/lymphoid cells (heterokaryons) in tissue culture, and further select those few fused cells secreting the specific antibody desired from the great majority of other heterokaryons. The strategy for selection of heterokaryons is based on the following principles.

1) Normal lymphocytes secreting antibody will not survive in tissue culture.
2) The tumor cells are genetic mutants that lack an enzyme (hypoxanthine phosphoribosyl transferase, HPRT) essential for the purine salvage pathway.
3) After fusion of normal lymphocytes and tumor cells, the whole mixture of cells is selectively poisoned, by the addition of methotrexate or its close relative aminopterin to the culture medium. This prevents nucleotide synthesis by the normal pathways, but cells that possess the purine salvage pathway can survive because hypoxanthine is also added to the medium (along with thymidine). Thus, unfused tumor cells die because they are poisoned and cannot synthesize all the needed nucleotides with

the added hypoxanthine and thymidine, and since normal lymphocytes also die in any case in tissue culture, only heterokaryons (hybridomas) can grow because the lymphocyte component provides the HPRT, and the tumor cell contribution provides the ability to grow in tissue culture.

The tumor cells also provide the immunoglobulin-synthesizing machinery, since they are plasma cell–derived lines, and some of the lines currently available for fusion have been further selected for loss of the ability to synthesize or secrete their own endogenous immunoglobulin. Thus, after a period ranging from a few days to 2–3 weeks, colonies of heterokaryons will grow selectively in the poisoned cultures of fused cells. A thousand or more clones can be expected from a single fusion with a mouse spleen. The hybridomas secreting the desired antibody are then selected by assaying culture supernatants for the appropriate antibody, generally by radioisotopic (RIA) or enzyme-linked (ELISA) immunoassays. The subsequent steps involve repeated cloning, expansion, and selection, as clearly described by Goding [1982], who gives excellent technical protocols for the whole process of hybridoma production.

Heterokaryons in general are unstable as regards chromosomal retention through cycles of division, and hybridomas are no exception. Since the antibody genes and those for HPRT are on separate chromosomes, hybridomas frequently lose antibody-producing properties without losing their ability to grow well, and other lines that produce good antibody may be subject to poor growth in culture owing to loss of HPRT synthesis or other undefined causes. However, repeated cloning usually yields a number of relatively stable hybridoma lines from a fusion, and these can be used to produce monoclonal antibody for use, either in large-scale tissue culture or by growth in ascites form in the peritoneal cavity of mice treated with pristane (tetramethyl pentadecane). The latter form of monoclonal antibody production has the disadvantage of producing ascites fluid that contains not only the monoclonal antibody, but also large quantities of normal, polyclonal mouse immunoglobulin. These normal immunoglobulins all have unknown reactivities which may give spurious test results. However, ascites-grown hybridomas do produce much higher titers of antibody than tissue culture–grown cells, which may be an advantage.

POTENTIAL USES OF MONOCLONAL ANTIBODIES

As discussed by Pressman [1980], several potential uses of immunological methods in the diagnosis and management of cancer have been evident for many years. Our newfound ability to prepare monoclonal antibodies of defined specificity has held out the tantalizing prospect that some of these approaches may now be realized, and it is likely that additional applications will soon become apparent. For convenience, these will be considered under three main headings.

Detection of Soluble Tumor Antigens

One of the more exciting potential applications for monoclonal antibodies concerns the detection of soluble tumor antigens in serum, a prospect which if realized would pave the way for the use of radioimmunoassay, ELISA, or comparable methods for mass screening and early diagnosis of individual tumors. This might be helpful, for example, in individuals at high risk of developing cancer, and also for tumors in sites other than the cervix which are not readily amenable to cytological examination. In addition, in the contexts of chemotherapy of gynecologic cancer, it is conceivable that appropriate screening for circulating tumor antigens might in the future provide a simple means of monitoring the efficacy of treatment and tumor recurrence in semiquantitative terms. Assays performed with conventional antisera for certain soluble "tumor-associated" antigens such as alpha-fetoprotein (AFP) and carcinoembyronic antigen (CEA) have already shown promise in this regard [Sikora, 1982]. The exquisite specificity of monoclonal reagents may allow the preparation of more discriminating antisera recognizing tumor-specific antigens. This in turn would greatly facilitate progress toward the theoretical goal of precise recognition of tumors from different organs, and possibly even their distinction by histological type.

Localization of Tumors

Recently, there has been considerable interest in the possibility of using immunological methods to aid in the localization of cancer. For example, after purification and attachment of a suitable label, antibodies could be injected and used to "target" tumors, perhaps allowing both accurate localization of primary tumors and detection of metastases. Several examples of the use of monoclonal antibodies for this purpose have been reported recently. Goldenberg et al. [1980] described successful localization of several tumors with radioiodinated antibodies, achieving positivity rates in ovarian and cervical cancer of 88% and 90% respectively. However, it should be stressed that the monoclonal antisera employed were directed toward the tumor-associated antigen CEA, and were not therefore specific for the tumors under investigation. A similar approach was taken by Epenetos et al. [1982a], who also showed specific uptake by tumors including ovarian cancer. The antibodies used were again tumor-associated rather than tumor-specific, and quite apart from some technical difficulties which remain to be solved, the numbers of patients examined to date are small. However, this approach appears to have promise as a powerful alternative or adjunct diagnostic method and compares very favorably with radiopharmaceuticals such as gallium-67 citrate and indium-111–labeled bleomycin, both of which are taken up by nonmalignant tissues at sites of infection. In addition, scintigraphy with a gamma camera is a relatively straightforward procedure, and the sensitivity appears to be adequate; tumors 2 cm in diameter were readily detected by Goldenberg et al. [1980], and with the use of ^{123}I as label, Epenetos and colleagues [1982c] were able in experimental animals to discriminate lesions as small as 1 mm. In this regard, it is of interest that Epenetos et al. [1982a] noted that this method can also yield positive results when other standard methods such as ultrasonography and computerized tomography are negative.

Monoclonal antibodies can also obviously be used to detect and localize tumor cells in vitro. For example, Epenetos et al. [1982b] demonstrated the ability of monoclonal antibodies when used in conjunction with standard immunocytochemical techniques to identify malignant cells, including carcinoma cells derived from the ovary, in serous effusions. These results indicate that immunological examination with monoclonal antibodies may be a useful alternative to standard cytological analysis. Similarly, monoclonal antibodies could be used to localize tumor cells in pathological specimens, a recent example of this being the demonstration of carcinoid tumors with an antiserum recognizing the major product of such cells—serotonin [Cuello et al., 1982]. Although the antisera currently available are directed to tumor-associated antigens which are not necessarily specific for individual tumors, these findings have clear implications. Thus, it is possible to speculate that we may one day be able to confirm positively the presence of suspected tumors, and to identify specifically and accurately the site of origin. Moreover, if antibodies with this degree of discriminatory ability were to become available, their capability to pinpoint malignant cells in tissue sections might prove to be a useful aid in staging and prognosis.

Treatment of Tumors

As with localization of tumors, a major potential contribution of monoclonal antibodies in treatment is to aid in the more precise targeting of known cytotoxic substances on to tumors. This approach has not yet been widely evaluated, but several points of practical importance have already emerged, of which the overriding concern is the specificity of the antibodies available. With rare exceptions, monoclonal reagents prepared to date still recognize tumor-associated antigens which, although present on tumor cells, are shared with other normal tissues. Clearly, precise localization of tumors with antibodies would be better achieved with antibodies that are tumor-specific. In other words, while cross reaction with normal tissues may be considered an acceptable risk when a single dose of antibody is given for diagnostic purposes, it may well not be for the large amounts or multiple administrations that may be required for damaging reactive tumors. This is one reason why most clinical trials reported to date have involved tumors in which more detailed information concerning antigenic structure, or a wider selection of monoclonal reagents, is available. These include particularly leukoproliferative disorders [Deng et al., 1982; Dillman et al., 1982; Ritz and Schlossman, 1982] and melanoma [Koprowski et al., 1978]. Another approach which might under certain circumstances provide helpful information is to transplant human tumors into immunodeficient nude mice, so that some estimate may be made of the tissue specificity of new and untried antisera before these are used in humans [Koprowski et al., 1978; Sears et al., 1982]. However, the aim in the long term remains to develop truly tumor-specific reagents. Previous attempts to prepare such reagents by conventional methods have not been notably successful, and the hope is that hybridoma technology will permit the preparation of such specific antibodies.

Once tumors have been pinpointed by appropriately specific antisera, several approaches could be used to induce tissue damage. For example, since antibodies can be detected within tumors after intravenous injection, it might be anticipated that such attachment would initiate several damaging immunological mechanisms including lysis mediated by complement, antibody-dependent cellular cytotoxicity (ADCC), and elimination by phagocytic cells. In fact, monoclonal antibodies tend not to function well in this regard, the net result being that the hybridoma antisera produced to date are not nearly as toxic as are conventional antisera. However, this difficulty does not prevent the use of specific antibodies for the delivery of known cytotoxic substances. Candidates suggested to date include toxins such as ricin and diphtheria, cytotoxic drugs and immunomodulating agents [Baldwin, 1982], and no doubt the list will grow. Some studies have already been performed in animal models with monoclonal antibodies conjugated with adriamycin and Vindesine [Baldwin, 1982; Embleton et al., 1983], and the results thus far are seen to be encouraging.

Viewed objectively, there remain, perhaps predictably, a number of difficulties. One problem which compounds the inherent difficulties of achieving specific localization to the tissue in question is the possibility that depending on such factors as the vascularization of the tumor, delivery of antibody from the bloodstream may be poor. Weinstein and colleagues [1982] have suggested one alternative route of administration, namely by subcutaneous injection, so that antibody is taken up by the lymphatics into the regional nodes. This may be advantageous in the case of tumors that grow or spread primarily in the lymphatics. Administration of monoclonal reagents causes release of antigens from the cell membrane of target cells, and it is possible that blocking factors including soluble tumor-derived antigens might interfere with the targeting of injected antibodies [Ritz and Schlossman, 1982]. However, a more serious problem is the occurrence in some studies of anaphylactoid reactions following administration of monoclonal antibodies. For example, Dillman et al. [1982] found that infusion of > 10 mg antibody was associated with systemic effects. Other investigators have experienced fewer difficulties with such reactions, even with larger amounts of antiserum [Ritz and Schlossman, 1982]. The precise cause remains unknown, although some affected patients have been noted to develop antibodies to mouse immunoglobulin [Dillman et al., 1982]. Possibly this problem can be circumvented in the future with the use of monoclonal antibodies of human origin. The final point concerns the state of host defenses locally at the site of the tumor. Very little information is currently available, but the balance of evidence suggests at least some impairment [Ritz and Schlossman, 1982]. This has stimulated interest in "cotargeting" immunomodulators to the tumor by coupling them onto monoclonal antibodies. One example of this is the attempted delivery of interferon to the lesion with the aim of augmenting natural killer function locally [Baldwin, 1982].

CONCLUDING REMARKS

Whereas some enthusiasm for the potential uses of monoclonal antibodies in the detection of tumor antigens and the diagnosis of tumors appears justified, considerable caution is necessary in considering their potential as primary therapeutic agents. There are several reasons for this, chief among which is our limited knowledge of the tissue distribution of the antigens recognized by individual monoclonal antibodies to date. However, if the difficulties with specificity of targeting discussed above can be resolved, and particularly if tumor-specific antibodies can be produced, then a number of cytotoxic agents could be delivered directly to selected tumor tissues. Even if complete specificity cannot be achieved, the concentration of tumor-associated antigens on tumor cells may be sufficiently high that the inherently poor selectivity of most targeted cytotoxic agents can still be usefully improved. Thus, although much research must still be done before this approach can be properly tested in clinical trials, the next few years could signal several major changes in the management of gynecological malignancy related to the use of monoclonal antibodies.

ACKNOWLEDGMENTS

Publication No. 642 from the Department of Basic and Clinical Immunology and Microbiology, Medical University of South Carolina. R.M.G. was the recipient of NIH Research Career Development Award CA-00611.

REFERENCES

Baldwin RW (1982): Monoclonal antibodies in the diagnosis, detection and therapy of cancer. Proc R Soc Edinb 81B:261–276.

Cuello AC, Wells C, Chaplin AJ, Milstein C (1982): Serotonin immmunoreactivity in carcinoid tumors demonstrated by a monoclonal antibody. Lancet 1:771–773.

Deng C-T, Terasaki P, Chia J, Billing R (1982): Monoclonal antibody specific for human T acute lymphoblastic leukemia. Lancet 1:10–11.

Dillman RO, Shawler DL, Sobol RE, Collins HA, Beauregard JC, Wormsley SB, Royston I (1982): Murine monoclonal antibody therapy in two patients with chronic lymphocytic leukemia. Blood 59:1036–1045.

Embleton MJ, Rowland GF, Simmonds RG, Jacobs E, Marsden CH, Baldwin RW (1983): Selective cytotoxicity against human tumor cells by a Vindesine–monoclonal antibody conjugate. Br J Cancer 47:43–49.

Epenetos AA, Britton KE, Mather S, Shepherd J, Granowska M, Taylor-Papadimitriou J, Nimmon CC, Durbin H, Hawkins LR, Malpas JS, Bodmer WF (1982a): Targeting of iodine-123–labelled tumor-associated monoclonal antibodies to ovarian, breast, and gastrointestinal tumors. Lancet 2:999–1006.

Epenetos AA, Canti G, Taylor-Papadimitriou J, Curling M, Bodmer WF (1982b): Use of two epithelium-specific monoclonal antibodies for diagnosis of malignancy in serous effusions. Lancet 2:1004–1006.

Epenetos AA, Nimmon CC, Arklie J, Elliott AT, Hawkins LA, Knowles RW, Britton KE, Bodmer WF (1982c): Detection of human cancer in an animal model using radiolabelled tumour-associated monoclonal antibodies. Br J Cancer 46:1–8.

Goding JW (1982): Production of monoclonal antibodies by cell fusion. In Marchalonis JJ, Warr GW (eds): "Antibody As A Tool: The Applications of Immunochemistry." Chichester: John Wiley, pp 273–289.

Goldenberg DM, Kim EE, DeLand FH, Bennett S, Primus FJ (1980): Radioimmunodetection of cancer with radioactive antibodies to carcinoembryonic antigen. Cancer Res 40: 2984–2991.

Köhler G, Milstein C (1976): Derivation of specific antibody-producing tissue culture and tumour lines by cell fusion. Eur J Immunol 6:511–519.

Koprowski H, Steplewski Z, Herlyn D, Herlyn M (1978): Study of antibodies against human melanoma produced by somatic cell hybrids. Proc Natl Acad Sci USA 75:3405–3409.

Kozbor D, Rodor JC (1983): The production of monoclonal antibodies from human lymphocytes. Immunol Today 4:72–79.
Milstein C (1980): Monoclonal antibodies. Sci Am 243:66–74.
Pillemer E, Weissman IL (1981): A monoclonal antibody that detects a V_k-TEPC15 idiotypic determinant cross-reactive with a Thy-1 determinant. J Exp Med 153:1068–1079.
Pressman D (1980): The development and use of radiolabeled antitumor antibodies. Cancer Res 40:2960–2964.
Ritz J, Schlossman SF (1982): Utilization of monoclonal antibodies in the treatment of leukemia and lymphoma. Blood 59:1–11.
Sears HF, Atkinson B, Mattis J, Ernst C, Herlyn D, Steplewski Z, Hayry P, Koprowski H (1982): Phase-I clinical trial of monoclonal antibody in treatment of gastrointestinal tumors. Lancet 1:762–765.
Sikora K (1982): Monoclonal antibodies in oncology. J Clin Pathol 35:369–375.
Weinstein JN, Parker RJ, Keenan AM, Dower SK, Morse HC, Sieber SM (1982): Monoclonal antibodies in the lymphatics: Toward the diagnosis and therapy of tumor metastases. Science 218:1334–1337.

Second-Look Surgery in Gynecologic Malignancies

Vinay Malviya and Gunter Deppe

Division of Gynecologic Oncology, Department of Obstetrics and Gynecology, Wayne State University School of Medicine, Detroit, Michigan 48201

The concept of second-look surgery for assessment of disease status following treatment was introduced in 1948 by Wangensteen et al. for a patient with cancer of the cecum. It was employed to diagnose early recurrence in asymptomatic patients. Subsequently, the technique was carried out in patients with ovarian cancer and other gynecologic malignancies. Indications for a second look operation include: 1) staging of the referred patient in whom the initial laparotomy findings were unclear and/or tumor reduction was inadequate prior to institution of therapy; 2) monitoring the efficacy of the treatment regimen in order to assess regression of tumor and to allow definitive removal of tumor; and 3) surveying at specified intervals following therapy the patient with no clinical evidence of disease, or after prophylactic therapy to determine if residual disease is present.

The time interval between the initial and the second-look surgery has been a matter of speculation. There is considerable variability in the rate at which residual cancer will grow large enough to produce symptoms. Intervals at 6 months have been recommended for stomach cancers and 8 months of cancers of the colon [Wangensteen et al., 1954].

There is always concern of a false-negative second-look exploration which could occur either by failure of the surgeon to recognize residual cancer or failure of the pathologist to find small areas of cancer in histologic specimens. Therefore, at each reexploration, all suspicious tissues should be removed. The specimens should be identified, locations meticulously marked, and multiple histologic sections of each specimen made. It is common to have as many as 30 specimens from a single patient at reexploration.

Chemotherapy of Gynecologic Cancer, pages 341–350

It has been speculated that the liberal use of second-look surgery would result in incomplete, suboptimal, primary resection of tumor. However, this has not been upheld and in fact has encouraged more radical primary surgery, often with regional lymphatic excision [Gilbertson et al., 1962].

OVARIAN CARCINOMA

As the result of more effective chemotherapy for ovarian carcinoma, more patients are achieving remissions. Given the dose-limiting toxicity of many of the agents and the risk of developing serious sequelae after prolonged therapy, the concept of second-look surgery has rapidly evolved in patients with ovarian cancer. It is essential to accurately determine the resultant chemotherapeutic response and a safe treatment interval. The management of patients with epithelial tumors of the ovary is often hampered by lack of diagnostic tests that are sensitive enough to detect residual or recurrent tumor after initial therapy. Serologic tests, diagnostic radiography, ultrasound, and computerized axial tomography have not been uniformly reliable in demonstrating the presence of residual tumor or its response to therapy [Samaan et al., 1976; Samuels et al., 1975].

Residual tumor is often missed on the basis of clinical examination and diagnostic radiography. In a series of 128 patients, 64 who were found to have residual tumor at second look had no physical findings suggestive of disease prior to surgery [Schwartz and Smith, 1980]. Conversely, five patients who had palpable masses believed to be tumor had no evidence of disease at surgery.

In a series of 26 patients with stage III or IV ovarian cancer, the results of pelvic and abdominal ultrasound were correlated with second-look surgery [Pussel et al., 1980]. It was found that ultrasound had an 84% correlation with laparotomy in detecting the presence of ovarian tumor in the pelvis, and a 92% correlation in detecting liver and right diaphragmatic metastases. However, it was not sensitive in detecting intraperitoneal spread and detected only 36% of those found at laparotomy. This is probably due to the small size of intraperitoneal deposits. Thus, though ultrasound has an important role in the management of advanced ovarian cancer, it has its limitations. CAT scans and directed needle biopsies also share these limitations.

With more frequent use of combination chemotherapy for ovarian cancer most patients tolerate only 6–12 courses of therapy. Long-term chemotherapy has been associated with chronic leukopenia and thrombocytopenia. The cardiotoxicity of adriamycin has been well documented. Cis-platinum–

containing regimens have neurotoxicity and nephrotoxicity as the dose-limiting factors. Furthermore, there is a significant risk of developing leukemia after prolonged therapy with alkylating agents [Reimer et al., 1977]. This makes discontinuation of these agents at the appropriate time imperative. Second-look laparotomy has been the usual method of intraperitoneal evaluation, and the operative and histologic findings have been the basis for discontinuation, modification, or reinstitution of both chemotherapy and radiation therapy.

The timing for second-look surgery following chemotherapy for ovarian carcinoma has varied from 6 to 24 months [Schwartz and Smith, 1980; Smith et al., 1976; Wallach and Blinick, 1970]. Early reexploration may endanger complete chemotherapeutic response. Conversely, delay may risk escape of tumor leading to loss of surgical advantage.

In one series of 109 patients with complete clinical response, the 5-year survival rate was directly proportional to the number of courses of chemotherapy [Smith et al., 1976]. Patients who underwent second-look laparotomy after four or fewer monthly cycles of chemotherapy had a 5-year survival of only 9%, as compared to 32% for patients who had 5–9 courses of chemotherapy, and 80% for those who had ten or more courses. All patients who had 12 or more courses of chemotherapy were alive at the time of their report. This study suggests that second look should be delayed until a minimum of 12 courses of chemotherapy has been administered.

Second-look exploration in patients with ovarian carcinoma should be a well-planned systematic operation. On the basis of the findings at surgery, treatment may be modified and subsequent therapy planned. Chemotherapy should be discontinued if no disease is found.

TECHNIQUE OF SECOND-LOOK LAPAROTOMY

1) A vertical midline incision is made, extending approximately 6 cm, above the umbilicus.

2) Cytologic washings must be obtained upon entering the peritoneal cavity from a) the pelvis, b) the right and left paracolic spaces, and c) the right and left hemidiaphragms.

3) Adhesolysis must be performed to allow adequate examination of all parietal and visceral surfaces.

4) Examination of the peritoneal surfaces may be palpatory and, when possible, visual. A laparoscope or sigmoidoscope may be used to visualize areas not accessible to direct visual examination such as the superior surface of the liver, or the right and left hemidiaphragms. Both lobes of the liver

must be palpated. The mesentery and serosa of the bowel should be carefully inspected in all cases. The remaining abdominal viscera should be carefully inspected including stomach, gall bladder, spleen, and kidneys.

5) Attention is next directed to the pelvis, where the peritoneum and viscera are examined. The pelvic peritoneum should be biopsied for metastatic implants. The pelvic side walls should be opened and lymph-node–bearing areas examined. All adhesions or plaques on the parietal and visceral peritoneum should be biopsied.

6) If no gross disease is present multiple biopsies should be taken. These include the known areas of residual tumor recorded at the initial operation. It usually includes lateral pelvic peritoneum, cul-de-sac peritoneum, serosa of the sigmoid colon, anterior bladder peritoneum, lateral paracolic spaces, and the inferior surface of the diaphragm. Residual round ligaments and infundibulo pelvic ligaments should also be biopsied.

7) The uterus, ovaries, and omentum if present are removed. Routine appendectomy is recommended by a few centers, as this may be the occult site of a primary mucinous adenocarcinoma indistinguishable from a mucinous carcinoma of the ovary.

8) Selective lymph node biopsies should be performed from the common and external iliac lymph nodes as well as the periaortic lymph nodes up to the level of the renal arteries. Approximately 25–30 biopsy specimens and 6–10 cytologic specimens are obtained for study from most patients.

9) If residual disease is present, cytoreductive surgery should be performed. The aim should be to reduce the size of the largest residual tumor to less than 2 cm in diameter. Resection of parts of the gastrointestinal or urinary tract can be justified only if all residual tumor can be removed. The benefits of urinary or fecal diversion must be weighed against the risk of recurrence.

A properly conceived and performed second-look operation should be a part of the pretreatment plan in patients with ovarian cancer. The mortality and morbidity of surgery in such patients, even those who have received radiation therapy, are low, and the benefits far outweigh the risk.

Complications associated with the greatest morbidity are related to the gastrointestinal tract and include bowel injury, intestinal obstruction, and prolonged ileus. Urinary tract injuries and infections add to the morbidity. Other complications, such as pulmonary atelectasis, hemorrhage requiring blood transfusion, and wound infections occur as commonly as with other surgical procedures. Table I summarizes the experience of several institutions with second-look laparotomy in ovarian carcinoma. Of 376 patients who underwent a second-look operation, 147 (39%) had no evidence of malignancy. The recurrence rate following the negative second look was 20%.

TABLE I. Second-Look Laparotomy Results in Ovarian Carcinoma

No. patients[a]	Negative second look %	Recurrence after second look %	Reference
63	(36) 57	(6) 16	Roberts et al., 1982
63	(21) 33	(12) 19	Berek et al., 1983
37	(15) 40	(2) 13	Stuart et al., 1982
186	(58) 31	(7) 22	Schwartz and Smith, 1980
27	(17) 62	(3) 17	Curry et al., 1981
Totals 376	(147) 39	(30) 20	

[a]Number of patients who underwent a second-look operation.

The recurrence rate may actually be greater owing to short follow-up in some studies. These reports from the literature are inconclusive because of lack of a consistent definition of second-look procedures. They are further clouded because the numbers are too small to determine the impact of type of treatment, duration, and cell differentiation.

The diameter of the largest tumor nodule remaining after the initial surgery still remains the most important prognostic factor. Smith et al. [1976] suggested, however, that the total quantity of tumor remaining after surgery is not important if the largest single tumor mass not resected is less than 1 cm in diameter. Hence, it is more important to remove all tumor masses larger than 1 cm than to reduce total tumor volume by a fixed percentage such as 80% or even 95%. The patient will do poorly if the surgeon takes out 95% of tumor but leaves a single tumor nodule of 2 cm or larger. In contrast, if the whole peritoneal cavity is covered with small tumor nodules and only 50% of tumor is removed, then many patients will respond to chemotherapy with subsequent 5-year survivals having been reported. However, the Mount Sinai, New York, experience has demonstrated that the size of residual disease, after the completion of a first laparotomy, did not have an impact on complete clinical remission with eligibility for surgical end-staging laparotomy [Cohen et al., 1983]. This may indicate that an effective chemotherapeutic regimen can overcome the disadvantage of bulky, residual disease and affect a cure. In this respect, regimens containing Cisplatin and Adriamycin are not restricted in their chemotherapeutic efficacy as are the alkylating agents.

The rate of survival after a second-look procedure varies directly with the volume of tumor found and amount of tumor left behind at the second-look operation. The 5-year survival rate after second-look operation for patients with no evidence of disease was 72%. For patients with only microscopic tumor the 5-year survival was 35%. Patients with gross residual disease of 2 cm or greater at the time of second look had a 5-year survival rate of only 15%. Patients with no change in status of the tumor from initial operation had a survival rate of 18% [Griffiths et al., 1979].

The absence of palpable tumor has been associated with an appreciable prolongation of survival in stage III disease. However, relapse is inevitable unless effective chemotherapy can be carried to a point at which repeated intraperitoneal biopsy fails to reveal microscopic foci or residual tumor.

SECOND-LOOK LAPAROSCOPY

Sixty to seventy percent of patients found to be in clinical remission following chemotherapy for advanced ovarian carcinoma will have residual tumor at the time of second-look laparotomy. This major surgical procedure may be avoided by preliminary second-look laparoscopy. In a summary of the literature persistent tumor was detected in 32 (29%) of 109 patients by laparoscopy (Table II).

The incidence of complications with laparoscopy in various series has ranged from 6% to 21% [Berek et al., 1981; Mangioni et al., 1979; Rosenoff et al., 1975]. No mortalities were noted. The complication with the highest morbidity has been injury to the bowel. Hemorrhage from trauma to the inferior epigastric vessel as well as intra-abdominal bleeding is known to occur. Pneumothorax from diaphragmatic biopsies usually responds to conservative management [Roberts et al., 1982].

The incidence of complications was found to be significantly reduced by the use of a needlescope prior to insertion of the conventional laparascope. In one series this reduced the complication rate to 2.2% [Berek et al., 1981]. However, treatment should not be discontinued on the basis of a negative laparoscopy. Piver et al. [1977] have described a quick method of cytological evaluation via laparoscopy which takes approximately 30 min. They injected 50 cc of saline through the laparoscope, retrieved it, and sent the washings for immediate evaluation. All specimens were stained with a

TABLE II. Second-Look Laparoscopy in Ovarian Carcinoma

No. patients	Persistent tumor (%)	Reference
16	5 (31)	Rosenoff et al., 1975
22	8 (36)	Piver et al., 1980
24	8 (33)	Smith et al., 1977
47	11 (23)	Spinelli et al., 1976
Totals 109	32 (29)	

modified technique of the classic Papanicolaou stain. The presence of malignant cells in the washings ranged from a few individual cells to numerous clusters of cells. The absence of visible tumor and malignant cells in the cytologic washings permitted the use of second-look laparotomy while the patient was still under anesthesia.

Laparoscopy is not an alternative to second-look laparotomy but is a useful adjunct for determining presence of resectable, unresectable, or diffuse disease after chemotherapy. It may allow safe biopsy and confirmation of amount and extent of residual disease without subjecting the patient to a laparotomy.

OTHER GYNECOLOGIC MALIGNANCIES

Experience with second-look laparotomy in other gynecologic malignancies is limited but increasing. Recently, Roberts et al. [1982] published a series of second-look procedures in nonepithelial cancer of the ovary and cancer of the uterine corpus. All patients with nonepithelial cell cancer of the ovary had stage IA disease except for one patient with dysgerminoma who had stage III disease. All patients had second-look surgery and all were treated with VAC except for one patient with immature teratoma who refused any further therapy. The only positive second-look laparotomy was in the patient with dysgerminoma, who was treated with radiation therapy. In the negative group there were no recurrences with follow-up from 6 months to 9 years. Two patients with stage I carcinosarcoma and Sertoli-Leydig cell tumor of the ovary had negative second-look laparotomies after chemotherapy and were free of disease 1 and 4 years after laparotomy.

Six patients with uterine sarcoma (four carcinosarcomas and two leiomyosarcomas) underwent a second-look laparotomy. Five of the six with intraperitoneal disease initially had a negative second-look operation. The patient with positive laparotomy died 7 months later. Two of the five with negative laparotomy developed recurrence, one intraperitonally and the other in the lung. Both are, however, alive with disease.

Two patients with stage I adenocarcinoma of the uterus had second-look laparotomy, one of which was negative. The patient with positive laparotomy had a single focus of disease in the pelvis and is now free of disease after external pelvic radiation. The patient with negative laparotomy is free of disease after 6 months. Deppe et al. [1980] performed second-look laparotomy in three patients with advanced endometrial carcinoma who had been in clinical remission after at least 1 year of chemotherapy. Two of these three patients had no evidence of residual tumor at second-look laparotomy and one patient had a microscopic tumor.

THIRD-LOOK SURGERY

Patients found to have residual tumor after second-look laparotomy face the possibility of long-term complications, including chronic leukopenia, thrombocytopenia, and leukemia when chemotherapy is continued. It is often impossible to assess the tumor response to chemotherapy on the basis of clinical findings alone. In these patients a third look in search of gross tumor remnants or, in their absence the ability to biopsy various suspicious sites, may be indicated.

Microscopic disease at second look always presents a dilemma for further management. According to a study conducted at the M.D. Anderson Hospital [Copeland et al., 1983], third-look surgery has a limited role in the management of these patients. A careful appraisal of the tumor grade, the second-look surgical findings, and tumor-reductive aspects should provide sufficient information in patients with microscopic disease and may be more predictive of the ultimate outcome.

In this series the survival rates for patients with microscopic disease at second look were the same as the negative group except for one chemotherapy-related death due to bone marrow toxicity. These favorable survival rates could be attributed to one or more biological characteristics of the tumor: 1) microscopic disease foci represent residual portions of the tumor that have low malignant potential and are unresponsive to chemotherapy; 2) these foci represent nonclonogenic chemotherapy altered cell aggregates; 3) owing to short follow-up, these submacroscopic foci have not yet had time to become macroscopic and/or clinically recognizable; 4) chemoconversion to tissue of low malignant potential.

Patients who had tumor-reductive surgery at second look with continuation of chemotherapy may benefit from a third-look operation. In these patients further therapeutic decisions can be made on the basis of their third-look findings. Mortality as high as 23% has been reported with 24 or more courses of melphalan therapy [Copeland et al., 1983]. The technique and complications of third-look laparotomy are no different from those of second look.

CONCLUSION

Second-look surgery will remain the most sensitive method of detecting residual disease until more specific tumor markers or more sensitive radiographic techniques are developed. It has a definite role in management of epithelial cancer of the ovary. Its use in other gynecologic cancers is limited at the present time but is on the rise.

A modest but significant number of patients have been rendered free of disease with no evidence of malignancy after a final negative look. The benefits achieved by the ability to excise and delineate areas of residual cancer far outweigh the risks of surgery and justify the effort from the point of view of both patient and surgeon.

REFERENCES

Berek JS, Griffiths T, Leventhal JH (1981): Laparoscopy for a second-look evaluation in ovarian cancer. Obstet Gynecol 58:192–198.

Berek J, Hacker N, Lagasse L, Resnick B, Hunter T, Neiberg R, Elashoff R (1983): Second-look laparotomy for epithelial ovarian cancer. Proc Am Assoc Cancer Res 2:157.

Cohen CJ, Bruckner HW, Goldberg JD, Holland JF (1983): Improved therapy with cisplatin regimens for patients with ovarian carcinoma (FIGO III and IV) as measured by surgical end staging (second look surgery). The Mount Sinai experience. Clin Obstet Gynecol 10:307–324.

Copeland LJ, Wharton JT, Rutledge FN, Gershenson DM, Seski JC, Herson J (1983): Role of "third look" laparotomy in the guidance of ovarian cancer treatment. Gynecol Oncol 15:145–153.

Curry SL, Zembo MM, Nahas WA, Jahsan AE, Whitney CW, Mortel R (1981): Second look laparotomy for ovarian cancer. Gynecol Oncol 11:114–118.

Deppe G, Jacobs AJ, Cohen CJ (1980): Second-look operation in endometrial cancer. Diagn Gynecol Obstet 2:193–195.

Gilbertson VA, Wolder A, Wangensteen OH (1962): Palliation associated with second look failure: Cancers primary in the rectum, stomach and colon. Surg Gynecol Obstet 51:163–168.

Greco FA, Julian CG, Richardson RL, Burnett L, Hande KR, Oldham RK (1981): Advanced ovarian cancer: Brief intensive combination chemotherapy and second look operation. Obstet Gynecol 58:199–205.

Greene MH, Boice JD Jr, Greer BE, Blessing JA, Dembo AJ (1982): Acute non-lymphocytic leukemia after therapy with alkylating agents for ovarian cancer. N Engl J Med 307:1416–1421.

Griffiths CF, Parker LM, Fuller AF (1979): Role of cytoreductive surgical treatment in the management of advanced ovarian cancer. Cancer Treat Rep 63:235–240.

Jones Soo, Khoo K, Whitaker SV (1981): Evaluation of ovarian cancer by second look laparotomy after treatment. Aust NZ J Surg 51:30–33.

Kapadia SB, Krause JR (1978): Ovarian carcinoma resulting in acute leukemia following alkylating agent therapy. Cancer 41:1676–1679.

Keettel WC, Pixley EE, Buchsbaum HJ (1974): Experience with peritoneal cytology in the management of gynecologic malignancies. Am J Obstet Gynecol 120:174–182.

Mackman A, Ansfield J (1974): A second look at the second look operation in colonic cancer after the administration of 5-fluorouracil. Am J Surg 128:763–766.

Mangioni C, Bolis G, Molteni P, Belloni C (1979): Indications, advantages and limits of laparoscopy in ovarian cancer. Gynecol Oncol 7:47–55.

Piver MS, Lele SB, Barlow JJ, Gamarra M (1980): Second look laparoscopy prior to proposed second look laparotomy. Obstet Gynecol 55:571–573.

Piver MS, Lopez RC, Xymos F, Barlow JJ (1977): The value of pretherapy peritoneoscopy in localized ovarian cancer. Am J Obstet Gynecol 127:288–290.

Pussel SJ, Cosgrove DC, Hinton J, Wiltshaw E, Barker GH (1980): Carcinoma of the ovary—Correlation of ultrasound with second look laparotomy. Br J Obstet Gynaecol 87:1140–1144.

Reimer RR, Hoover R, Fraumeni JF, Young RC (1977): Acute leukemia after alkylating agent therapy of ovarian cancer. N Engl J Med 297:177–181.

Roberts WS, Hodel K, Rich WM, DiSaia PJ (1982): Second-look laparotomy in the management of gynecologic malignancy. Gynecol Oncol 13:345–355.

Rosenoff SH, DeVita VT, Hubbard S, Young RC (1975): Peritoneoscopy in the staging and follow-up of ovarian cancer. Semin Oncol 2:223–228.

Rosenoff SH, Young RC, Chabner B, Hubbard S, DeVita VT, Schein PS (1975a): Use of peritoneoscopy for initial staging and post-therapy evaluation of patients with ovarian carcinoma. Natl Cancer Inst Monogr 42:81–86.

Rosenoff SH, Young RC, Anderson T, Bagley C, Chabner B, Schein PS, Hubbard S, DeVita VT (1975b): Peritoneoscopy: A valuable staging tool in ovarian carcinoma. Ann Intern Med 83:37–41.

Samaan NA, Smith JP, Rutledge FN, Schultz PN (1976): The significance of measurement of human placental lactogen, human chorionic gonadotropin and carcinoembryonic antigen in patients with ovarian carcinoma. Am J Obstet Gynecol 126: 186–189.

Samuels BI, Novy S, Hevezi J, Smith J, Wallace S, Dodd GD (1975): Ultrasound as an aid in the diagnosis and management of ovarian carcinoma: Preliminary report. Natl Cancer Inst Monogr 42:87–97.

Schwartz PE, Smith JP (1980): Second look operation in ovarian cancer. Am J Obstet Gynecol 138:1124–1130.

Smith JP, Delgado G, Rutledge F (1976): Second look operation in ovarian carcinoma. Cancer 38:1438–1442.

Smith WG, Day TG, Smith JP (1977): The use of laparoscopy to determine the results of chemotherapy for ovarian cancer. J Reprod Med 18:257–260.

Spinelli P, Luini A, Pizzeti P (1976): Laparoscopy in staging and restaging of 95 patients with ovarian carcinoma. Tumori 62:493-500.

Stuart GCE, Jeffries M, Stuart JL, Anderson RJ (1982): The changing role of "second look" laparotomy in the management of epithelial carcinoma of the ovary. Am J Obstet Gynecol 142:612–616.

Wallach RC, Blinick G (1970): The second look operation for carcinoma of the ovary. Surg Gynecol Obstet 131:1–5.

Wangensteen OH, Lewis JF, Arhelger SW, Muller JJ, Maclean LD (1954): An interim report upon the "second look" procedure for cancer of the stomach, colon and rectum and for limited intraperitoneal carcinosis. Surg Gynecol Obstet 99:257–267.

Cancer Chemotherapy During Pregnancy

Allan J. Jacobs

Department of Obstetrics and Gynecology, Washington University School of Medicine, St. Louis, Missouri 63110

Chemotherapy assumes an ever increasing role in efforts to control or palliate malignant disease. DeVita et al. estimate that 420,000 patients a year present with disease beyond the capacity of localized treatment to control, or else with recurrent disease [1] (additional patients will benefit from adjuvant chemotherapy). Approximately half these patients have tumors that either are potentially curable by chemotherapy, or in whom appropriate use of chemotherapy will demonstrably improve survival.

Many of these tumors occur in women of reproductive age. The five types of cancer with the highest mortality in women between 15 and 34 years of age are leukemia, breast, brain, uterus, and Hodgkin's disease [2]. Table I demonstrates that many of the malignancies most receptive to treatment with chemotherapy may occur in women with reproductive potential.

Clearly, a number of women will be pregnant with a simultaneous malignancy which, if pregnancy were not present, would optimally be treated with chemotherapy. It is the objective of this essay to aid the clinician in managing these patients.

Information regarding the effects of chemotherapeutic agents on the fetus and pregnancy is scant and, for the most part, does not permit ready deduction of reliable generalizations for use of the drugs. Because of the small number of pregnant patients with cancer, most publications about human use of antineoplastic drugs comprise clinical case reports with small numbers. Rarely is the fetal pharmacology of the drug studied. Most patients taking the drug also have an advanced malignancy, which may effect the high rate of prematurity and inappropriately low birth weight observed in

Chemotherapy of Gynecologic Cancer, pages 351–362

TABLE I. Cancer in Women of Reproductive Age

Occur in women aged 15–40	Rarely, if ever, occur in women aged 15–40
Cancer in which a fraction of patients with advanced disease can be cured with chemotherapy	
Choriocarcinoma	Embryonal rhabdomysarcoma
Acute lymphocytic leukemia	Wilms tumor
Hodgkin's disease	
Ovarian carcinoma	
Non-Hodgkin's lymphoma	
Ewing sarcoma	
Cancers in which improved survival is demonstrable with chemotherapy	
Breast carcinoma	Chronic lymphocytic leukemia
Chronic myelogenous leukemia	Small cell carcinoma, lung
Soft-tissue sarcomas	Multiple myeloma
Malignant insulinoma	Gastric carcinoma
Glioblastoma	Endometrial carcinoma
	Adrenal cortical carcinoma
	Polycythemia vera
	Medulloblastoma
	Neuroblastoma

From DeVita et al. [1].

these patients. Few patients now receive a single agent, and many have received radiation therapy as well as chemotherapy during their pregnancy. There is a low natural rate of serious fetal malformations, with 1.25% of all babies having a gross malformation that can be recognized at birth [3]. It is therefore often difficult to attribute specific problems to a specific pharmacologic agent. Furthermore, since many cases of drug use in pregnancy are not reported, it is difficult to establish the magnitude of a potential teratologic problem.

Animal teratological studies do not provide clinically reliable information. There is an interspecific difference in teratogenic susceptibility which is both quantitative and qualitative. Thus, carmustine has little or no teratogenic effect in the rabbit, although it causes numerous skull, skeletal, cardiac, and other abnormalities in rats [4]; the same circumstance holds true for several other antineoplastic drugs [5]. Mustine administration during organogenesis results in limb defects and cleft palate in rats, but produces anophthalmia and tail defects in ferrets [6].

Little is known of the fetoplacental pharmacology of these agents in animals or man. In the case of most drugs, it has not been established to what extent they cross the placenta, or how the drug is distributed in the fetus.

It will be useful to summarize existing knowledge regarding the effect of chemotherapeutic drugs in pregnancy before presenting recommendations regarding their use.

EFFECTS OF DRUGS ON ORGANOGENESIS

Essentially all cytotoxic antineoplastic drugs demonstrate teratogenicity in an animal system. The effect of these drugs on human fetuses is less clear.

Antimetabolites

Methotrexate and aminopterin inhibit the reduction of folic acid by the enzyme folate reductase. Aminopterin produces teratogenic effects in chicks [7], as does methotrexate in rabbits [8]. Both agents produce deformities in humans when administered in the first trimester.

At one time, aminopterin was used as a first trimester abortifacient. It was not always successful in this regard, so that a number of exposed fetuses came to term and were born with deformities. These comprised skull malformations, shortened forearms, and missing digits [9–14]. In addition, neural tube defects have been observed [9–12]. Children followed past infancy had short stature [13] and borderline to subnormal intelligence [13,14].

Similar deformities have been noted following the first trimester administration of methotrexate [15,16], although there is no report of a mentally defective child being born in this circumstance. Following a course of MOPP (methotrexate, vincristine, procarbazine, and prednisone) in first trimester, a fetus delivered by therapeutic abortion demonstrated hypoplastic kidneys.

6-Mercaptopurine (6-MP, Purinethol) inhibits the generation of useful purine nucleotides from inosinic acid. It is teratogenic in rats and several other animals [18]. Its use in first trimester was associated with microphthalmia, cleft palate, and corneal opacities [6]. The patient also received 400 rads of external radiation to the spleen in first trimester, and additional 200 rads in second trimester, and busulfan from the second month until delivery [19]. At least 19 other women have been exposed to 6-MP, and 35 to azathioprine (which is metabolized to 6-MP) in first trimester, with subsequent delivery of morphologically normal children [20]. It appears that 6-MP and azathioprine rarely, if ever, cause disordered organogenesis in man.

Cystosine arabinoside (Ara-C, Cytarabine, Cytosar-U) acts as an inhibitor of DNA polymerase. It is teratogenic in rats [21] and mice [22], causing facial, skeletal, and CNS abnormalities. A fetus exposed to Ara-C in the first trimester was born with microtia, atresia of the left auditory canal, and deformities of upper and lower extremities [23]. Another offspring so exposed had deformities of the distal upper and lower limbs [24]. At least four additional normal babies were born to mothers who received Ara-C in the first trimester [25–27].

Other Drugs

6-Thioguanine (6-TG) causes limb anomalies in rats [18]. One patient delivered a fetus with limb deformities following administration of 6-TG and Ara-C. Another such patient had a normal baby [25].

There are no reports of a live baby being delivered following first trimester exposure to 5-fluorouracil (5FU). However, a fetus was aborted in this circumstance that had multiple limb deformities, pulmonary hypoplasia, esophageal, duodenal, and ureteral aplasia, and other abnormalities [28]. It is teratogenic in rats [21].

Alkylating Agents

Cyclophosphamide (CTX, Cytoxan) is teratogenic in rats [29] and mice [30]. There are three reports of teratogenicity in man possibly attributable to CTX. One involved minor lesions [31]. Another entailed missing digits, palatine grooves, and bilateral inguinal hernias [32]. Another patient aborted spontaneously with many defects following CTX and radiation therapy in first trimester [33]. The estimated fetal dose was less than 25 rads. There have been several reports of delivery of normal babies at term following CTX administration.

Nitrogen mustard (HN_2, mechlorethamine, Mustargen) induces a number of deformities in rats [18]. Two women have had normal babies after receiving NH_2 in the first trimester [34,35]. However, one patient receiving multiple drugs including HN_2 had lower limb defects [36].

Busulfan (Myleran) is teratogenic in rats [18]. Twenty-two offspring have been born to patients treated in the first trimester, two of whom exhibited congenital deformities [20].

Chlorambucil (Leukeran) causes urogenital abnormalities in rat fetuses [37]. The only report of its first-trimester use in humans describes a case of an induced abortion at 18 weeks in which the fetus demonstrated unilaterally absent kidney and ureter [38].

The use of Thio-tepa and melphalan (Alkeran) in first-trimester women has not been reported. Thio-tepa produces limb deformities in mice [31].

Other Agents

At least six normal babies have been born to mothers taking doxorubicin (Adriamycin) in first trimester [40]. An additional normal baby was born to a woman who had received the related anthracycline antibiotic, daunorubicin (Cerubidine) in first trimester [11]. Intravenous doxorubicin, when given intravenously to a woman at 20 weeks' gestation, was found not to be present subsequently in amniotic fluid [42]. The use of other antineoplastic antibiotics has not been reported in that first trimester of pregnancy, although some are teratogenic in various animal species [43,44].

Vinca alkaloids are teratogenic in rodents [45]. One patient received vinblastine (Velban) in first trimester in combination with HN_2 and procarbazine, and delivered a fetus with limb deformities [36]. As with other recently released agents, reports of single-agent use in pregnancy are rare.

Procarbazine has been used in three first-trimester women, with one possible instance of teratogenicity.

Cisplatin (Platinol) is teratogenic in rats [46]. It was given to one woman in late first trimester before abortion. The only abnormality was a giant cell found in the fetal testis [47].

Dacarbazine (DTIC-Dome) is teratogenic in animals [48], but there are no reports of pregnant women receiving the compound.

Hormonal Agents

Fluoxymesterone (Halotestin) is an androgen used in mammary carcinoma. No fetal abnormalities associated with its use have been identified (personal communication, C. Vanderlinden, Upjohn Co.). Women occasionally develop virilizing conditions owing to spontaneous testosterone secretion, such as luteoma of pregnancy. In this circumstance, most female infants are born with virilization [49]. It might be expected, therefore, that fluoxymesterone might exhibit similar properties.

Medroxyprogesterone acetate (MPA, DMPA, Provera, Depo-Provera) is used in gynecologic and, occasionally, in other tumors. There may be low incidence of congenital anomalies of the "Vacterl" (vertebral, anal, cardiac, tracheal, esophageal, renal, and limb) group in patients receiving exogenous progestational hormone drug organogenesis [50]. This has been estimated as no more than seven in 10,000 births [51]. No teratogenic effect has been identified in rats or mice, but MPA causes cleft palates in rabbits [52].

Prednisone is frequently utilized in acute lymphocytic leukemia. There has been one report of a baby born with birth defects and ring G chromosome after first-trimester exposure (personal communication, C. Vanderlinden), but many patients have undoubtedly used this drug, mostly for nonneoplastic conditions. The drug is not considered to be teratogenic in man. Placental transfer is poor, and few cases of hypoadrenalism have occurred in babies born to patients on the drug [53].

Tamoxifen (Nolvadex) is an antiestrogen used against breast carcinoma. There are no data regarding its teratogenicity in humans.

PERINATAL EFFECTS OF ANTINEOPLASTIC DRUGS

Potential adverse effects of chemotherapy are not limited to fetal malformation. It should not seem strange that cells that interfere with cellular replication should result in stunted fetal growth or cause the death of the fetus. This might be due to a direct effect on the fetus, or to an effect on the mother's ability to sustain a pregnancy. Women receiving these drugs during pregnancy are, ipso facto, desperately ill; the primary disease may itself compromise the pregnancy.

If a drug crosses the placenta, it can produce the same specific toxic effects in the fetus as in the mother. Barber [54] observes that little is written about the hematologic profile in neonates of women who have received antineoplastic drugs.

Abortion, Prematurity, and Growth Retardation

Aminopterin is such an efficient abortifacient that it was at one time utilized clinically for this purpose [9]. Methotrexate is a poor abortifacient. Azathioprine (Imuran), which is metabolized to 6-MP, is associated with an abnormally high number of late spontaneous abortions [55]. 6-MP is even more efficient as an abortifacient; six of 18 patients who have received the drug in first trimester as a single agent have aborted spontaneously [56]. Among the alkylating agents, only HN_2 appears to be associated with a high rate of spontaneous abortions [57]. It is not known that other categories of antineoplastic compounds cause abortion.

Prematurity is a frequent accompaniment to treatment with cytotoxic drugs. Lee reported that four of 12 children born to leukemic women with various treatment regimens were born premature [58]. Single-agent 6-MP has been associated with three such cases [59–61]. Premature delivery has also occurred with melphalan [62]. There have been several reports of prematurity in babies born to women treated with intensive regimens of combination chemotherapy [63–67].

Nicholson [57] reported low birth weight in 40% of patients treated with cytotoxic drugs. This frequently occurs even when the baby is morphologically normal. Among drugs with a significant single-agent experience, busulphan stands out as being associated with this complication [68].

Neonatal Complications

Barber states that neonatal hematodepression probably occurs more commonly than the literature suggests [54]. There have been several reports of this complication [67,68]. Two babies delivered at term died of undeterminable causes [59,69]. Another, whose mother was receiving MTX, VBL, and ACT-D at the time of delivery, had focal seizures which were relieved by administration of folic acid [70].

Lactation

Studies of drug levels in milk are few, if they exist at all. A nursing baby whose mother was taking CTX developed thrombocytopenia and leukopenia, which reversed following cessation of lactation [71]. We could find no other information about lactation during chemotherapy.

LONG-TERM EFFECTS ON OFFSPRING

Four areas of concern present themselves regarding the long-term well-being of patients born to women receiving cytotoxic chemotherapy. The question of physical malformation has been addressed at length. Another concern involves the effect of treatment on the child's intelligence. Data already cited suggest a problem in this regard in children exposed to antifolate agents in first trimester. If the child is morphologically normal, present data do not predict whether or not he will be mentally normal. Most case reports have been submitted within a year of birth. Even when follow-up is longer, objective mental testing has rarely been obtained.

There is concern regarding the long-term health of these children, particularly with regard to the likelihood of their developing cancer. No such cases have been reported. Moe et al. [72] have followed 212 patients treated for acute lymphocytic leukemia. Six of these patients, treated for 4.5 to 10 years, have subsequently had a total of ten children with no malformations or cancer. A recent report suggests that women treated with alkylating agents for ovarian carcinoma have a 9.6% chance of developing acute nonlymphocytic leukemia within 7 years [73]. The risk remains constant over that time, and is related to the total cumulative dose of drug received. It is quite possible that children exposed in utero to alkylating agents will be at risk for development of leukemia. No such case has yet been reported, however. Few such patients have been treated in any center, and the children are not being followed systematically, so the true risk is difficult, if not impossible to ascertain.

The mutagenic potential of these drugs is difficult to establish. A wide variety of drugs produce chromosomal damage when given to humans, including HN_2, CTX, CMBL, melphalan, MTX, ARA-C, 6-MP, azathioprine, and bleomycin [74]. Fetuses with chromosomal damage have been identified following administration of ARA-C, 6-TG [75], and azathioprine [76]. The susceptibility of germ cells to such insults, and the likelihood of transmitting these defects, are unclear.

RECOMMENDATIONS AND SUMMARY

A substantial amount of clinical case data has accumulated regarding some of the older chemotherapeutic agents. The number of case reports has decreased in recent years. This may be because increasing awareness of teratogenicity has limited use of these drugs during pregnancy, or because the legality and increased acceptability of induced abortion have encouraged women who need chemotherapy in the first half of pregnancy to terminate their pregnancies. The trend toward the use of combination chemotherapy has curtailed the number of women receiving a single drug during pregnancy, so experience with newer agents in this regard is minimal.

It is clear that all cytotoxic agents share properties that suggest the possibility of deleterious effects. All are teratogenic in mammals, and all cause chromosomal damage in vitro or in vivo. Adverse effects have been documented for a number of drugs (Table II).

The following clinical recommendations can be made regarding cytotoxic chemotherapy. Every antimetabolic and alkylating agent for which significant experience exists is probably teratogen, an abortifacient, or both. Women in the first trimester of pregnancy who require such a drug should be informed of the dangers. Induction of abortion needs to be considered as an option.

The use of corticosteroids and progestagens for antineoplastic therapy is warranted at all stages of pregnancy and does not indicate interruption of pregnancy. Fluoxymesterone should be avoided with a coexisting female fetus. Long-term effects on the male fetus are not reported, so abortion is

TABLE II. Effects of Chemotherapeutic Drugs on the Fetus

Agent	Teratogen	Abortifacient
Methotrexate	Yes	?
6-Mercaptourine	No	Yes
Cytarabine	Yes	?
5-Fluorouracil	Probably	?
Cyclophosphamide	Yes	No
Nitrogen mustard	?	Yes
Busulfan	Yes	?
Chlorambucil	Probably	?
Doxorubicin	?	?

not an unreasonable option if the drug is to be used in the first half of pregnancy. It is probably unwise to administer tamoxifen to a pregnant woman.

Patients requiring chemotherapy late in pregnancy with drugs other than corticosteroids or progestational agents should be considered for delivery prior to treatment. Most of them have conditions requiring fairly prompt treatment. Therefore, undue delay to await fetal maturity or cervical inducibility is unwarranted. Obstetrical management should be conducted in a center with tertiary-level equipment and expertise, because of the likelihood of premature birth or fetal growth retardation. The child should be followed closely by a pediatrician for abnormal psychomotor development, so that rehabilitative efforts may be initiated as soon as they might be beneficial. Finally, the patient and her husband should receive adequate emotional support and counseling. These cases generally involve a family unit that will soon have a young widower and an orphan, and whose financial resources will have been depleted.

REFERENCES

1. De Vita VT, Henney JE, Hubbard SM: Estimation of the numerical and economic impact of chemotherapy in the treatment of cancer. In Burchenal JH, Oettgen HF (eds): "Cancer: Achievements, Challenges and Prospects for the 1980's." New York: Grune and Stratton, 1980, pp 859–880.
2. Barber HRK: Malignant disease in the pregnant women. In Coppelson M (ed): "Gynecologic Oncology: Fundamental Principles and Clinical Practice." Edinburgh: Churchill Livingstone, 1982, pp 795–805.
3. Pritchard JA, MacDonald PC, Williams N: "Obstetrics," 15 Ed. New York: Appleton-Century-Crofts, 1976, p 825.
4. Thompson DG, Molello JA, Strebing RJ, Dyke IL, Robinson VB: Reproduction and teratology studies with oncylytic agents in the rats and rabbit. I. 1,3-bis-(2-chloroethyl)-1-nitrosourea (BCNU). Toxicol Appl Pharmacol 30:422–439, 1974.
5. Thompson DG, Molello HA, LaBeau JE: Differential sensitivity of the rat and rabbit to the teratogenic and embryotoxic effects of eleven antineoplastic drugs. Toxicol Appl Pharmacol 45:353, 1978.
6. Beck F, Schon H, Mould G, Swidzinska P, Curry S, Grauwilger J: Comparison of the teratogenic effects of mustine hydrochloride in rats and ferrets. Teratology 13:151–160, 1976.
7. Karnofsky DA, Patterson PA, Ridgeway LP: Effects of folic acid "4-amino" folic acids, and related substances on the growth of the chick embryo. Proc Soc Exp Biol Med 71:447–452, 1949.
8. Adams CB, Hay ME, Lutwach-Mann C: The action of various agents upon the rabbit embryo. J Embryol Exp Morphol 9:468–491, 1961.
9. Thiersch JB: Therapeutic abortions with a folic antagonist, 4-aminopteroglutamic acid, administered by the oral route. Am J Obstet Gynecol 63:1298–1302, 1952.

10. Meltzer HJ: Congenital anomalies due to attempted abortion with 4-aminopteroglutamic acid. JAMA 161:1253, 1951.
11. Warkany J, Beaudry DH, Hornstein S: Attempted abortion with 4-aminopteroglutamic acid (Aminopterin): Malformations in the child. Am J Dis Child 97:274–281, 1959.
12. Emerson DJ: Congenital malformations due to attempted abortion with aminopterin. Am J Obstet Gynecol 84:356–357, 1962.
13. Howard NJ, Rudd NL: The natural history of aminopterin-induced embryopathy. Birth Defects 13:85–93, 1977.
14. Shaw EB, Steinbach HL: Aminopterin-induced fetal malformation: Survival of an infant after attempted abortion. Am J Dis Child 115:477–482, 1968.
15. Milunsky A, Graef JW, Graynor MF: Methotrexate-induced congenital malformations. J Pediatr 72:790–795, 1968.
16. Powell HR, Ekert H: Methotrexate-induced congenital malformations. Med J Aust 2: 1076, 1971.
17. Mennuti MT, Shepard TH, Mellman WJ: Fetal renal malformation following treatment of Hodgkin's disease during pregnancy. Obstet Gynecol 46:194–196, 1975.
18. Chaube S, Murphy ML: The teratogenic effects of drugs active in cancer chemotherapy. Adv Teratol 3:181–237, 1968.
19. Diamond I, Anderson MM, McCreadie A: Transplacental transmission of busulfan (Myleran) in a mother with leukemia. Pediatrics 25:85–90, 1960.
20. Sweet DL, Kinzie J: Consequences of radiotherapy and antineoplastic therapy for the fetus. J Reprod Med 17:241–246, 1976.
21. Takehira Y, Kameyama Y: Morphogenesis of reductional malformations of digit in rat fetuses induced by cytosine arabinosine or 5-fluorouracil. Congen Anom 21:105–118, 1981.
22. Manson JM, Dourson ML, Smith CC: Effects of cytosine and arabinoside on in vivo and in vitro mouse limb development. In Vitro 434–442, 1977.
23. Wagner VM, Hill JS, Weaver J, Baehner RL: Congenital abnormalities in baby born to cytarabine treated mother. Lancet 2:98–99, 1980.
24. Shafer I: Teratogenic effects of antileukemic compounds. Arch Intern Med 141:514–515, 1961.
25. Moreno H, Castleberry RP, McCann WP: Cytosine arabinoside and 6-thioguanine in the treatment of childhood actute myeloblastic leukemia. Cancer 40:988–1004, 1979.
26. Pizzuto J, Aviles A, Noriega L, Niz I, Morales M, Romero F: Treatment of acute leukemia during pregnancy: Presentation of nine cases. Cancer Treat Rep 64:679–683, 1980.
27. Alegre A, Chunchuretta R, Rodriguez-Alarcon J, Cruz E, Prada M: Successful pregnancy in acute promyelocytic leukemia. Cancer 45:152–153, 1982.
28. Stephens JD, Golbus MS, Miller TR, Wilber RR, Epstein CJ: Multiple congenital anomalies in a fetus exposed to 5-fluorouracil during the first trimester. Am J Obstet Gynecol 137:747–749, 1980.
29. Chaube S, Kury G, Murphy ML: Teratogenic effects of cyclophosphamide in the rat. Cancer Chemother Rep 51:363–376, 1967.
30. Gibson JE, Becker BA: The teratogenicity of cyclophosphamide in mice. Cancer Res 28:475–480, 1968.
31. Coates A: Cyclophosphamide in pregnancy. Aust NZ J Obstet Gynecol 10:33–34, 1970.
32. Greenberg KH, Ranaka KR: Congenital anomalies probably induced by cyclophosphamide. JAMA 188:423–426, 1964.
33. Toledo TM: Fetal effects during cyclophosphamide and irradiation therapy. Ann Intern Med 74:87–91, 1971.

34. Zoet AG: Pregnancy complicating Hodgkin's disease. Northwest Med 49:373–374, 1950.
35. Barry RM, Diamond HD, Crauen LF: Influence of pregnancy on the course of Hodgkin's disease. Am J Obstet Gynecol 84:445–454, 1962.
36. Garrett MJ: Teratogenic effects of combination chemotherapy. Ann Intern Med 80: 667, 1974.
37. Monie IW: Chlorambucil-induced abnormalities in the urogenital system of rat fetuses. Anat Rec 139:145–154, 1961.
38. Shotton D, Monie IW: Possible teratogenic effect of chlorambucil on a human fetus. JAMA 186:74–75, 1963.
39. Takano K, Tammura T, Nishimura H: The susceptibility of the offspring of alloxan-diabetic mice to a teratogen. J Embryol Exp Morphol 14:63–73, 1965.
40. Garcia V, San Miguel J, Lopez Borrasca A: Doxorubicin in first trimester of pregnancy. Ann Intern Med 94:547, 1981.
41. Sears HF, Reid J: Granulocytic sarcoma. Cancer 37:1808–1815, 1976.
42. Roboz J, Gleicher N, Wu K, Chahinian P, Kerenyi T, Holland J: Does doxorubicin cross the placenta? Lancet 2:1382–1383, 1979.
43. Wilson JG: Effects of acute and chronic treatment with actinomycin-D on pregnancy and the fetus in the rat. Harper Hosp Bull 47:109–118, 1966.
44. Kury G, Craig JR: The effect of mitomycin C on developing chicken embryos. J Embryol Exp Morphol 17:229–237, 1967.
45. Ferm VH: Congenital malformations in hamster embryos after treatment with vinblastine and vincristine. Science 141:426, 1963.
46. Lazar R, Conran PC, Dajmanov J: Embryotoxicity and teratogenicity of cis-diamminedichloroplatinum. Experientia 35:647–648, 1979.
47. Jacobs AJ, Marchevsky A, Gordon RE, Deppe G, Cohen CJ: Oat cell carcinoma of the uterine cervix in a pregnant woman treated with cis-diamminedichloroplatinum. Gynecol Oncol 9:405–410, 1980.
48. Chaube S, Swinyard CA: Congenital anomalies in fetal rats produced by the anticancer agent 4(5)-(3,3-dimethyl-1-Triazeno) imidazole-carboxamide. Anat Rec 186:461–470, 1976.
49. Thomas E, Mestman J, Henneman C, Anderson G, Hoffman R: Bilateral luteomas of pregnancy with virilization. Obstet Gynecol 39:577–584, 1972.
50. Wilson JG, Brent RL: Are female sex hormones teratogenic? Am J Obstet Gynecol 141:567–580, 1981.
51. Fraser IS, Weisberg E: A comprehensive review of injectable contraception with special emphasis on depot medroxyprogesterone acetate. Med J Aust Spec Suppl 1:1–20, 1981.
52. Andrew FD, Staples RE: Parental toxicity of medroxyprogesterone acetate in rabbits, rats and mice. Teratology 15:25–32, 1977.
53. Giacoia GP, Yaffe S: Perinatal pharmacology. In Sciarra JJ (ed): "Gynecology and Obstetrics," Vol 3, Ch 100. Philadelphia: Harper and Row, 1982.
54. Barber HR: Fetal and neonatal effects of cytotoxic agents. Obstet Gynecol 58:41S–47S, 1981.
55. Golby M: Fertility after renal transplantaion. Transplantation 10:201–207, 1970.
56. Stern JL, Johnson TRB: Antineoplastic drugs and pregnancy. In Niebyl JR (ed): "Drug Use in Pregnancy." Philadelphia: Lea and Febiger, 1982.
57. Nicholson HO: Cytotoxic drugs in pregnancy. J Obstet Gynecol Br Commonw 75:307–312, 1968.
58. Lee RA, Johnson CE, Hanlon DG: Leukemia during pregnancy. Am J Obstet Gynecol 84:455–458, 1962.

59. Mersky C, Rigal W: Pregnancy in acute leukemia treated with 6-mercaptopurine. Lancet 2:1268–1269, 1956.
60. Loyd HO: Acute leukemia complicated by pregnancy. JAMA 178:1140–1143, 1961.
61. Ravenna P, Stein PJ: Acute monocytic leukemia in pregnancy. Am J Obstet Gynecol 85:545–548, 1963.
62. Levin SR, Spaulding AG, Wirman JA: Multiple myeloma: Orbital involvement in a growth. Arch Ophthalmol 95:642–644, 1977.
63. Doney KC, Kraemer KF, Shepard TH: Combination chemotherapy for acute myelocytic leukemia during pregnancy: Three case reports. Cancer Treat Rep 63:369–371, 1979.
64. O'Donnell R, Costigan C, O'Connell LG: Two cases of acute leukemia in pregnancy. Acta Hematol 61:298–300, 1979.
65. Sanz MA, Rafecas FJ: Successful pregnancy during chemotherapy for acute promyelocytic leukemia. N Engl J Med 306:939, 1982.
66. Tobias SS, Morganstern G, Bloom HJG, Powles RL: Doxorubicin in pregnancy. Lancet 1:776, 1980.
67. Taylor G, Blom J: Acute leukemia during pregnancy. So Med J 73:1314–1315, 1980.
68. Dugdale M, Fort AT: Busulfan treatment of leukemia during pregnancy: Case report and review of the literature. JAMA 199:131–133, 1967.
69. Thomas PRM, Peckham MJ: The investigation and management of Hodgkin's disease in the pregnant patient. Cancer 38:1443–1451, 1976.
70. Hutchison JR, Peterson EP, Zimmerman EA: Coexisting metastatic choriocarcinoma and normal pregnancy. Obstet Gynecol 31:331–336, 1968.
71. Durodola JI: Administration of cyclophosphamide during late pregnancy and early lactation: A case report. J Natl Med Assoc 71:165–166, 1979.
72. Moe PJ, Lethinen M, Wegelius R, Friman S, Kreuger A, Berg A: Progeny of survivors of acute lymphocytic leukemia. Acta Paediat Scand 68:301–303, 1979.
73. Greene MH, Boice JD, Greer BE, Blessing JA, Dembo AJ: Acute lymphocytic leukemia after therapy with alkylating agents for ovarian cancer: A study of five randomized clinical trials. N Engl J Med 307:1416–1421, 1982.
74. Sieber SM, Adamson RH: Toxicity of antineoplastic agents in man: Chromosomal aberrations, antifertility effects, congenital malformations, and carcinogenic potential. Adv Cancer Res 22:57:153, 1975.
75. Mauer LH, Jackson FR, McIntyre OR, Benirschke K: Fetal group C trisomy after cytosine arabinoside and thioguanine. Ann Intern Med 75:809–810, 1971.
76. Leb DE, Weisskopf B, Kanovitz BS: Chromosome aberrations in the child of a transplant recipient. Arch Intern Med 128:441–444, 1971.

Immunotherapy of Gynecologic Cancer

Jonathan S. Berek and Neville F. Hacker

Division of Gynecologic Oncology, UCLA School of Medicine, Jonsson Comprehensive Cancer Center, Los Angeles, California 90024

Immunotherapy is a method of cancer treatment which seeks to utilize the body's immune defenses for tumor rejection. This can be accomplished either through augmentation of an existing host response or by the injection of activated immune cells or their biologic products into the host.

The complexity of immune regulatory mechanisms has made their thorough understanding elusive. Thus, therapeutic intervention has been based on empiric attempts to control a system defined by relatively insensitive serum assays or skin tests. A comprehensive discussion of immune regulatory processes will not be undertaken in this chapter; they will be referred to in the context of developing rational therapeutic modalities.

The primary immunotherapeutic agents utilized in the past have been "nonspecific"—i.e., agents which were introduced into the human system that were designed to elicit a generalized inflammatory reaction, including both humoral and cellular immune responses. Because of the diverse effects of the agents in vivo, they are often referred to as immunomodulators. The response by a given host depends on her immunocompetence—i.e., the ability of the treated individual to react to the agent with a generalized immune reaction. Some portions of the elicited response may, in fact, be counterproductive causing immune suppression.

In addition to humoral immunity, antibody produced by "B-cell" lymphocytes, and cell-mediated "T-cell" immunity, a group of natural cytotoxic effector lymphocytes, or natural killer (NK) cells, have been described [Herberman, 1980]. These cells are morphologically large granular lymphocytes (LGL), and possess inherent cytotoxic activity against foreign substances and tumor systems. Antibody-dependent, cell-mediated cytotoxicity

Chemotherapy of Gynecologic Cancer, pages 363–374

(ADCC), or "K-cell" function, represents a population of lymphocytes which require complement fixation and the presence of specific antibodies to stimulate destruction of foreign cells [Bast et al., 1983]. In addition, a variety of T-cell subpopulations can now be identified using monoclonal antibodies. Cells that principally possess "suppressive" and "helper" activity have been identified [Fujimoto et al., 1976]. T-lymphoid cells regulate B-cell function and hence control antibody production by means of the helper and suppressor T-cell subpopulations [Fahey, 1978]. Soluble factors are released from both suppressor and helper T-cells and mediate T-cell and B-cell maturation.

The concept of immune enhancement implies that the immunocompetent host is more likely to respond to cytotoxic drugs when immunotherapy and chemotherapies are combined. Experimental data in animals show that certain tumors can be more aggressively rejected by their host if they are exposed to a nonspecific immunostimulant prior to their injection with a chemotherapeutic agent [Hanna and Key, 1982]. This type of study provides the impetus for clinical trials that combine these modalities.

Specific immunity, typically performed by inoculation of the host and involving a late lymphocytic "memory," has been investigated as a treatment for cancer, but has not yet proved successful.

Specific immunotherapy, using a serum directed at a single antigenic determinant, has always been the goal of the immunologist. The development of monoclonal antibodies, the "hybridoma" [Köhler and Milstein, 1978], has encouraged considerable research in an attempt to discover antibodies raised against specific antigenic determinants of a tumor. These antibodies could serve to identify the presence of the abnormal cell, to follow its growth pattern, and perhaps to therapeutically destroy the cell. Some success has been achieved using monoclonal antibodies therapeutically in humans with B-cell lymphomas [Foon et al., 1982]. The development of these therapies relies on the principle that there are antigenic differences between cancer cells and their precursors. Tumor-associated antigens have been described in several systems [Bast et al., 1983; Order et al., 1975), but specificity has yet to be documented in gynecologic malignancies. Oncofetal antigens, such as carcinoembryonic antigen (CEA) and alpha-fetoprotein (AFP), are found in a variety of cell types.

A variety of tests have been employed to determine host immunocompetence, the most common of which has been the placement of mumpus, candida, or PPD skin tests to exclude anergy. DNCB (dinitrochlorobenzene) also produces an acute local inflammatory response in the immunocompetent host. Skin and serum assay have been shown to correlate well with tumor virulence (grade), burden, and host nutritional status [DiSaia, 1976].

BIOLOGIC RESPONSE MODIFIERS

The term "biologic response modifier" (BRM) is used to describe an agent, specific or otherwise, that can modulate or modify the immune system. Nonspecific immunotherapies have been the agents utilized in most of the previous trials for treatments of patients with gynecologic malignancies. They have typically involved inoculation of the host with an inactivated bacterium, such as *Corynebacterium parvum* (CP), which is a heat-killed, gram-negative anaerobic bacillus; bacillus Calmette-Guerin (BCG), which is a live, attenuated strain of *Mycobacterium bovis*; and Freund's complete adjuvant (FCA).

Modifications of these agents are usually made by biochemically extracting fractions of these organisms. Biochemical fractionation, typically via acid or phenol-extracted materials and their residues, can lead to the identification of active components, such as a glycolipid or carbohydrate, which might selectively be found on the cell wall membrane. The component might possess the antigenic determinants which more selectively elicit desirable immunological responses while sparing less desirable immune reactions and side effects [Muruhata et al., 1980]. MER is the methanol-extracted residue of BCG and retains significant immunomodulatory activity of BCG in a variety of animal systems, while avoiding potential problems associated with viable BCG.

Levamisole is a nonspecific immunomodulator which principally potentiates the expression of delayed hypersensitivity reaction in immunocompetent hosts [Gusdon et al., 1981]. It enhances the maturation of T-lymphocytes by an unknown mechanism.

C. parvum (CP) is an agent which induces a variety of immune regulatory mechanisms [Halpern, 1975]. CP induces a rapid inflammatory response, heralded by a mobilization of neutrophilic white cells. Macrophage attraction and cytotoxicity activation results from exposure to CP. Natural killer (NK) cytotoxicity is also enhanced, and T-lymphocyte activation occurs [Herberman, 1980]. CP has been shown to be active in many animal systems [Scott, 1974], and tumor rejection is temporally associated with cellular response. Studies of a murine teratocarcinoma in C3HeB/FeJ mouse comparing biochemically fractionated *C. parvum* revealed that tumor rejection in animals treated IP with the residue of pyridine-extractable *C. parvum*, a fraction that contains the cell walls [Berek et al., 1983b], is comparable to the rejection observed after IP administration of whole, unmodified *C. parvum*.

BCG has been widely used in many tumor systems and has been given either systemically, by intralesional injection, or excarification [Bast et al.,

1974]. These have occasionally been mixed with whole irradiated tumor cells and injected into the patient as a vaccine. In a large series [Borstein et al., 1973], intracutaneously injected melanoma lesions in patients with cutaneous recurrence demonstrated some active tumor rejection by BCG. Visceral or parenchymal metastatic disease, however, has been resistant to this type of therapy. While there have been some preliminary results using BCG as an adjuvant in children with acute lymphocytic leukemia and with stage II melanoma, randomized studies have not yet revealed significant results. In ovarian cancer, BCG has been used in combination with cytotoxic agents in a randomized prospective study [Alberts et al., 1978], and an apparent increase in survival was detected, but this has not yet been substantiated.

Interferons have recently received considerable attention because of their ability to react as immunomodulators in various biologic systems. These are a group of small glycoproteins, occurring as single-chain polypeptides, which are natural cellular by-products that have been shown to be elicited by a variety of stimuli, particularly viral infections. Interferon is a potent stimulator of natural cytotoxicity (NK) cells in vitro and in vivo, and this has been associated with antitumor activity in several animal models [Stewart, 1979]. The precise role of interferon in relation to other components of the immune mechanism has not been elucidated, but most likely these molecules represent intermediary modulating molecules. Clinical trials have been undertaken with a variety of different types of interferon in different tumor systems, but limited information is currently available on the effectiveness of interferon in gynecologic malignancies. However, there are several studies that are ongoing which will be discussed below.

TREATMENT OF OVARIAN CANCER

There has been considerable interest in the potential for immunotherapy in ovarian cancer. This is in part due to the fact that long-term survival in patients with epithelial malignancies is poor, and that most patients present with metastatic disease. It has long been felt that the patients with advanced disease are significantly immunocompromised, and a variety of studies in the past have confirmed this conclusion [Khoo and MacKay, 1974].

Studies using vaccines in ovarian cancer have produced only occasional responses. Graham and Graham [1962] treated 232 patients with gynecologic malignancies, 48 of whom had ovarian cancer, with Freund's complete adjuvant. FCA was mixed either with DNA-protein extract of the tumor or viable tumor cells. While systemic reactions to the agents were low in most patients who had tumor progression, the vaccine did not control tumor proliferation.

More recently, tumor cell vaccines have been developed [Hudson et al., 1976; Crowther and Hudson, 1977] utilizing injection of sonicated tumor cell walls into rabbits to develop a heterologous antiserum. BCG combined with an allogeneic tumor cell vaccine was given to ten patients with stage III or IV ovarian cancer. Administration of alkylating agents along with the BCG and a vaccine of 10^7 irradiated allogeneic tumor cells resulted in a prolonged survival compared retrospectively to historical controls [Hudson et al., 1976]. While these reports suggested some improvement in survival in a very small number of patients, they were all uncontrolled and retrospective.

Patients have been treated by one group [Julliard et al., 1978] with irradiated tumor cells injected intralymphatically, a technique referred to as active specific intralymphatic immunotherapy (ASILI). One complete response with the patient free of clinical evidence of disease at 13 months was reported in seven patients with epithelial ovarian carcinoma treated with ASILI. Unfortunately, most of these patients have bulky, persistent tumors located in the peritoneal cavity, and these patients did not respond to this type of therapy.

Most studies in metastatic ovarian cancer have utilized nonspecific immunotherapies, most commonly *C. parvum* and BCG, the agents that have been used in the largest single retrospective series to date.

Phase I studies of *C. parvum* in oncology patients has demonstrated that toxicity generally includes systemic chills, fever, malaise, nausea, and vomiting in most patients [Alberts et al., 1978; Webb et al., 1978; Bast et al., 1983; Montavani et al., 1981; Rao et al., 1977; Gall et al., 1978]. Serious toxicity, including hypotension, prolonged elevated temperatures, and chest pain, is uncommon. Early studies of subcutaneously administered *C. parvum* in patients with ovarian cancer [Rao et al., 1977] combined escalating doses with cyclophosphamide, doxorubicin, and 5-fluorouracil (CAF) administered monthly. Pretreatment immune parameters were good in patients who were responders to therapy compared to those who were not, but immune function was not augmented by therapy. In a randomized trial of chemoimmunotherapy with CAF with or without intravenously administered *C. parvum* [Wanebo et al., 1977], the treatment groups showed no difference in response rates, disease progression-free intervals, or survival.

Creasman et al. [1979] reported a retrospective series of patients treated with either melphalan alone or melphalan plus *C. parvum* administered simultaneously. The study evaluated 108 patients with untreated stage III ovarian epithelial malignancies. The combination group had 53% total response rate compared to 29% in the group treated with melphalan alone. However, a prospective randomized study attempting to confirm these findings has shown no significant differences thus far between melphalan alone 7 mg/m^2 day × 5 days PO given every 4 weeks and the same regimen plus C. *parvum* 4 mg/m^2 given IV on day 7 following chemotherapy [GOG Statistical Report, 1983, GOG Protocol 25]. It is interesting to note that in most experimental animal systems when immunotherapy and chemotherapy are combined, the tumor rejection is only augmented when the immunostimulant precedes the administration of cytotoxic agents by sufficient interval to permit some positive immunomodulation [Hanna and Key, 1982].

In a study by the Gynecologic Oncology Group, melphalan and levamisole were combined to treat 23 patients with stages III and IV ovarian cancer [Gusdon et al., 1981]. Four of these patients (17%) had negative second-look laparotomies, and there was no serious toxicity. A randomized trial comparing this agent with and without chemotherapy has not been undertaken.

In a randomized prospective study by Alberts et al. [1978], 66 patients with stages III and IV epithelial ovarian carcinomas were treated with either a combination of adriamycin and Cytoxan, or adriamycin, Cytoxan plus concomitant intravenous BCG. Adriamycin was given at 40 mg/m^2 on day 1, cyclophosphamide at 200 mg/m^2 on days 3–6, and BCG was given on day 8 and day 15. This cycle was repeated every 4 weeks. Of the 32 patients who were treated with a combination of chemoimmunotherapy, the total response rate was 56%, with two of 32 evaluable patients having a complete response. The median duration of response was 45 weeks, the median survival 93 weeks. This is compared to the 34 patients treated with adriamycin, Cytoxan alone where only 11 patients had a partial response (32% response rate). Median duration of response in this group was 26 weeks with a median survival of 59 weeks. While these investigators concluded that immunotherapy combined with chemotherapy might improve the results for ovarian carcinoma, we are awaiting the results of a GOG study which compares adriamycin, Cytoxan, and cis-platinum with or without BCG administered by escarification in a prospective randomized approach for patients with suboptimal stage III disease.

In a recent development, patients have been treated with intraperitoneal immunotherapy. In patients with minimal residual, epithelial ovarian carcinoma following treatment with combination cytotoxic chemotherapy, Bast et al. [1983] reported 12 patients so treated at the Dana-Farber Cancer

Institute and the UCLA Jonsson Comprehensive Cancer Center. Of the 12 evaluable patients there were five responders, including two complete responses. All of the responding patients had macroscopic disease of 4 mm or less maximum tumor diameter at the initiation of therapy. Antibody-dependent, cell-mediated cytotoxicity (ADCC) is significantly augmented during the course of therapy [Bast et al., 1983] as is NK cytotoxicity [Berek et al., 1983a; Lichtenstein et al., 1983]. The increase of cytotoxic effectors in the peritoneal cavity correlates well with the response to the agent C. *parvum* is administered through an indwelling IP dialysis catheter (Tenchkoff catheter) and administered every 2 weeks in escalating doses starting at 0.25 mg/m^2 and rising to 4 mg/m^2. Because of the responses observed in the phase I toxicology study, a phase II study of intraperitoneally administered C. *parvum* has been undertaken for those patients who have minimal residual carcinomas (< 5 mm maximum tumor diameter) documented at second-look laparotomy.

The intraperitoneal administration of C. *parvum* has been noted by Montavani et al. [1981] to be useful for the palliation of ascites in women with advanced ovarian cancer. In eight patients, IP administration of 7 to 14 mg of C. *parvum* on days 0, 7, and 28 resulted in complete disappearance of ascites in three patients, and a marked reduction of the effusion in two others. The palliative effect was noted to be sustained for 6 to 13+ months.

Hernandez et al. [1981] reported the treatment of nine patients with advanced ovarian epithelial malignancies who were given IP installation of a sterile, pyrogen-free, rabbit-derived human ovarian antitumor serum (HOATS). Although the study is very preliminary, the clinical response rate was 80%, with a 1-year survival of 87%. A trial of passive serotherapy utilizing the rabbit heteroantiserum is being studied prospectively [Order et al., 1981]. Patients are being treated with intraperitoneal ^{32}P, total abdominal irradiation, and melphalan, with or without 150 to 200 ml of serum. After a 2-year follow-up in 13 patients, there is no difference in survivals between the two groups.

While there are no significant studies using interferon in patients with ovarian cancer, there are two GOG pilot studies using intravenous and intraperitoneally administered interferon which have been recently initiated.

A group of researchers from Tokyo [Ohkawa et al., 1981] studied the use of intraperitoneal administration of semisynthesized acid polysaccharides, BCG and OK432 (Picibanil, which is a streptococcal preparation). For 4 days in a row, these agents were administered intraperitoneally with weekly intraperitoneal injections of adriamycin, 5FU, Endoxan, bleomycin, and mitomycin C. While this is an uncontrolled study, the 60 evaluable patients treated between 1970 and 1977 had a 5-year survival of 40%. These results further suggest that locoregional immunotherapy combined with chemotherapy may play a role in the control of ovarian cancer confined to the peritoneal cavity.

Because in many animal models the most successful immunomodulators are those that can be brought into direct contact with regional tumors, the intraperitoneal administration of such agents has great appeal.

TREATMENT OF CERVICAL CANCER

A study undertaken by the Gynecologic Oncology Group [1983] (Protocol 24) evaluated the treatment of women with cervical carcinoma, clinical stages IIB, IIIB, and IVA confined to the pelvis and/or para-aortic lymph nodes. Radiotherapy to the pelvis alone was compared to the same therapy plus intravenous C. *parvum*. The most common and limiting toxicity was moderate to severe chills and fever in the patients receiving C. *parvum* and occasional elevations of the total white count. In a study of 132 patients taking C. *parvum*, only nine patients had no significant adverse effects and dose modification was required in 47 cases. A preliminary analysis of these data suggest that C. *parvum* does not add any therapeutic effect as an adjuvant to radiotherapy in this particular patient population [GOG Statistical Report, 1983].

A phase I–II trial of intracervical injection of C. *parvum* in patients with stage IB and IIA carcinoma of the cervix has been undertaken [Minot et al., 1981]. This is a prospective randomized trial which indicated a relapse rate of only 5% (1 of 22) patients who received both an intralesional injection of 2 mg C. *parvum* 10 days prior to a radical hysterectomy compared to 29% of (6 of 21 patients) in those patients who had a radical hysterectomy only ($P < 0.05$). These data have not been confirmed in a subsequent analysis and the incidence of lymph node involvement and lesion size in each group have not been controlled. Although there are theoretical reasons to suggest that it might be an appropriate means of therapy, primarily because of the direct intralesional injection of the agent into a locally grown tumor, other BRM have not been tested as an adjuvant in stage I disease.

Several agents have been used for the treatment of intraepithelial neoplasia which can be easily eradicated by the intracervical injection of human leukocyte interferon [Ikic et al., 1981] and cis-retinoic acid [Surwit et al., 1982]. There is some interest as to whether or not these agents might be prophylactic against the development or worsening of dysplasia in the cervix.

In addition, 15 patients with invasive squamous cell carcinoma of the cervix (stages IA, IB, and IIA) have been treated with topical human leukocyte interferon 3 weeks prior to surgery, and nine of these patients received IM interferon concomitantly [Ikic et al., 1981]. The authors claim tumor shrinkage of about two-thirds in most patients and complete disappearance of tumor in three, although accurate dimensions were not reported.

TREATMENT OF VAGINAL AND VULVAR CANCER

Vaginal intraepithelial neoplasia has been shown to regress following local exposure to DNCB treatment [Guthrie and Way, 1975]. Six women without evidence of invasive cancer were treated with DNCB, and all patients had normal cytology after 2 to 35 months follow-up.

Another report [Freedman and Bowen, 1980] studied the use of a virus-modified homologous tumor cell extract in eight patients with invasive vulvar carcinoma and two or more positive groin lymph nodes. The patients were initially vaccinated three times a week and then twice a week for up to 2 years. All patients studied were free of disease 2 to 24 months later, whereas historical controls treated with surgery alone had a median time to recurrence of 14.8 months. Delayed hypersensitivity and antiviral antibody titers were elevated in most patients. These findings have not yet been confirmed by a controlled study.

GESTATIONAL TROPHOBLASTIC NEOPLASIA (GTN)

While extensive research using immunotherapy has not been performed in patients with GTN, principally because most tumors respond to cytotoxic chemotherapies, the immunobiology of trophoblastic tissue has been the subject of considerable interest. Paternal histocompatibility antigens have been noted to be present in metastatic GTN and this has prompted the notion that immunotherapy may play a role in the treatment of patients whose tumors are refractory to chemotherapy or as an adjunct in chemotherapy "high-risk" metastatic GTN. One study utilized systemic immunization with paternal leukocytes and induced a complete resolution of pulmonary metastasis in a patient with choriocarcinoma [Cinander et al., 1961]. Also, spontaneous regression of metastasis of choriocarcinoma has been reported to occur following surgical resection of the primary tumor, suggesting that cytoreduction may enhance the ability of the host mechanisms to reject metastatic lesions [Goldstein and Berkowitz, 1982].

PROSPECTS FOR SPECIFIC IMMUNE ENHANCEMENT

Adoptive Transfer

Adoptive specific immunotherapy means the transfer of active lymphoid cells from a specifically immunized donor to a tumor-bearing recipient, typically a syngeneic or allogeneic variety. While adoptive transfer has been observed in a variety of animal tumor models, it has not been widely used in human subjects. In early trials, many human recipients developed severe reactions, most commonly graft versus host (GVH). There may be a role for regional adoptive transfer in ovarian cancer, similar to the use of nonspecific therapies as outlined above.

Monoclonal Antibodies

Since the pioneering work of Köhler and Milstein [1978], considerable interest has been generated in the development of monoclonal antibodies against ovarian tumors that could be used for tumor detection, monitoring, and, more specifically, for therapy. A monoclonal antibody raised against epithelial ovarian carcinoma (OC-125) in the human has been reported [Bast et al., 1983]. Another antibody is currently being tested as a possible means of diagnosing and monitoring patients [Epenetos et al., 1982]. Considerable work needs to be accomplished in order to utilize monoclonal antibodies for this purpose, with the identification and isolation of tumor-specific antigens. Perhaps this will become a reality in the near future.

CONCLUSION

Immunotherapy for gynecologic malignancies has been disappointing thus far. However, preliminary studies indicate that immune enhancement leading to tumor rejection can most likely occur when the various BRM are brought into direct contact with the tumors, when the tumor burden is minimal, such as in an adjuvant setting, or when it is combined in the appropriate temporal relationship with cytotoxic chemotherapy.

REFERENCES

Alberts DS, Salmon ES, et al. (1978): Chemoimmunotherapy for advanced ovarian carcinoma with adriamycin-cyclophosphamide ± BCG: Early report of a Southwest Oncology Group study. Recent Results Cancer Res 68:160–165.

Bast RC, Zbar B, et al. (1974): BCG and cancer. N Engl J Med 290:1413–1420, 1458–1469.

Bast RC, Feeney M, et al. (1981): Reactivity of a monoclonal antibody with human ovarian carcinoma. J Clin Invest 68:1331–1337.

Bast RC, Berek JS, et al. (1983): Intraperitoneal immunotherapy of human ovarian carcinoma with *Corynebacterium parvum*. Cancer Res 43:1395–1401.

Bast RC, Klug T, et al. (1983): Monitoring growth of human ovarian carcinoma with a radioimmunoassay for antigen(s) defined by a murine monoclonal antibody (OC125). N Engl J Med 309:83–87.

Berek JS, Bast RC, et al. (1983a): Functional and phenotypic characterization of lymphocytes from the peritoneal effluents of patients with advanced stage ovarian cancer. Obstet Gynecol (in press).

Berek JS, Hacker NF, et al. (1983b): Tumor rejection in the peritoneal cavity of a murine ovarian cancer model using immunotherapy with biologic response modifiers. Proc Soc Gyn Onc 14:5.

Borstein RS, Mastrangelo MJ, et al. (1973): Immunotherapy of melanoma with intralesional BCG. Natl Cancer Inst Monogr 39:213–220.

Cinander B, Hayler MA, et al. (1961): Immunotherapy of a patient with choriocarcinoma. Can Med Assoc J 84:306.

Creasman WT, Gall SA, et al. (1979): Chemoimmunotherapy in the management of primary stage III ovarian cancer: A Gynecologic Oncology Group study. Cancer Treat Rep 68:319–323.

Crowther ME, Hudson C (1977): Experience with a pilot study of active specific immunotherapy in advanced ovarian cancer. Clin Oncol 3:397.

DiSaia PJ (1976): Overview of tumor immunology in gynecologic cancer. Cancer 38:566–580.

Epenetos AA, Britton KE, et al. (1982): Targeting of iodine-123–labelled tumor-associated monoclonal antibodies to ovarian, breast and gastrointestinal tumors. Lancet Nov 6:999–1004.

Fahey JL (1978): "Principles of Immunology With Relevance to Immunotherapy in Immunotherapy of Human Cancer." New York: Raven, pp 31–39.

Foon KA, et al. (1982): Treatment of B-cell lymphoma with monoclonal anti-idiotype antibody. N Engl J Med 307:686–687.

Freedman RS, Bowen JM (1980): Virus-modified homologous tumor cell extract in the treatment of vulvar cancer. Cancer Immunol Immunother 8:33.

Fujimoto S, Green MI, et al. (1976): Regulation of the immune response to tumor antigens. II. The nature of immunosuppressor cells in tumor-bearing hosts. J Immunol 116(3):800–806.

Gall SA, Blessing JA, et al. (1978): Toxicity manifestation following intravenous *Corynebacterium parvum* administration to patients with ovarian and cervical carcinoma. Am J Obstet Gynecol 132:555–560.

Goldstein DD, Berkowitz RS (1982): "Gestational Trophoblastic Neoplasms: Clinical Principles of Diagnosis and Management." Philadelphia: WB Saunders.

Graham JB, Graham RM (1962): The effect of vaccine on cancer patients. Surg Gynecol Obstet 114:1.

Gusdon JP, Homesley HD, et al. (1981): Chemotherapy of advanced ovarian epithelial carcinoma with melphalan and levamisole: A pilot study of the Gynecologic Oncology Group. Am J Obstet Gynecol 141:65–70.

Guthrie D, Way S (1975): Immunotherapy of non-clinical vaginal cancer. Lancet 2:1242.

Gynecologic Oncology Group (GOG) Statistical Report (1983).

Halpern B (1975): "*Corynebacterium parvum*: Applications in Experimental and Clinical Oncology." New York: Plenum.

Hanna MG, Key ME (1982): Immunotherapy of metastases enhances subsequent chemotherapy. Science 217:367–369.

Herberman RB (1980): "Natural Cell-mediated Immunity Against Tumors." New York: Academic, pp 973–984.

Hernandez E, Rosenshein NB, et al. (1980): IP immunotherapy and chemotherapy in advanced epithelial ovarian cancer. Cancer Treat Rep 66:1981–1982.

Hudson CN, Levin L, et al. (1976): Active specific immunotherapy for ovarian cancer. Lancet 2:877–879.

Ikic D, Kirhmajer V, et al. (1981): Application of human leukocyte interferon in patients with carcinoma of the uterine cervix. Lancet 9:1027–1030.

Julliard GJF, Boyer PJJ, et al. (1978): A phase I study of active specific intralymphatic immunotherapy (ASILI). Cancer 41:2215–2225.

Khoo SK, Mackay EV (1974): Immunologic reactivity of female patients with genital cancer: Status in preinvasive, locally invasive and disseminated disease. Am J Obstet Gynecol 119:1018–1025.

Köhler G, Milstein C (1978): Continuous cultures of fused cells secreting antibody of predefined specificity. Nature 256:495–497.

Lichtenstein A, Berek JS, et al. (1983): Activation of peritoneal lymphocyte cytotoxicity in patients with ovarian cancer by intraperitoneal treatment with *Corynebacterium parvum*. J Biol Response Modifiers (in press).

Minot MH, Len JW, et al. (1981): Lower relapse rate after neighbourhood injection of *Corynebacterium parvum* in operable cervical carcinoma. Br J Cancer 44(6):856–62.

Montavani A, Sessa C, et al. (1981): Intraperitoneal administration of *Corynebacterium parvum* in patients with ascitic ovarian tumors resistant to chemotherapy: Effects of cytotoxicity of tumor associated macrophages and NK cells. Int J Cancer 27:437–446.

Muruhata RI, Cantrell J, et al. (1980): Dissociation of biological activities of *Corynebacterium parvum* by chemical fractionation. Int J Immunopharm 2:47–53.

Ohkawa K, Ohkawa R, et al. (1981): Locoregional immunotherapy and chemotherapy in advanced ovarian cancer cytotoxicity. Asian Oceania Fed Obstet Gynecol, Oct:352.

Order SE, Thurston J, et al. (1975): Ovarian tumor antigens: A new potential for therapy. Natl Cancer Inst Monogr 42:23–43.

Order SE, Rosenshein N, et al. (1981): The integration of new therapies and radiation in management of ovarian cancer. Cancer 48:590–596.

Rao B, Wanebo HJ, et al. (1977): Intravenous *C. parvum*: An adjuvant to chemotherapy for resistant advanced ovarian cancer. Cancer 39:514–526.

Scott MT (1974): *Corynebacterium parvum* as an immunotherapeutic anti-cancer agent. Semin Oncol 1:367–378.

Stewart WE (1979): "The Interferon System." New York: Springer-Verlag.

Surwit EA, Meyskens FL, et al. (1982): Chemoprevention of intraepithelial neoplasia of the cervix with locally applied B-trans-retinoic acid: A phase I/II trial. Proc W Assn Gyn Oncol 10:10.

Wanebo HJ, Ochoa M, et al. (1977): Randomized chemoimmunotherapy trial of CAF and intravenous *C. parvum* for resistant ovarian cancer—Preliminary results. Proc Am Assoc Cancer Res 18:225.

Index